THE AMERICAN SOCIETY OF ADDICTION MEDICINE HANDBOOK ON PAIN AND ADDICTION

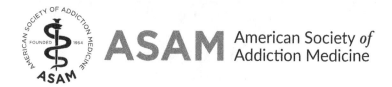

This is a publication of the American Society of Addiction Medicine (ASAM).

ASAM is a member-driven organization, representing over 3,200 physicians and associated professionals dedicated to increasing access and improving the quality of addiction treatment; educating physicians, other medical professionals and the public; supporting research and prevention; and promoting the appropriate role of physicians in the care of patients with addictions.

Learn more and get connected at www.asam.org.

The American Society of Addiction Medicine Handbook on Pain and Addiction

Edited by

Ilene R. Robeck, M.D., FASAM

Herbert L. Malinoff, M.D., FACP, DFASAM

Melvin I. Pohl, M.D., DFASAM

R. Corey Waller, M.D., M.S., DFASAM

Michael F. Weaver, M.D., DFASAM

Mark A. Weiner, M.D., DFASAM

William F. Haning, III, M.D., DFASAM, DFAPA

Managing Editor

Bonnie B. Wilford, M.S.

OXFORD
UNIVERSITY PRESS

OXFORD
UNIVERSITY PRESS

Oxford University Press is a department of the University of Oxford. It furthers
the University's objective of excellence in research, scholarship, and education
by publishing worldwide. Oxford is a registered trade mark of Oxford University
Press in the UK and certain other countries.

Published in the United States of America by Oxford University Press
198 Madison Avenue, New York, NY 10016, United States of America.

Library of Congress Cataloging-in-Publication Data
Names: Robeck, Ilene R., editor. | American Society of Addiction Medicine.
Title: The American Society of Addiction Medicine handbook on pain and
addiction / edited by Ilene R. Robeck, Herbert L. Malinoff, Melvin I. Pohl,
R. Corey Waller, Michael F. Weaver, Mark A. Weiner, William F. Hanning III.
Other titles: Handbook on pain and addiction
Description: Oxford ; New York : Oxford University Press, [2018] |
Includes bibliographical references.
Identifiers: LCCN 2017040393 | ISBN 9780190265366 (pbk. : alk. paper)
Subjects: | MESH: Pain Management | Opioid-Related Disorders—
complications | Chronic Pain—complications
Classification: LCC RB127 | NLM WL 704.6 | DDC 616/.0472—dc23
LC record available at https://lccn.loc.gov/2017040393

CONTENTS

Section II. Diagnosing and Treating Pain and Addiction: Common Principles | 81

Section III. Treating Pain in Patients Diagnosed with, or at Risk for, Co-Occurring Addiction | 161

Section IV. Treating Opioid Use Disorder in Patients Diagnosed with Chronic Pain | 219

Section V. Adapting Treatment to the Needs of Specific Patient Populations | 279

Editors of the Handbook

Ilene R. Robeck, M.D., FASAM
Co-Chair, National Veterans Affairs
Primary Care Pain Champions
Initiative
Director of Virtual Pain Care
Hunter Holmes McGuire Veteran
Affairs Medical Center
Richmond, VA

**Herbert L. Malinoff, M.D.,
FACP, DFASAM**
Clinical Assistant Professor,
Department of Anesthesiology
University of Michigan
Medical Center
Ann Arbor, MI
Attending Physician, St. Joseph
Mercy Hospital
Ypsilanti, MI

Melvin I. Pohl, M.D., DFASAM
Chief Medical Officer
Las Vegas Recovery Center
Las Vegas, NV

**R. Corey Waller, M.D.,
M.S., DFASAM**
Senior Medical Director for
Education and Policy
National Center for Complex Health
and Social Needs
Camden, NJ

Michael F. Weaver, M.D., DFASAM
Professor, Department of Psychiatry
and Behavioral Sciences
Medical Director, Center for
Neurobehavioral Research on
Addiction
University of Texas Health
Science Center
Houston, TX

Mark A. Weiner, M.D., DFASAM
Medical Director of Substance Use
Disorders
Section Head, Addiction Medicine
Program Director, Addiction
Medicine Fellowship
Medical Director, Integrated Health
Associates Pain Management
Consultants
St. Joseph Mercy Hospital
Ann Arbor, MI

**William F. Haning, III, M.D.,
DFASAM, DFAPA**
Professor of Psychiatry and Director,
Addiction Programs
John A. Burns School of Medicine,
University of Hawaii
Honolulu, HI

Bonnie B. Wilford, M.S.
Executive Vice President
Coalition on Physician Education in
Substance Use Disorders (COPE)
Easton, MD

Acknowledgments

Patients with substance use disorder (SUD) are at increased risk of developing chronic pain. When certain medications are used to treat chronic pain, it is essential that the treating clinician understand the potential for development of dependence or addiction. To help health care professionals meet this responsibility, the *ASAM Handbook on Pain and Addiction* reviews and analyzes the interplay between pain and addiction and provides clinically relevant information and guidance.

The Handbook would not have been possible without the contributions and strong dedication of many individuals. Foremost among these are the editors, Ilene R. Robeck, M.D., FASAM, Herbert Malinoff, M.D., FACP, DFASAM, Melvin I. Pohl, M.D., DFASAM, R. Corey Waller, M.D., M.S., DFASAM, Michael F. Weaver, M.D., DFASAM, Mark A. Weiner, M.D., DFASAM and William F. Haning, III, M.D., DFASAM, DFAPA. We also are deeply indebted to Bonnie B. Wilford, M.S., whose expertise as both managing editor and specialist in the field of addiction medicine has served us well in making this Handbook a reality. Special thanks also go to the authors whose work appears in this Handbook for their intellectual contributions to this endeavor.

ASAM also expresses special gratitude to members of the Publications Council: William F. Haning, III, M.D., DFAPA, DFASAM, Randall Brown, M.D., Ph.D., DFASAM, Chris A. Cavacuiti, M.D., CCFP, DFASAM, Lori D. Karan, M.D., FACP, DFASAM, Karen A. Miotto, M.D., DFASAM, Peter Selby, MBBS, CCFP, FCFP, MHSc, DFASAM, Alan A. Wartenberg, M.D., FACP, DFASAM, and Michael F. Weaver, M.D., DFASAM, for their guidance to and support of the Handbook.

Finally, ASAM is enormously grateful to the publisher, Oxford University Press, whose staff worked diligently with the ASAM publication staff: Brendan McEntee, Director of Quality and Science, and Yemsrach Kidane, Manager of Quality and Science, to bring this project to a successful conclusion.

ASAM Publications Council

William F. Haning III, M.D., DFAPA, DFASAM, *Chair*
Randall Brown, M.D., Ph.D., DFASAM
Chris A. Cavacuiti, M.D., CCFP, DFASAM
Lori D. Karan, M.D., FACP, DFASAM
Karen A. Miotto, M.D., DFASAM
Peter Selby, MBBS, CCFP, FCFP, MHSc, DFASAM
Alan A. Wartenberg, M.D., FACP, DFASAM
Michael F. Weaver, M.D., DFASAM

Editors of the Handbook

Ilene R. Robeck, M.D., FASAM, *Editor in Chief*
Herbert L. Malinoff, M.D., FACP, DFASAM
Melvin I. Pohl, M.D., DFASAM
R. Corey Waller, M.D., M.S., DFASAM
Michael F. Weaver, M.D., DFASAM
Mark A. Weiner, M.D., DFASAM
William F. Haning III, M.D., DFASAM., DFAPA

Authors of the Handbook

Sharone Abramowitz, M.D., FASAM
Louis E. Baxter, Sr., M.D., FASAM
Abigail Brooks, Pharm.D., BCPS
Emily Brunner, M.D.
Nelly A. Buckalew, M.D., N.D., M.S., M.S.L.
Lucile Burgo-Black, M.D., FACP
Christopher Cavacuiti, M.D., CCFP, MHSc, FASAM
Jacqueline Cleary, Pharm.D., BCACP
Marianne Cloeren, M.D., M.P.H., FACOEM, FACP
Stephen Colameco, M.D., M.Ed., DFASAM
Robert L. DuPont, M.D.
Steven Eraker, M.D.
Jason Baker Fields, M.D., DABAM
James W. Finch, M.D.
Marc J. Fishman, M.D.
Jeffrey Fudin, Pharm.D., DAIPM, FCCP, FASHP
Stephen F. Grinstead, A.D., LMFT, ACRPS, CADC-II
Ross Halpern, Ph.D.
Steven R. Hanling, M.D.
John A. Hopper, M.D.

Stephen C. Hunt, M.D., M.P.H.
Lori D. Karan, M.D., DFASAM, FACP
Courtney Kominek, Pharm.D., BCPS, CPE
Robert Levy, M.D., FASAM
Herbert L. Malinoff, M.D., FACP, DFASAM
Zachary Marcum, Ph.D., Pharm.D.
Rachel Maree, M.D., M.P.H.
Anthony J. Mariano, Ph.D.
Jeremiah McKelvey, Pharm.D.
David Mee-Lee, M.D.
Michael M. Miller, M.D., DFASAM, DLFAPA
Karen Muchowski, M.D., FAAFP
Stephen Mudra, M.D.
Vivek H. Murthy, M.D., M.B.A.
Yngvild Olsen, M.D., M.P.H., FASAM
James A. D. Otis, M.D., FAAN, DABPM
Sanjog S. Pangarkar, M.D.
Theodore V. Parran, Jr., M.D.
Thien C. Pham, Pharm.D.
Melvin I. Pohl, M.D., DFASAM
Peter Przekop, D.O., Ph.D.
Ilene R. Robeck, M.D., FASAM
Edwin A. Salsitz, M.D., FACP, DFASAM
Gerald R. Shulman, Ph.D.
Afreen Siddiqui, M.D.
Christopher J. Spevak, M.D., FASAM
Mishka Terplan, M.D., M.P.H., FACOG, FASAM
R. Corey Waller, M.D., M.S., DFASAM
Alan A. Wartenberg, M.D., FACP, FASAM
Michael F. Weaver, M.D., DFASAM
Debra K. Weiner, M.D.
Mark A. Weiner, M.D., DFASAM
Bonnie B. Wilford, M.S.
Bernd Wollschlaeger, M.D.
Martha J. Wunsch, M.D., FAAP, DFASAM
Penelope P. Ziegler, M.D., FASAM

Content Reviewers

Anthony H. Dekker, D.O.
Marc J. Fishman, M.D.
William F. Haning, M.D., DFASAM, DFAPA
John A. Hopper, M.D.

Herbert L. Malinoff, M.D., FACP., DFASAM
Jane C. Maxwell, Ph.D.
Theodore V. Parran, Jr., M.D.
Melvin I. Pohl, M.D., DFASAM
Ilene R. Robeck, M.D., FASAM
R. Corey Waller, M.D., M.S., DFASAM
Michael F. Weaver, M.D., DFASAM
Mark A. Weiner, M.D., DFASAM
Stephen A. Wyatt, D.O.

ASAM Staff and Consultants

Yemsrach Kidane, M.A., ASAM Manager, Quality and Science
Brendan McEntee, ASAM Director, Quality and Science
Bonnie B. Wilford, M.S., Managing Editor,
ASAM Handbook on Pain and Addiction

Oxford University Press

Andrea L. Knobloch, Senior Editor, Medicine
Tiffany X. Lu, Assistant Editor, Clinical Medicine

Introduction: The Clinical Challenge of Pain and Addiction

ILENE R. ROBECK, M.D., FASAM

Our understanding of pain and addiction have evolved dramatically over the past decade, leading to significant changes in the treatment of both medical disorders. Perhaps none has been more dramatic than the revolution in attitudes toward use of opioid analgesics for pain.

Ten years ago, responsible scientists and clinicians focused on the problem of inadequate diagnosis and management of pain. To address this very real problem, they led a movement to promote wider and more intensive use of opioid analgesics.

However, over the past five years, clinicians, policymakers, and society as a whole have witnessed the adverse results of this approach, as evidenced by dramatic increases in the rates of opioid use disorder, overdose, and death, all accompanied by startling growth in the nonmedical use of prescription opioids as well as consumption of illicit opiates such as heroin.

These developments confront physicians and other health professionals with a dual challenge. On one hand, safe and adequate treatment of pain remains a high priority, especially as the population ages and more individuals are diagnosed with and treated for conditions accompanied by pain. This effort to provide better pain management encompasses patients who are suffering from a substance use disorder or who are in recovery from such a disorder.

On the other hand, the dramatic escalation in the number of individuals of all ages who use opiates in ways that are dangerous to themselves and others must be considered as part of the overall effort to treat pain appropriately.

The last five years also have witnessed an evolution from a biomedical to a biopsychosocial approach to pain. In a biomedical model, the patient assumes a passive role in his or her care. Treatment primarily addresses the nociceptive pain generator through the use of medications and/or procedures. In contrast, the biopsychosocial approach to pain engages the patient as an active partici-pant in pain care and takes into account all aspects of the patient's life. The biopsychosocial approach also incorporates an understanding that medical and mental health comorbidities, functional improvement, movement, and cogni-tive approaches are as important to the treatment of pain as medications and procedures.

To help encourage and guide this evolution in our understanding of pain and its treatment, a number of public and private sector organizations have developed guidelines for safe prescribing of opioids, and are urging—or some-times requiring—practitioners to learn more about how to manage pain safely and effectively while also preventing, diagnosing, and treating adverse out-comes such as opioid misuse, addiction, overdose, and death. For example, the Centers for Disease Control and Prevention (CDC), the Office of the Surgeon General of the United States, the Federation of State Medical Boards (FSMB), the Veterans Administration (VA), and a growing number of state governments have published or are developing guidelines and model policies for pain man-agement. In addition, the Food and Drug Administration (FDA), the Substance Abuse and Mental Health Services Administration (SAMHSA), and other agen-cies within the U.S. Department of Health and Human Services (HHS) have supported the development and delivery of continuing medical education courses on the safe and effective management of pain (as discussed in online Appendix C of this Handbook).

This flood of advice and information, while well-intended and welcome, has led to confusion and frustration on the part of many health care professionals as they work to deliver optimal care to individual patients. In recognition of this dilemma, the American Society of Addiction Medicine (ASAM) has enlisted an outstanding group of physicians, pharmacologists, researchers, and medical educators in the development of this *ASAM Handbook on Pain and Addiction*. Their goal has been to produce a concise guide to the prevention, identification, and management of both pain and addiction, organized in a way that answers the specific needs of individual caregivers in their daily interactions with real patients.

Importantly, the *ASAM Handbook* is designed to reflect the growing evi-dence base as well as to comport with guidance provided in other ASAM publications, such as ASAM's textbooks, *Principles of Addiction Medicine* and *Essentials of Addiction Medicine*, the *ASAM Patient Placement Criteria*, and the *ASAM Handbook on Addiction*, all of which are widely used by practitioners to guide patient-specific decisions about appropriate components and intensity of care.

The authors, editors, and publisher of the *ASAM Handbook on Pain and Addiction* recognize that options for treating pain while preventing addiction are changing so rapidly that there is no "perfect" time to create a publication such as this one, because there is a persistent risk that some of the advice it contains may become obsolete even before the book is published.

Although keenly aware of that risk, ASAM's leaders decided to publish the Handbook now because the need for concise, accurate information grows more urgent by the day.

The *ASAM Handbook* thus attempts to outline the state of the art as we know it today. It also provides a conceptual framework for understanding the need for a comprehensive approach to the management of pain and the prevention of addiction—a framework that incorporates self-management, cognitive approaches, movement approaches, and carefully selected evidence-based procedures—all integrated with carefully prescribed opioid analgesics. The authors and editors also are committed to sharing information on key resources that will enable readers to keep pace with this rapidly evolving field.

The editors of this handbook and the leaders of ASAM (including its very active Publications Council) gratefully acknowledge the many contributions to this publication—and the research on which it is based—by ASAM members and other experts and organizations.

We also extend our gratitude to readers for their interest in pain and addiction and their commitment to advancing patient care. We welcome their feedback, which will help us "fine tune" the handbook so that it responds to the real-world needs and concerns of health care providers, as well as the patients to whom they deliver life-changing, life-saving care.

Foreword: Advancing Our Understanding of Pain and Addiction

Dear Colleague,

I am asking for your help to solve an urgent health crisis facing America: the opioid epidemic. Everywhere I travel, I see communities devastated by opioid overdoses. I meet families too ashamed to seek treatment for addiction. And I will never forget my own patient whose opioid use disorder began with a course of morphine after a routine procedure.

It is important to recognize that we arrived at this place on a path paved with good intentions. Nearly two decades ago, we were encouraged to be more aggressive about treating pain, often without enough training and support to do so safely. This coincided with heavy marketing of opioids to doctors. Many of us were even taught—incorrectly—that opioids are not addictive when prescribed for legitimate pain.

The results have been devastating. Since 1999, opioid overdose deaths have quadrupled, and opioid prescriptions have increased markedly—almost enough for every adult in America to have a bottle of pills. Yet the amount of pain reported by Americans has not changed. Now, nearly 2 million people in America have a prescription opioid use disorder, contributing to increased heroin use and the spread of HIV and hepatitis C.

I know solving this problem will not be easy. We often struggle to balance reducing our patients' pain with increasing their risk of opioid addiction. But, as clinicians, we have the unique power to help end this epidemic. As cynical as times may seem, the public still looks to our profession for hope during difficult moments. This is one of those times.

That is why I am asking you to pledge your commitment to turn the tide on the opioid crisis. Together, we will build a national movement of clinicians to do three things: *First*, we will educate ourselves to treat pain safely and effectively. A good place to start is the *TurnTheTideRx Pocket Guide* with the Centers for

Disease Control (CDC) Opioid Prescribing Guideline. *Second,* we will screen our patients for opioid use disorder and provide or connect them with evidence-based treatment. *Third,* we can shape how the rest of the country sees addiction by talking about and treating it as a chronic illness, not a moral failing.

Years from now, I want us to look back and know that, in the face of a crisis that threatened our nation, it was our profession that stepped up and led the way. I know we can succeed because health care is more than an occupation to us. It is a calling rooted in empathy, science, and service to humanity. These values unite us. They remain our greatest strength.

Thank you for your leadership.

Rear Admiral Vivek H. Murthy, M.D., M.B.A
19th Surgeon General of the United States, 2014–2017

THE AMERICAN SOCIETY
OF ADDICTION MEDICINE
HANDBOOK ON
PAIN AND ADDICTION

ADDRESSING PAIN AND ADDICTION

Core Concepts

The chapters in **Section I** lay the groundwork for the sections that follow by focusing on the core knowledge that undergirds the fields of pain management and addiction treatment.

- In **Chapter 1**, the authors review current data on the incidence and prevalence of pain and addiction, with special attention to substance use problems involving opioids. This reflects the widespread use of opioids to treat pain, as well as the presence of pain and substance use disorders in a large number of patients.
- **Chapter 2** summarizes current research into the neurophysiology of pain and addiction, with a focus on the characteristics of the human brain that create—or increase—a particular individual's vulnerability to chronic pain and/or addiction.
- In **Chapter 3**, the author reviews the psychosocial aspects of pain and addiction, which play a significant role in increasing or reducing vulnerability to both of these disorders.
- In addition to discussing current terms used to describe pain and addiction, the author of **Chapter 4** considers how the language we use illuminates personal and societal attitudes toward those disorders.
- The author of **Chapter 5** addresses the challenges involved in providing integrated care for pain and addiction, which often involves multiple institutions and caregivers, posing challenges with communication (among clinicians and with the patient) and coordination of services.
- The care of patients with co-occurring pain and addiction raises a number of ethical issues, such as those involving informed consent to treatment and disclosure of information to family members, employers, the courts, and other entities. These and other issues are explored in **Chapter 6**.
- As with ethical issues, pain and addiction each raise specific considerations around compliance with legal and regulatory standards. These issues are explored in **Chapter 7**.

Chapter 1

The Epidemiology of Pain and Addiction

EMILY BRUNNER, M.D. AND
ROBERT LEVY, M.D., FASAM

Public health experts increasingly agree that "the misuse of and addiction to opioids—including prescription pain medicines, heroin, and synthetic opioids such as fentanyl—is a serious national problem that affects public health as well as social and economic welfare" [1]. This statement is supported by recent data from the Centers for Disease Control and Prevention (CDC), which recently estimated that the total economic burden of prescription opioid misuse in the United States is $78.5 billion per year, which includes the costs of health care, lost productivity, addiction treatment, and criminal justice involvement [1].

In 2015, more than 33,000 Americans died as a result of an opioid overdose [2]. In the same year, an estimated 2 million persons in the United States suffered from substance use disorders related to prescription opioid analgesics, and 591,000 suffered from a heroin use disorder (note that these populations are not mutually exclusive) [3].

The issue of opioid misuse and addiction has become a public health epidemic with devastating consequences, including not only increases in opioid abuse and related fatalities from opioid overdose, but also the rising incidence of neonatal abstinence syndrome due to opioid use during pregnancy and the increased spread of infectious diseases, including human immunodeficiency virus (HIV) and hepatitis C [4,5]. (Note that "prescription drug abuse" or "nonmedical use" includes the use of medications without a prescription, for purposes other than those for which they were prescribed, or simply for the experience or feeling that the drugs can cause.)

Although misuse and abuse of opioids affects many Americans, certain populations—such as young people, older adults, and women—appear to be at special risk [2]. Recent research has found a significant increase in mid-life mortality in the United States, particularly among white Americans with less education. Increasing death rates from drug and alcohol poisoning are believed to have played a significant role in this change (Table 1.1) [6].

Some Epidemiological Principles

Epidemiology has been defined in several different ways, but is characterized most simply as the study of how diseases are distributed in populations, as well as the study of the determinants of disease and health [7,8]. Some basic terms used in epidemiology deserve attention in this chapter because they are helpful in understanding the literature of epidemiology and some of the studies reported here (Box 1.1).

Prevalence generally is used to describe the ratio of the total number of cases of a particular disease, divided by the total number of individuals in a particular population at a specific time. *Incidence* refers to the occurrence of new cases of a disease, divided by the total number at risk for the disorder during a specified period of time [7].

Prevalence takes into account both the incidence and duration of a disease, because it depends not only on the rate of newly developed cases over time, but also on the length of time the disease exists in a given population. In turn, the duration of the disorder is affected by the degree of recovery vs. death from the disease. Incidence generally is taken to represent the risk of contracting a disease, whereas prevalence is an indicator of the public health burden the disease imposes on the community [7,8].

The strength of association between a particular characteristic and the development of a disease generally is described as the *relative risk*, which describes the incidence of disease among individuals who have a particular characteristic (such as a family history of opioid addiction), divided by the incidence of disease among those who do not have that characteristic. If there is no difference in the incidence among those with and without the characteristic, the ratio is equal to one.

The *odds ratio* also is a measure of the strength of an association between a characteristic and a disease. A relative risk or odds ratio greater than one indicates a positive association of disease with a given characteristic. A relative risk or odds ratio less than one signifies a negative association, which may indicate the existence of a protective effect associated with the characteristic [9].

Types of Epidemiological Studies

For the purposes of this chapter, epidemiological studies can be divided into two types: (1) observational or (2) experimental.

TABLE 1.1 Trends in Prevalence of Various Drugs Among Persons Age 12 and Older, Ages 12–17, Ages 18–25, and Ages 26 and Older; 2013–2015 (in Percentages)*

Drug	Time Period	Ages 12 or Older			Ages 12–17			Ages 18–25			Ages 26 or Older		
Pain Relievers	Lifetime	[13.50]	13.60	-	[7.30]	7.30	-	[20.80]	20.00	-	13.00	13.30	-
	Past Month	1.70	1.60	**1.40**	[1.70]	1.90	1.10	[3.30]	2.80	2.40	1.50	1.40	1.30
Heroin	Lifetime	1.80	1.80	**1.90**	0.20	0.10	0.10	1.80	2.00	1.80	2.00	2.00	2.10
	Past Month	0.10	[0.20]	**0.10**	0.10	0.10	0.00	0.30	0.20	0.30	0.10	[0.20]	0.10
Tranquilizers	Lifetime	9.00	9.40	-	[2.30]	2.70	-	12.00	12.50	-	9.20	9.70	-
	Past Month	[0.60]	0.70	**0.70**	[0.40]	0.40	0.70	1.20	1.20	1.70	0.60	0.70	0.50
Sedatives	Lifetime	2.90	3.00	-	[0.50]	[0.80]	-	1.30	1.30	-	3.40	3.50	-
	Past Month	0.10	0.10	**0.20**	0.10	0.20	0.10	0.10	0.20	0.20	0.10	0.10	0.20

Source: Excerpted from Substance Abuse and Mental Health Services Administration (SAMHSA). *National Survey on Drug Use and Health: Trends in Prevalence of Various Drugs for Ages 12 or Older, Ages 12 to 17, Ages 18 to 25, and Ages 26 or Older; 2013—2015 (in percent), 2016.* Rockville, MD: SAMHSA, U.S. Department of Health and Human Services; 2017.

BOX 1.1 Terminology

Incidence refers to the number of *new* cases of an indexed disease that develop in a specified interval of time in a particular population.

Point incidence is the number of *new* cases of an indexed disease identified at a specified point in time.

Prevalence indicates the proportion of a population that is diagnosed with an indexed disease or characteristic at a specified point in time.

Lifetime prevalence is the proportion of a population that has experienced the index disease at some point in their lifetimes.

Relative risk indicates the strength of association between a particular characteristic and the development of disease.

Observational studies include cross-sectional, case-control, and cohort studies. In cross-sectional studies or surveys, individuals are evaluated at a particular point in time through use of interviews or physical examination [8]. Whether classified as case-control (retrospective) or cohort (longitudinal, prospective), such studies generally test a hypothesis that an association exists between a particular exposure (risk factor) and a disease or other outcome. In all observational studies, the investigator observes the study participants and gathers information for analysis [9].

Experimental studies, such as randomized clinical trials, are designed by the investigator, who selects the study groups. An intervention (such as a new type of treatment) is given to one group of participants but not another. The study participants are followed, and the outcomes of each group are measured and compared [9].

Data on the Use of Opioids to Treat Chronic Pain

In the general population, the prevalence of regional or widespread chronic musculoskeletal pain syndrome is about 30% [10].

Incidence and Prevalence of Centralized Pain Syndrome

Centralized pain syndrome is seen in patients who have chronic pain and in whom the repeated experience of pain leads to changes in the pain processing pathways in the brain so that, over time, a heightened experience of pain develops.

Centralized pain states may be related to specific organ systems—such as irritable bowel syndrome, chronic headache, endometriosis, temporomandibular joint (TMJ) syndrome, interstitial cystitis, and failed back syndrome—although more generalized pain phenomena also occur. The prototypical syndrome of ongoing generalized pain is fibromyalgia, which involves multiple organ systems (see Chapter 26 of this Handbook).

The prevalence of fibromyalgia is estimated at 2–8%. The prevalence of fibromyalgia increases with age, with peak prevalence occurring between the ages of 60 and 70 [11].

Centralized pain states have similar epidemiology across different organ systems, with the following commonalities. The ratio of women to men is 2 to 1 across the majority of centralized pain states [12]. The prevalence does not vary significantly across different cultures, countries of origin, or ethnic groups [11]. Centralized pain syndromes are likely to be underdiagnosed in men, possibly because of gender differences in describing or minimizing pain. Twin studies show that genetics determine about 50% of the risk of developing a centralized pain syndrome [12].

Trends in Prescribing Opioids for Chronic Pain

The United States has only 4.6% of the world's population, but U.S. residents consume 99% of all the hydrocodone and 81% of all the oxycodone prescribed worldwide [1]. Since 1999, the amount of prescription opioids sold in the United States has nearly quadrupled [1-3], even though there has not been a significant change in the amount of pain reported by patients (Figure 1.1) [2].

In 54% of all cases of nonmedical use of a prescription medication, the drug was obtained from a friend or relative [13]. Looking specifically at opioids intended for nonmedical use, the drugs were obtained directly from a single physician in only 18% of cases and from multiple physicians in fewer than 2% of cases; in another 1% of cases, the source was the Internet [1]. Thus, although it is extremely helpful to have controlled substance registries at the state level (known as prescription drug monitoring programs or PDMPs), the data they collect do not cover all sources of prescription opioids (Figure 1.2) [1].

Morbidity and Mortality Associated with the Use of Opioids to Treat Chronic Pain

Drug overdose deaths in general, and opioid-involved deaths in particular, continue to increase in the United States, and multiple studies show that overdoses related to prescription opioids are a driving factor in the 15-year increase [1]. Specifically, the number of overdose deaths involving opioids (both prescription opioids and heroin) has quadrupled since 1999 (Figure 1.3). Between 2000 and 2015, more than half a million persons died of overdoses—a figure that equals 91 overdose deaths per day [2].

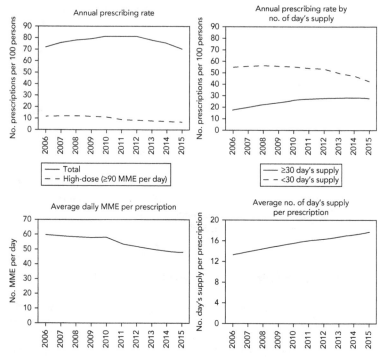

Figure 1.1 *Annual Prescribing Rates of All Opioids vs. High-Dose Opioids, 2006-2015*

Source: Guy Jr. GP, Zhang K, Bohm MK, et al. Vital Signs: Changes in opioid prescribing in the United States, 2006–2015, Figure 1. MMWR. 2017 Jul 7;66(26):699.

Data on Opioid Use Disorder

An issue with which many clinicians struggle is determining the difference between physiological *opioid dependence* and the disease of *opioid use disorder* (OUD). The majority of patients on long-term opioid medications develop a physiological dependence on opioids, as evidenced by the emergence of withdrawal symptoms (such as diarrhea, flushing, and nausea) if the opioid therapy is stopped. Patients who are physically dependent on opioids also demonstrate *tolerance*, meaning that—over time—they require higher doses of medication to achieve an effect similar to that induced by a lower dose when opioid use was initiated [10].

While an emotional response to the prospect of running out of opioid medication (dependence) and requests for higher doses (tolerance) always should raise red flags and indicate the need for further discussion between

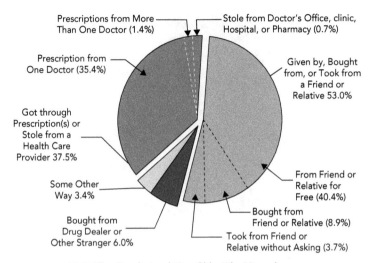

11.5 Million People Aged 12 or Older Who Misused
Prescription Pain Relievers in the Past Year

Figure 1.2 *Sources of Prescription Opioids Among Past-Year Non-Medical Users, 2016*

Source: Substance Abuse and Mental Health Services Administration (SAMHSA). Key substance use and mental health indicators in the United States: Results from the 2016 National Survey on Drug Use and Health, Figure 34 (HHS Publication No. SMA 17-5044, NSDUH Series H-52). Rockville, MD: SAMHSA, Center for Behavioral Health Statistics and Quality, Sep. 2017. (Accessed at: https://www.samhsa.gov/data/.)

physician and patient, these cautions are not necessarily indicative of addiction [14,15].

In fact, the definition of physical dependence has been separated from that of opioid use disorder in the *Diagnostic and Statistical Manual of Mental Disorders*, 5th edition (DSM-5), and its presence no longer is required for a diagnosis of opioid use disorder (addiction) [16]. This change is designed to reduce the confusion between dependence on and tolerance for opioid medications and true opioid addiction.

Prevalence of Opioid Use Disorder in Patients with Chronic Pain

At present, there is very little high-quality research on long-term treatment of chronic nonmalignant pain with long-term opioids. Many of the randomized

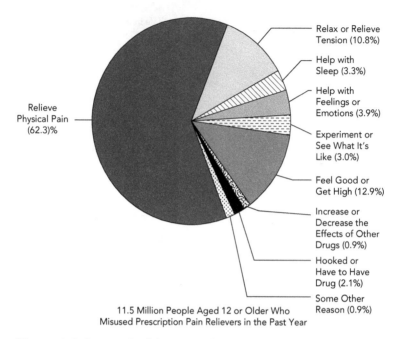

Relax or Relieve Tension (10.8%)

Help with Sleep (3.3%)

Help with Feelings or Emotions (3.9%)

Experiment or See What It's Like (3.0%)

Feel Good or Get High (12.9%)

Increase or Decrease the Effects of Other Drugs (0.9%)

Hooked or Have to Have Drug (2.1%)

Some Other Reason (0.9%)

Relieve Physical Pain (62.3)%

11.5 Million People Aged 12 or Older Who Misused Prescription Pain Relievers in the Past Year

Figure 1.3 *Reasons Cited for Misuse of Prescription Pain Relievers, 2016*

Source: Substance Abuse and Mental Health Services Administration (SAMHSA). Key substance use and mental health indicators in the United States: Results from the 2016 National Survey on Drug Use and Health, Figure 33 (HHS Publication No. SMA 17-5044, NSDUH Series H-52). Rockville, MD: SAMHSA, Center for Behavioral Health Statistics and Quality, Sep. 2017. (Accessed at: https://www.samhsa.gov/data/.)

studies that do exist specifically exclude patients with a history of substance use or mental disorder. This does not reflect actual medical practice, as these are the very patients who are most likely to receive opioid treatment in routine care [17].

For a long time, opioid addiction was thought to be a rare phenomenon. In one early study, charts were pulled for patients who had been given opioids for a variety of indications, with no specificity of dosing or duration of treatment. The investigators concluded that only four of the 11,882 persons treated with an opioid medication while in an inpatient setting were subsequently diagnosed with "addiction" [1]. Unfortunately, over a period of time, this study was widely cited as "proof" that there was only about a 1% risk that a patient treated with opioids in an outpatient setting would develop addiction.

More recently, it has been recognized that the real prevalence of opioid use disorder is significantly higher [2,3]. The prevalence of opioid use disorder that develops as a result of long-term use of opioids to treat chronic pain varies widely, with estimates ranging from 3.2–27% [18]. The preponderance of estimates are in the range of 20–25% [10,13].

Mortality Associated with Opioid Use Disorder

Data from the 2015 National Survey on Drug Use and Health (NSDUH) [13] support an estimate that 22.6 million persons, or 8.9% of Americans ages 12 and older, had used opioids for nonmedical purposes in the preceding month. The NSDUH survey found that, of this group, 5.1 million had used opioid analgesics, which was second only to the rate of marijuana use [13].

As a result of this widespread use, the number of deaths attributed to drug poisoning and overdose has surpassed the mortality resulting from motor vehicle crashes as the leading cause of accidental death in the United States, and half of these deaths are attributed to opioid analgesics [18]. Overdose deaths involving prescription opioid pain relievers have more than tripled in the past 20 years [18].

A comprehensive review in 2010 calculated that opioid use increases the risk of death by almost 15-fold [19]. This increased risk of death is attributed to overdose (the most common cause), suicide, and trauma. In contrast, protective factors were identified as receiving addiction treatment (including medication management with either methadone or buprenorphine), being HIV-seronegative, and having a lower number of episodes of injection drug use [20].

Mortality Associated with Specific Opioids

Overall, the recent escalation in heroin use and the resulting increase in cases of heroin overdose have occurred in tandem with a dramatic increase in misuse and abuse of opioid analgesics. Of particular concern has been the rise in new populations of heroin users, particularly young people [1].

Heroin

Abuse of heroin in the United States increased by 63% from 2002 through 2013 [21]. Over the same time period, the rate of heroin-related overdose deaths increased by 286% (from 0.7 per 100,000 to 2.7 per 100,000) (Figure 1.4) [21].

The rate of heroin initiation among persons with a history of nonmedical use of opioid analgesics has been found to be 19 times greater than in persons who have no history of nonmedical use of prescription opioids [21].

Some studies show that heroin use is increasing most sharply among women, regardless of income level. Nevertheless, the demographics of persons who are at greatest risk of heroin use disorder remain males age 18–25,

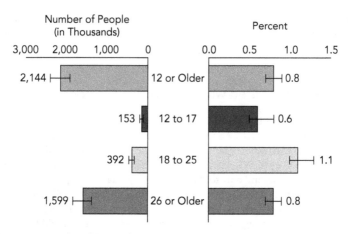

Figure 1.4 *Opioid Use in the Past Year, by Age Group, 2016*

Source: Substance Abuse and Mental Health Services Administration (SAMHSA). Key substance use and mental health indicators in the United States: Results from the 2016 National Survey on Drug Use and Health, Figure 41 (HHS Publication No. SMA 17-5044, NSDUH Series H-52). Rockville, MD: SAMHSA, Center for Behavioral Health Statistics and Quality, Sep. 2017. (Accessed at: https://www.samhsa.gov/data/.)

non-Hispanic whites, those with less than $20,000 annual household income, Medicaid recipients, and the uninsured [21].

Oxycodone

Among opioid analgesics that are subject to nonmedical use, oxycodone has been found to be particularly popular, probably because oxycodone crosses quickly into the brain and creates a more intense "high" than other opioids [19]. As a result, some have described oxycodone as a "gateway drug" to heroin.

Studies have found that increases in the number of hospitalizations for overdoses and other problems with opioid analgesics are predictive of an increase in the number of heroin overdose hospitalizations in subsequent years [20].

Fentanyl and Other Synthetic Opioids

The emergence of illicitly manufactured synthetic opioids—including fentanyl, carfentanyl, and their analogues—represents an escalation of the ongoing opioid epidemic. Fentanyl is a mu-opioid receptor agonist that is 80 times more potent than morphine in vivo. While fentanyl is available as a prescription medication—primarily for use as an anesthetic, for the treatment of post-surgical pain, or for the management of pain in opioid-tolerant patients—it is the illicitly manufactured versions that have been largely responsible for the tripling of overdose deaths related to synthetic opioids in just two years, from 3,105 in 2013 to 9,580 in 2015 [2].

A variety of fentanyl analogues and synthetic opioids are included in these numbers, such as carfentanyl (which is approximately 10,000 times more potent than morphine), acetyl-fentanyl (about 15 times more potent than morphine), butyrfentanyl (more than 30 times more potent than morphine), U-47700 (about 12 times more potent than morphine), and MT-45 (roughly equivalent to morphine in potency), among others [17].

Conclusion

The opioid crisis began in the mid-to-late 1990s, prompted by a number of factors that led to a dramatic increase in opioid prescribing. These factors included a regulatory, policy, and practice focus on opioid medications as the primary treatment for many types of pain; [22] a widespread (albeit subsequently discredited) belief that that opioids prescribed for pain would not lead to addiction; [23] the release of American Pain Society guidelines in 1996 that encouraged providers to assess pain as "the fifth vital sign" at each clinical encounter; and the initiation of aggressive marketing campaigns by pharmaceutical manufacturers, who promoted the notion that opioids do not pose a significant risk for misuse or addiction, and that they are appropriate as "first-line" treatments for chronic pain [24].

The sale of prescription opioids more than tripled between 1999 and 2011 [25], and this was paralleled by a more than fourfold increase in treatment admissions for opioid abuse and a nearly fourfold increase in overdose deaths related to prescription opioids [26]. Federal and state efforts to curb opioid prescribing resulted in a leveling off of opioid prescriptions, beginning in 2012 [27]. However, heroin-related overdose deaths had already begun to rise in 2007 and continued to increase from just over 3,000 in 2010 to nearly 13,000 in 2015 [28].

We now know that the misuse of prescription opioids is a significant risk factor for heroin use, and that 80% of heroin users begin with misuse of prescription opioids [29]. While only about 4% of those who misuse prescription opioids go on to initiate heroin use within five years, this subset of individuals who prefer heroin as the less expensive, easier-to-obtain street drug are emblematic of the progression of opioid addiction [30].

The opioid overdose crisis continues to escalate, with a striking increase in deaths related to illicitly manufactured synthetic opioids such as fentanyl. In fact, the population of individuals who use and overdose on fentanyl looks very similar to the population who use heroin. However, the drivers of fentanyl use can be complicated, as the drug often is sold in counterfeit pills—designed to look like common prescription opioids or benzodiazepines such as alprazolam (Xanax)—or added as an adulterant to heroin or other drugs, unbeknownst to the user [29]. Thus, market forces support the proliferation of higher-potency opioids, as individuals who are addicted to opioids develop tolerance and seek increasingly potent agents [30].

Epidemiological research into the origins and progression of the opioid epidemic can help improve our understanding of etiological mechanisms, identify appropriate targets for interventions, and ultimately, reduce the prevalence and adverse outcomes of opioid and other substance use disorders [1].

For More Information on the Topics Discussed:

American Society of Addiction Medicine (ASAM):

Crum R. The epidemiology of substance use disorders (Chapter 2). In RK Ries, DA Fiellin, SC Miller, R Saitz, eds. *The ASAM Principles of Addiction Medicine, Fifth Edition*. Philadelphia, PA: Wolters Kluwer; 2014.

Wedde M, Kokotailo PK. Epidemiology of adolescent substance use (Chapter 100). In RK Ries, DA Fiellin, SC Miller, R Saitz, eds. *The ASAM Principles of Addiction Medicine, Fifth Edition*. Philadelphia, PA: Wolters Kluwer; 2014.

National Institute on Drug Abuse (NIDA). NIDAMED:

Resources to increase physicians' awareness of the effect of substance use on patients' health and to help identify drug use early and prevent it from escalating to abuse or addiction. (Access at: drugabuse.gov/nidamed)

Substance Abuse and Mental Health Services Administration (SAMHSA):

National Survey on Drug Use and Health (NSDUH) Report. Rockville, MD: SAMHSA, U.S. Department of Health and Human Services; 2017. (Access at: https://nsduhweb.rti.org/respweb/homepage.cfm)

Acknowledgment

The authors express their gratitude to Jane C. Maxwell, Ph.D., recently retired Director of the Center for Excellence in Epidemiology at the University of Texas at Austin, for her thoughtful contributions to this chapter.

References

1. Compton WH. *Research on the Use and Misuse of Fentanyl and Other Synthetic Opioids: Testimony Before the House Committee on Energy and Commerce, Subcommittee on Oversight and Investigations.* Washington, DC: U.S. House of Representatives; March 14, 2017.

2. Rudd RA, Seth P, David F, et al. Increases in drug and opioid-involved overdose deaths—United States, 2010–2015. *MMWR.* 2016 Dec 16;65:1445–1452.

3. Substance Abuse and Mental Health Services Administration (SAMHSA). *National Survey on Drug Use and Health: 2015 Detailed Tables.* Rockville, MD: SAMHSA, U.S. Department of Health and Human Services; 2016.

4. Patrick SW, Davis MM, Lehmann CU, et al. Increasing incidence and geographic distribution of neonatal abstinence syndrome: United States 2009 to 2012. *J Perinatol.* 2015;35:650–655.

5. Peters PJ, Pontones P, Hoover KW, et al., for the Indiana HIV Outbreak Investigation Team. HIV infection linked to injection use of oxymorphone in Indiana, 2014–2015. *NEJM.* 2016;375:229–239.

6. Zibbell JE, Iqbal K, Patel RC, et al. Increases in hepatitis C virus infection related to injection drug use among persons aged ≤30 years—Kentucky, Tennessee, Virginia, and West Virginia, 2006–2012. *MMWR* 2015;64:453–458.

7. Gordis E. *Epidemiology, 4th Edition.* Philadelphia, PA: Saunders Elsevier; 2009.

8. Lilienfeld DE, Stolley PD. *Foundations of Epidemiology, 3rd Edition.* New York: Oxford University Press; 1994.

9. Porta M, ed. *A Dictionary of Epidemiology, 5th Edition.* New York: Oxford University Press, 2008.

10. National Institute on Drug Abuse (NIDA). *Misuse of Prescription Drugs.* Bethesda, MD: NIDA, National Institutes of Health; August 2016. (Accessed at: https://www.drugabuse.gov/publications/research-reports/misuse-prescription-drugs/)

11. Clauw D. Fibromyalgia and related conditions. *Mayo Clin Proc.* 2015 May;90(5):680–692.

12. Vincent A, Lahr BD, Wolfe F, et al. Prevalence of fibromyalgia: A population-based study in Olmsted County, Minnesota, utilizing the Rochester Epidemiology Project. *Arthritis Care Res.* 2013 May;65(5):779–786.

13. Substance Abuse and Mental Health Services Administration (SAMHSA). *National Survey on Drug Use and Health: Misuse of Prescription Pain Relievers and Other Prescription Psychotherapeutics Among People Aged 12 or Older Who Were Current Misusers of Any Prescription Psychotherapeutics: 2015.* Rockville, MD: SAMHSA, U.S. Department of Health and Human Services; 2017.

14. Compton WM, Boyle M, Wargo E. Prescription opioid abuse: Problems and responses. *Prev Med.* 2015 Nov;80:5–9.

15. Crum R. The epidemiology of substance use disorders. In RK Ries, DA Fiellin, SC Miller, R Saitz, eds. *The ASAM Principles of Addiction Medicine, Fifth Edition.* Philadelphia, PA: Wolters Kluwer; 2014:19–35.

16. American Psychiatric Association (APA). *Diagnostic and Statistical Manual of Mental Disorders, Fifth Edition (DSM-5)*. Washington, DC: American Psychiatric Association Publishing; 2013.

17. Deyo R, Von Korff M, Duhrkoop D, et al. Opioids for low back pain. *BMJ*. 2015 Jan 5;350:g6380.

18. Pohl M. Chronic pain and addiction: Challenging co-occurring disorders. *J Psychoactive Drugs*. 2012;44(2):119–124.

19. Degenhardt L, Bucello C, Mathers B, et al. Mortality among regular or dependent users of heroin and other opioids: A systematic review and meta-analysis of cohort studies. *Addiction*. 2011 Jan;106(1):32–51.

20. Andersson H. Increased mortality among individuals with chronic widespread pain relates to lifestyle factors: A prospective population-based study. *Disabil Rehabil*. 2009;31(24):1980.

21. Jones C, Logan J, Gladden RM, et al. Vital signs: Demographic and substance use trends among heroin users: United States 2002–2013. *MMWR*. 2015 Jul 10;64(26):719–725.

22. Rosenblum A, Marsch LA, Joseph H, et al. Opioids and the treatment of chronic pain: Controversies, current status, and future directions. *Exp Clin Psychopharm*. 2008;16:405–416.

23. Van Zee A. The promotion and marketing of Oxycontin: Commercial triumph, public health tragedy. *Am J Public Health*. 2009;99:221–227.

24. Morone NE, Weiner DK. Pain as the fifth vital sign: Exposing the vital need for pain education. *Clin Ther*. 2013;35:1728–1732.

25. Cicero TJ, Inciardi JA, Munoz A. Trends in abuse of Oxycontin and other opioid analgesics in the United States: 2002–2004. *J Pain*. 2005;6:662–672.

26. Centers for Disease Control and Prevention (CDC). Vital signs: Overdoses of prescription opioid pain relievers—United States, 1999-2008. *MMWR Morb*. 2011;60:1487–1492.

27. Dart RC, Surratt HL, Cicero TJ, et al. Trends in opioid analgesic abuse and mortality in the United States. *NEJM*. 2015;372:241–248.

28. Compton WM, Jones CM, Baldwin GT. Nonmedical prescription-opioid use and heroin use. *NEJM*. 2016;374:1296.

29. Carlson RG, Nahhas RW, Martins SS, et al. Predictors of transition to heroin use among initially non-opioid dependent illicit pharmaceutical opioid users: A natural history study. *Drug Alcohol Depend*. 2016;160:127–134.

30. Kerr T, Small W, Hyshka E, et al. "It's more about the heroin": Injection drug users' response to an overdose warning campaign in a Canadian setting. *Addiction*. 2013;108:1270–1276.

Chapter 2

The Neuroscience of Pain and Addiction

R. COREY WALLER, M.D., M.S., DFASAM

If you are distressed by anything external, the pain is not due to the thing itself,
but to your estimate of it; and this you have the power to revoke at any moment.
— MARCUS AURELIUS, *Meditations*

The neurological architecture of pain, as well as that of addiction, is vast and extremely detailed. It involves the injury or exogenous chemicals ingested, neurochemicals released in response, the receptors that are bound, the cells that are depolarized, the nuclei that sense and interpret the signal, the integrated systems and physiological changes involved in a response, and the behavior that occurs as a result. It is impossible to discuss all of these issues in a single chapter. Therefore, this chapter will focus on the basic neuroscience of pain and addiction, as well as how the interplay between the two disorders can affect patients who suffer from both.

Progress in Understanding Pain and Addiction

Over the past several decades, considerable progress has been made in understanding the nature of pain and addiction. The initial protein targets for almost all substances of abuse have been identified. In addition, several circuits in the brain containing those targets are now known to mediate the addicting actions of drugs of abuse [1].

We now know that, over time, repeated drug exposure causes adaptations in the brain's reward pathways that seem to have two major consequences. First, during periods of active drug use or shortly after stopping drug intake, the ability of natural rewards to activate the reward pathways is diminished, and the individual experiences depressed motivation and mood. Taking more drugs is the quickest, easiest way for such an individual to feel "normal" again.

Second, drug use causes long-lasting memories related to the drug experience, to an extent that even after prolonged periods of abstinence (months or years), stressful events or exposure to drug-associated cues can trigger intense craving and relapse, in part by activating the brain's reward pathways.

Reward pathways are very old from an evolutionary point of view. Presumably they evolved to mediate an individual's response to natural rewards, such as food, sex, and social interaction. Drugs of abuse activate these reward pathways with a force and persistence that is not seen under ordinary conditions [2].

Neuroimaging studies of humans and gene targeting of other animals have identified specific neurological substrates, receptor agonists and antagonists [3]. Neuroimaging has allowed researchers to measure neural effects following drug exposures as they occur, as well as how they change and persist in the brains of individuals with substance use disorders and how they remit after periods of abstinence.

Substances that are neurotoxic with chronic use (such as opioids) induce changes that are evident at a gross structural level. Affected brain areas include:

- The *brain stem,* which controls basic functions critical to life, such as heart rate, breathing, and sleeping.
- The *limbic system,* which contains the brain's reward circuit, linking multiple brain structures that control and regulate humans' ability to feel pleasure. Feeling pleasure motivates humans to repeat certain behaviors (such as eating) that are critical to survival. The limbic system is activated when we perform these activities, as well as by drugs of abuse. In addition, the limbic system is responsible for humans' perception of other emotions, both positive and negative, which explains the mood-altering properties of many drugs.
- The *cerebral cortex,* which is divided into areas that control specific functions. Different areas also process information from our senses, enabling us to see, feel, hear, and taste. The front part of the cortex—the frontal cortex or forebrain—is the thinking center of the brain, which powers our ability to think, plan, solve problems, and make decisions [2].

Alcohol, opioids, and other substances that are misused or abused act by enhancing specific brain neurochemical pathways in a manner similar to that induced by other natural rewards (such as food and sex), but in a more intense and prolonged manner. Dopamine-containing projections from the ventral tegmental area to the nucleus accumbens are key components of brain reward circuitry. Activity in this dopamine pathway plays a pivotal role in coding reward (and its saliency), predicting reward, and generating the motivation to pursue reward. The same pathway is involved in priming cortical regions that exert inhibitory control and executive function (choice), and in conditioned or learned responses [3]. By mimicking the brain effects of natural rewards— which serve biological needs—certain drugs exert a capacity to shape human behavior [4].

Although initial activation of the neural pathway is a critical step in reinforcing behavior and promoting substance misuse, it is the long-term changes in brain circuitry in the higher cortical pathways that are most closely associated with addiction. In fact, repeated administration of the substance of abuse triggers long-term synaptic changes in higher brain regions and excitatory neuropathways, as learned associations with drug-related events are formed [5].

Ultimately, these changes modify (diminish) the way in which the brain perceives the value of natural rewards. They also diminish the capacity of the prefrontal cortex to exert cognitive control over drug-seeking behavior, while at the same time enhancing the brain's response to drug-related cues and stimuli [6].

At a behavioral level, the individual transitions from experiencing the acute effects of a drug, to patterns of recreational use, and then to pathological states of abuse or addiction. The persistence of addiction is based on the remodeling of synapses and brain circuits, similar to the process of long-term associative memory, in which drug-associated environmental stimuli or cues have inordinate power to direct behavior [7].

The persistence of changes in brain activity of persons who are addicted to an opioid helps to explain the persistence of their drug-related behaviors, their altered motivational hierarchies, and their responses to cues and craving, all of which can persist for long periods after substance use has stopped [8]. Such changes have obvious implications for the required course and effectiveness of treatment in addicted individuals.

Addiction should be viewed as distinct from *physical dependence*, in which individuals develop tolerance and experience withdrawal if opioid administration is stopped abruptly [1]. Physical dependence per se is neither necessary nor sufficient to cause addiction: some drugs of abuse do not cause physical dependence, while opioids and some other drugs used for medical conditions can cause physical dependence in the absence of addiction. Moreover, physical dependence and withdrawal syndromes are largely mediated by different regions of the central nervous system (CNS) than those important to addiction.

Issues That Confound Basic Neuroscience

Despite the exciting research studies that have been completed and are currently under way, many issues in the neurophysiology of pain and addiction are not yet completely understood. One reason is that the majority of knowledge obtained about the structure and function of the nervous system is obtained through laboratory studies rather than "real life." Sadly, we are in something like the dark ages in terms of true functional neuroscience. However, we also are at the precipice of understanding how actual life events significantly affect both brain structure and function.

One of the areas that is most often studied is the effect of trauma in early life on the development of cognitive capabilities, memory allocation, and overall emotional stability [9,10]. Another area of great interest is the impact of organic mental illness on the behaviors and brain function of a patient with chronic pain. Other issues—such as social instability, genetic predisposition, and the overall inadequacies of the current health care system—significantly affect every patient.

Brain Structures and Their Functions

The major areas of the brain and the principal functions of each include the following (Figure 2.1):

- **Amygdala (Amyg):** This central matrix within the limbic system (i.e., the emotional brain):
  - Contains more than a dozen different nuclei;
  - Is the target of more than 1,000 different connections from all over the brain;
  - Belongs to the *visual system* (which is responsible for reading the emotions on people's faces);
  - Is part of the *autonomic system* and thus is responsible for arousal (as well as the lack of arousal in pathological or aversive states);
  - Is part of the *value network* through its connections with the orbitofrontal cortex, and thus is responsible for helping determine the relative value of an action in terms of either immediate gratification or future gratification. This function is close to—but different from—brain reward. It is bypassed in the pathological state of addiction.
  - Is a site of pathology in post-traumatic stress disorder (PTSD), producing aberrant emotional responses to pain and possibly personality disorders through conditioned aversive response memory [11,12,13].
- **Lateral amygdala (L-Amyg):** The sensory and aversive learning amygdala projects mostly to and from the *prefrontal cortex* (the home of complex thought). The lateral amygdala:

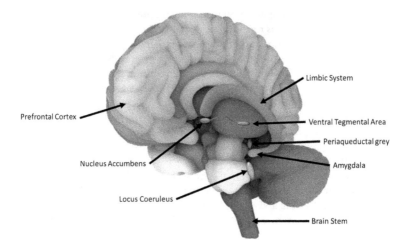

Figure 2.1 *Major Areas of the Brain Affected by Substance Use and Pain*

- Is the fear and anxiety center of the brain;
- Takes in many pieces of information and "decides" whether or not to be motivated in response to such information; and
- If motivated, sends a signal to the central nuclei to perform the emotional response of freeze, flight, or startle.
- **Central Amygdala (C-Amyg):** The central amygdala (which produces emotional responses) has most of its connections to the hypothalamus, periaqueductal gray (PAG), and other brain stem structures. It:
  - Instigates the "freeze" response mediated by the PAG;
  - Instigates the "flight" response mediated by the hypothalamus and the locus coeruleus (LC);
  - Connects with the ventral tegmental area (VTA) to release dopamine when under conditioned stress; and
  - Can modulate arousal and/or attention if guided by the lateral amygdala.
- **Locus Coeruleus (LC):** The locus coeruleus is the unsung nuclei of pain and addiction. It is:
  - The major site of central production of norepinephrine;
  - Involved in the sleep/wake cycle;
  - A major component of opioid withdrawal and, to a lesser extent, thanol (EtOH) withdrawal.
  - This structure also may play a significant role in the stress response to chronic pain [11,14,15].
- **Hypothalamus:** The hypothalamus plays a larger role in pain and addiction than is generally recognized. For example, it is

- responsible for motivation to seek something, but not responsible for liking it if it is forced upon it (that is, the hypothalamus is the not involved in the *feeling* of reward, but rather generates the need to *seek* reward. In addition, the hypothalamus is responsible for the major neuro-endocrine responses to chronic pain and addiction [11,12].
- **Periaqueductal Gray** (PAG). Major structure involved in descending pain modulation:
  - Major central producer of opioids and is mostly responsible for central control of analgesia;
  - Also produces enkephalin (endorphin) and oxytocin;
  - Has connections to the prefrontal cortex and may modulate copulatory behavior and maternal bonding [11,12,16].
- **Nucleus Accumbens (NAc, a.k.a. the ventral striatum):** Made up of a core and a shell and is the structure responsible for translating an emotional stimulus into behaviors. Lovingly referred to as the "pleasure center":
  - Mostly responsible for behavioral sensitization after repetitive drug use;
  - Is the functional interface between the limbic system and the motor system;
  - Has reciprocal innervations with the whole of the limbic system and the prefrontal cortex.
  - Ultimately, it "informs" us what is pleasurable [11,12,17].
- **Ventral Tegmental Area (VTA):** The site that initiates behavioral sensitization to a drug via release of dopamine to the NAc and the PFC:
  - Responsible for male ejaculation (Holsteg);
  - Responsible for the signal for the rat to "press the lever" to get more drug [11,12,17].
- **Hippocampus (Hipp):** Responsible for memory allocation and understanding "context":
  - One of the few sites that creates new cells.
  - This creation is significantly decreased with drug use, leading to the "not learning from my mistakes" phenomenon in substance use disorder.
  - This learning is generally modulated by the VTA, which is why we remember stimulating and rewarding information better than the boring stuff. Again, however, more stimulation is not "better" as already described [11,12,18,19].
- **Raphe Nuclei (RN):** Primarily release serotonin (5-HT) and acts as a modulator for aggression, emotion, and mood, and are impacted by drugs of abuse and pain:
  - Mainly impacted by alcohol, opioids, cocaine, amphetamines, and 3,4-Methylenedioxymethamphetamine (MDMA).
  - When affected, can lead to violent and impulsive behavior [11,12,20].

- **Dorsal Horn of the Spinal Cord:** Receives the pain signal input from Aδ and C fibers:
  - These are then modulated by interneurons that send signals up the ascending pathways;
  - Produces endogenous opioids to modulate pain [12,21,22].
- **Spinothalamic/Cervicothalamic Tract:** Ascending tract that sends the pain signal from the dorsal horn to the thalamus:
  - Pain → spinothalamic tract → thalamus → sensory cortex [16,21,23,24].
- **Spinoreticular Tract**: Ascending tract that ends a pain signal to the alertness centers of the brain:
  - Pain → spinoreticular tract → reticular formation → locus coeruleus [16,21,23,24].
- **Spinomesencephalic Tract:** Ascending tract responsible for connection with the limbic system and instigating the emotional response to pain:
  - Pain → spinomesencephalic tract → PAG → limbic system [16,21,23,24].
- **Spinohypothalamic Tract**: Ascending tract responsible for the signal causing the endocrine response to pain:
  - Pain → spinohypothalamic tract → hypothalamus → endocrine response [16,21,23,24].
- **Descending Modulatory Pain Tracts:** Two major tracts responsible for modulating pain at the spinal cord, based on our perception of pain and the situation:
  - Pain → ascending tract information assessed → PAG (opioid) → locus coeruleus (norepinephrine [NE]) → dorsal horn → decrease in pain;
  - Pain → ascending tract information assessed → raphe magnus (5-HT, enkephalin) → dorsal horn → decrease in pain [16,21,23-26].

Addiction Pathways

The contemporary understanding of the chronic brain disease that is addiction has coalesced over the past 15 years into a consistent yet evolving set of known facts [11,12,17,20,25,27,28].

The first is that the VTA and the NAc are the center of our reward system and, when significantly altered, they orchestrate behaviors that manifest as the patterns described by the DSM-5. The second fact is that early-life trauma lowers the threshold of substance use needed to develop these alterations. Third, if the dopamine axis can be stabilized pharmacologically, then persistent behavioral therapy can undo the old conditioned response to the cues associated with substance use, thus stabilizing the behaviors. Sounds simple, right?

While we know that the VTA and the NAc play a vital role in reward eval-uation and realization, there are also many other structures involved in the pathological aspects of addiction. For instance, the dopamine projections passing through the lateral hypothalamus have been shown to be responsible for the craving of reward and to increase the hedonic tone of the brain [29]. While dopamine neurons in the VTA, NAc, and hypothalamus play the most significant roles in reinforcement of drug craving and use, these behaviors can be altered by the external emotional centers. For instance, the amygdala can regulate fear or anxiety about the absence of a drug. One pathway shows that as the LC senses an acute lack of opioid, it will start to release norepinephrine. This sends a signal to the C-amyg, instigating a flight response and signal-ing the VTA that reward is needed for survival [30]. This in turn signals the L-amyg, which then signals the prefrontal cortex, the PAG, the hippocampus (for a memory of where to find said drug), and the hypothalamus to trigger the craving.

This becomes persistent pathology at the point at which constant drug use creates a permanent lack of dopamine in the VTA and NAc. When this occurs, the system is in a constantly heightened state of arousal, and any small cue or outside stress, or the smallest dose of a related drug, will set off the cascade. Behaviors will become more and more survival-related as the dopamine level drops and the LC, C-amyg, L-amyg, and hypothalamus are less and less capable of compensating for the learned nature of this response [31].

Pain Pathways

In order to better understand the way that pain is transmitted, identified, and acted upon, we will consider three different scenarios of a pain response [11–13,15,16,19,21,29–31].

1. *Normal response in a person with average to high pain tolerance:* Imagine a patient has acute or chronic pain, such as twisting a chronically painful back. The first signals will arise from the dorsal horn, move through the ascending pathways, be received by the appropriate structures, and then modulate the pain signal through the descending pathways. So it will look something like this: Emotionally assess, and if all is good, then → **Increase** descending **inhibition** → thus **decreasing** the ascend-ing **pain signal** → all happening while we produce our own endorphins from the dorsal horn and the PAG → This in turn equals less pain and greater function.

2. *Normal response in a person with "low" pain tolerance:* In this scenario, a patient with a low pain tolerance experiences the same acute or chronic pain (twisting a chronically painful back).

Emotionally assess, and all **not good** → **Increase** in descending **excitatory** pathway (less norepinephrine from the LC and less 5-HT and ENK from the raphe magnus and PAG) → **Decrease** in **inhibitory** pathway → **Increase** in perceived **pain** followed by agitation and tachypnea → This changes the pH in the serum and thus increases the amount of endorphin released in response from PAG and Zone II and III of the dorsal horn → Then, after the panic-like state, pain normalizes.

3. Exogenous opioids are added, triggering the following effects:
   - Reduced production of endogenous opioids in the PAG and the dorsal horn;
   - The body "ramps up" the frequency of pain signals;
   - A greater signal emanates from ascending tracts (spinothalamic, spinoreticular, and spinomesencephalic), resulting in more pain in a widened area;
   - Endorphin production from PAG and the dorsal horn is reduced;
   - The patient experiences worsened sleep patterns;
   - The patient also exhibits more emotional lability from the opioid's effects on the limbic system.

The persistence of changes in brain activity of persons who are addicted to an opioid helps to explain the persistence of their drug-related behaviors, their altered motivational hierarchies, and their responses to cues and craving, all of which can persist for long periods after substance use has ceased [8]. Such changes have obvious implications for the required course and effectiveness of treatment in individuals with opioid use disorder.

Conclusion

Understanding the neuroscience of pain and addiction matters, because that is what physicians are treating. As the emotional pathology of a patient with chronic pain accumulates, so does the risk of addiction. Given this fact, trauma-informed care should be the rule rather than the exception.

Understanding all of this also helps clinicians understand why treatments for pain, suffering, and addiction are very similar in terms of the approaches employed. Taking the emotion (but not the empathy) out of the treatment of pain and addiction allows neuroscience to dictate the appropriate steps in treatment.

It also is clear that overlap of neurologic structures involved in pain and addiction is immense when the pain signal is correctly interpreted and acted upon. Therefore, the clinician's initial response to "drug seeking" in patients with pain ought to be to address the pain. It is now clear that, if the pain is not addressed, the patient's drug-seeking behaviors will persist even after the pain is gone. Thus, the patient's initial effort to find relief from pain will evolve into the pathology of addiction.

For More Information on the Topics Discussed:

American Society of Addiction Medicine (ASAM):

Volkow ND, Warren KR. Drug addiction: The neurobiology of behavior gone awry (Chapter 1). In RK Ries, DA Fiellin, SC Miller, R Saitz, eds. *The ASAM Principles of Addiction Medicine, Fifth Edition*. Philadelphia, PA: Wolters Kluwer; 2014.

Beveridge TJR, Roberts DCS. The anatomy of addiction (Chapter 3). In RK Ries, DA Fiellin, SC Miller, R Saitz, eds. *The ASAM Principles of Addiction Medicine, Fifth Edition*. Philadelphia, PA: Wolters Kluwer; 2014.

Gallagher RM, Koob G, Popescu A. The pathophysiology of chronic pain and clinical interfaces with addiction (Chapter 93). In RK Ries, DA Fiellin, SC Miller, R Saitz, eds. *The ASAM Principles of Addiction Medicine, Fifth Edition*. Philadelphia, PA: Wolters Kluwer; 2014.

In the Literature:

Fenton BW, Shih E, Zolton J. The neurobiology of pain perception in normal and persistent pain. *Pain Manag*. 2015;5(4):297–317.

Wise RA, Koob GF. The development and maintenance of drug addiction. *Neuropsychopharmacology*. 2014 Jan;39(2):254–262.

References

1. O'Brien CP, Chair, for the SAMHSA-NIDA Consensus Panel on New Pharmacotherapies for Opioid Use Disorders. *Clinical Guidance on the Use of Extended-Release Injectable Naltrexone in the Treatment of Opioid Use Disorders and Related Comorbidities*. Rockville, MD: Substance Abuse and Mental Health Services Administration (SAMHSA) and Bethesda, MD: National Institute on Drug Abuse (NIDA), U.S. Department of Health and Human Services; 2013.
2. National Institute on Drug Abuse (NIDA). *Drugs, Brains, and Behavior: The Science of Addiction*. Bethesda, MD: NIDA, National Institutes of Health; July 2014. (Accessed at: https://www.drugabuse.gov/publications/drugs-brains-behavior-science-addiction)
3. Kalivas PW, Volkow ND. The neural basis of addiction: A pathology of motivation and choice. *Am J Psychiatry*. 2005 Aug;162(8):1403–1413.
4. Frew AK, Drummond PD. Negative affect, pain and sex: The role of endogenous opioids. *Pain*. 2007 Nov;132(Suppl 1):S77–S85.
5. Nestler EJ. From neurobiology to treatment: progress against addiction. *Nat Neurosci*. 2002 Nov;5(Suppl):1076–1079. Review.
6. Kalivas PW, Volkow ND. The neural basis of addiction: A pathology of motivation and choice. *Am J Psychiatry*. 2005 Aug;162(8):1403–1413.

7. Kauer JA. Learning mechanisms in addiction: Synaptic plasticity in the ventral tegmental area as a result of exposure to drugs of abuse. *Annu Rev Physiol.* 2004;66:447–475. Review.

8. Nestler EJ. Is there a common molecular pathway for addiction? *Nat Neurosci.* 2005 Nov;8(11):1445–1449. Review.

9. Faulx D, Baldwin J, Zorrah Q, et al. Adverse childhood events in the mental health discussion. *Am J Public Health.* 2011;101(7):1156–1157.

10. Violence Prevention. 2016; April 01. (Accessed at: https://www.cdc.gov/violenceprevention/acestudy/index.html)

11. Kandel ER. *Principles of Neural Science, 5th ed.* New York: McGraw-Hill; 2012.

12. Conn PM. *Conn's Translational Neuroscience.* London, UK: Academic Press; 2017.

13. Yassa MA, Hazlett RL, Stark CE, et al. Functional MRI of the amygdala and bed nucleus of the stria terminalis during conditions of uncertainty in generalized anxiety disorder. *J Psychiatr Res.* 2012;46(8):1045–1052.

14. Isenberg-Grzeda E, Ellis J. Supportive care and psychological issues around cancer (editorial). *Curr Opin Support Palliat Care.* 2015;9(1):38–39.

15. Llorca-Torralba M, Borges G, Neto F, et al. Noradrenergic locus coeruleus pathways in pain modulation. *Neuroscience.* 2016;338:93–113.

16. Deer TR, Leong MS, Buvanendran A. Comprehensive treatment of chronic pain by medical, interventional, and integrative approaches. *The American Academy of Pain Medicine Textbook on Patient Management.* New York: Springer; 2013.

17. Volkow ND, Warren KR. Drug addiction: The neurobiology of behavior gone awry. In RK Ries, DA Fiellin, SC Miller, R Saitz, eds. *The ASAM Principles of Addiction Medicine, Fifth Edition.* Philadelphia, PA: Wolters Kluwer; 2014:3–18.

18. Kranzler HR, Ciraulo DA, Zindel LR. *Clinical Manual of Addiction Psychopharmacology.* Washington, DC: American Psychiatric Publishing; 2014.

19. Fairbanks CA. *Neurobiological Studies of Addiction in Chronic Pain States.* New York: Springer-Verlag; 2016.

20. Stahl S, Muntner N. *Stahl's Essential Psychopharmacology: Neuroscientific Basis and Practical Application.* Cambridge, UK: Cambridge University Press; 2013.

21. Bear MF, Connors BW, Paradiso MA. *Neuroscience: Exploring the Brain.* Philadelphia, PA: Wolters-Kluwer; 2016.

22. Wilson JH, Hunt T. *Molecular Biology of the Cell, 6th Edition.* New York: Garland Science; 2015.

23. Ossipov MH. The perception and endogenous modulation of pain. *Scientifica.* 2012;1–25.

24. Ossipov MH, Morimura K, Porreca F. Descending pain modulation and chronification of pain. *Curr Opin Support Palliat Care.* 2014 Jun 15;8(2):143–151.

25. Yarnitsky D. Role of endogenous pain modulation in chronic pain mechanisms and treatment. *Pain.* 2015 Apr;156 Suppl 1:S24–31. doi:10.1097/01.j.pain.0000460343.46847.5826.

26. Roeder Z, Chen Q, Davis S, et al. Parabrachial complex links pain transmission to descending pain modulation. *Pain.* 2016;157(12):2697–2708.

27. Stein EA, Pankiewicz J, Harsch HH, et al. Nicotine-induced limbic cortical activation in the human brain: A functional MRI study. *Am J Psychiatry.* 1998;155(8):1009–1015.
28. Shilliam CS, Heidbreder CA. Gradient of dopamine responsiveness to dopamine receptor agonists in subregions of the rat nucleus accumbens. *Eur J Pharmacol.* 2003;477(2):113–122.
29. Lalanne L, Ayranci G, Kieffer BL, et al. The kappa opioid receptor: From addiction to depression, and back. *Front Psychiatry,* 2014 Dec 8. doi:10.3389/fpsyt.2014.00170
30. Brightwell J, Taylor B. Noradrenergic neurons in the locus coeruleus contribute to neuropathic pain. *Neuroscience.* 2009;160(1):174–185.
31. Emery MA, Bates ML, Wellman PJ, et al. Differential effects of oxycodone, hydrocodone, and morphine on activation levels of signaling molecules. *Pain Med.* 2016 May 1;17(5):908–914. doi:10.1111/pme.12918. Epub 2015 Sep 9

Chapter 3

Psychosocial Aspects of Pain and Addiction

ROSS HALPERN, PH.D.

Cultural stigma associated with pain treatment and drugs has been on the decline since the 1950s. The stoic heroism of the World War II period led to "beat generation" experimentation with many substances in the late 1950s, opening the door for the social revolution of the 1960s [1].

The Vietnam War produced a generation of physically and emotionally wounded men coming home to a society that was unwelcoming and in turmoil. As a result, many treated their pain with alcohol and drugs. This new generation of fathers was less able to "stow it away" (stoicize it) without the help of numbing agents [2].

Greater openness and experience with drugs, along with a multimillion-dollar promotional effort, set the stage for a pharmaceutical approach to dealing with chronic pain. However, whether that actually *is* the best way to deal with pain has proved to be another question entirely.

Why Focus on Chronic Pain?

All pain has an emotional component. The circumstance and interpretation of pain affect the experience of pain. For example, if a soldier in Afghanistan is shot during a mission, but immediately sees it as a means to go home and be with his wife and daughters, the pain may be more tolerable. If once he arrives home and reunites with his family, he finds a job and feels self-respect, it is less likely that his injury will become a source of chronic pain. On the other hand, if a man struggling to support his family through a small business is injured or diagnosed with a disease and sees as it as the end of his ability to function, the physical pain is more likely to be expressed as both physical and emotional pain and may lead to intolerable or chronic pain.

Many physicians have worked with patients suffering with chronic pain that appears to be out of proportion to the assumed source or that has no clearly defined physical cause. Treatment in the form of pills, shots, and surgery may have been provided, but the pain continues. This supports the author's belief that chronic physical pain that is out of proportion to the diagnosed cause, or that has no diagnosable cause, usually is the result of unconscious emotional pain. Research clearly shows that *unconscious interpretations of experience* suggesting that a person is unsafe, not "good enough," alone, or at fault will create or exacerbate pain [3].

The idea that an individual's mind has the ability to create pleasure or pain is rooted in ancient Eastern philosophy. Considering the power and complexity of the unconscious to govern our lives, self-blame often becomes a key variable in preventing us from expressing pain emotionally rather than physically. Events in our lives (such as our own experience of abuse or trauma) often are too unbearable to feel directly. When they are informed by guilt, we somehow interpret the abuse or trauma as our fault, so it is expressed as physical pain.

The Patient's Experience of Pain

When a pain diagnosis is elusive at best, and treatment with pills, shots, or surgical interventions has been unsuccessful, gaining an understanding of the emotional components of the patient's experience of pain is the next order of business.

Although each patient's experience is unique, one can make certain assumptions about the human emotional experience overall. For example, it is certain that anyone who suffers from long-term, life-destroying feelings of low self-worth was abused, neglected, or abandoned as a child. It is equally certain that a person who recently lost a loved one, or who has been in an unhappy relationship of many years, or who is unable to connect to the world in a meaningful way, is hurting inside [4].

However, because we function as individuals, we perceive stimuli and feel the complexity of our own emotions as unique. No two people experience the same circumstance in the same way. Each of us lives in and has experienced a different world, and our unique interpretations of that world are affected by our emotional experience from moment to moment.

Emotions and Physiology

With research-based identification of a clear connection between the brain and the body's organs in the normal functioning of both the autonomic nervous system and the immune system, the biological (bodily) impact of emotional experience under conditions of extreme stress has been revealed [5]. Disruptions along the pathways of these normal biological processes, based on emotional experience, have been found to influence the creation of a variety of chronic conditions.

An important discovery in recent research has been the impact on the body of the inflammatory responses of the immune system. As the immune system identifies and attacks pathogens in the body, there always is some impact on healthy tissue, usually in the form of inflammation [6]. If the immune system's response, managed by the hypothalamic-pituitary-adrenal (HPA) axis, isn't shut down, a variety of conditions can result. Overreactions of the immune system, known as *dysregulation,* can result in damaged tissue, often leading to arthritis, some cancers, diabetes, Alzheimer's disease, heart disease, allergies, and asthma, among other chronic conditions [7]. Similarly, a link between post-traumatic stress disorder (PTSD) and various somatic ailments has been observed for a long time [8].

Whether an emotional trauma results from a sudden, unanticipated event such as a vehicle crash or war, or is a result of abuse, deprivation, or abandonment as a child, the impact can be severe and unmanageable. One's understanding of the experience can be confused by guilt and anger, or accompanied by such debilitating panic that it needs to be repressed and as a result is expressed indirectly. Sudden overpowering loss can render the biological and emotional systems unable to cope, leading to significant expressions of pain in both body and mind.

Despite the findings in support of a biological effect of emotional experience on chronic pain, efforts to approach chronic pain "scientifically" must be attempted with caution so as not to compromise treatment by overlooking the uniqueness and specificity of any particular person's experience. To apply a standardized diagnosis and treatment plan, as though each person's illness is the same as every other person's, is to undermine our best chance of delivering humane and effective care. Psychological understanding reveals subtle as well as significant differences from one patient to another in terms of the meaning of an event and how it is being processed and expressed.

Psychosomatic Expression

Sigmund Freud referred to the transition of emotional pain into a physical symptom as a "conversion" [9]. Through his clinical research, Freud learned that the repression of painful memories was a potential precursor to physical symptoms, often including disabling levels of pain [10]. Psychosomatic symptoms and illness have been documented and understood for a long time. Nevertheless, as contemporary medicine becomes more and more responsive to emotional experience, it is just beginning to shift its focus to a psychological understanding of chronic pain (Box 3.1).

Sources of chronic pain often involve an emotion such as anger or even rage toward the person or persons depended on for survival [3]. These feelings, perceived as "self-destructive," create an unconscious conflict. This unconscious process "converts" the emotion into illness or pain rather than risking a direct expression of anger sabotaging a relationship on which the patient depends.

Painful experiences that need to be repressed can be the result of emotional and physical abuse, or trauma at an age when the patient was too young and too powerless to comprehend or cope with it. Interpretations often include mistaken self-blame, creating an intolerable emotional pain based on guilt. If the message delivered through parental abuse, neglect, rejection, or shaming is that the child is not deserving of the care, love, and nurture the parent is supposed to provide, then the child inevitably blames himself or herself. A self-definition evolves that can include a painful sense of unworthiness, an

---

BOX 3.1 Psychosocial Considerations in Evaluating a Pain Patient

- There is always an emotional component to pain. As you interview the patient, be aware of any significant imbalance between the level of pain and distress expressed by the patient and the presumed diagnosis.
- Spinal disc degeneration is a condition of aging and in most adults is not a cause of chronic pain.
- High levels of emotional stress, as in PTSD, can directly cause an inflammatory condition.
- Overreactions of the immune system can directly cause an inflammatory condition.
- Gaining insight from previous psychological factors may involve:
  1. Correlation between childhood abuse, trauma, deprivation, and adult onset of chronic pain.
  2. Chronic pain may reproduce or mimic a parent's pain or condition, triggered unconsciously for a variety of emotional reasons. For example, unresolved grief can manifest in this way, with the onset of pain often linked to a significant anniversary, such as the date of a parent's diagnosis or death.
  3. A correlation between having to "walk on eggshells" and fibromyalgia.
  4. Living in a hypercritical environment as a child or adult, as in an emotionally abusive or alcoholic home. The child absorbs so much tension that the body can break.

emotional interpretation that we do not deserve love (i.e., that we are not "good enough," that it is our fault, that we are flawed in some basic way, or that we are left with the understanding that we are unlovable). As a result, we learn to expect rejection and mistreatment in all of our relationships, which is a scenario that generates pain.

The unconscious belief that we have nothing of value to offer does not remove our need for love and acceptance. In fact, it stimulates efforts to compensate for the flaw in some way. Such compensation can take many forms, going so far as to include a belief that punishment is the answer because it is somehow deserved. In order to survive, we believe unconsciously that we will always have to do something extra. This belief becomes an important aspect of who we are and how we function [11].

Conclusions

Pain is a form of communication. If the pain is heard and its warning heeded, further injury can be prevented. In the case of chronic pain, paying close attention usually reveals where the injury lies, whether in the emotions or elsewhere, and possibly the appropriate treatment as well.

Psychologists' ability to listen to both conscious and unconscious expression is their most valuable skill. The therapist listens for patterns of thought, feelings, or beliefs, which provide insight into the individual's consciousness but might not be apparent. Often internal connections are revealed that help a person understand aspects of themselves or their experience that form an unresolved area, possibly a conflict of emotion or unconscious belief that has resulted in something difficult and perhaps too painful to look at or feel directly. Painful emotions, unless understood and accepted as real, inevitably express themselves one way or another.

For example, unconscious grief often expresses itself in pain, headache, backache, accidents, rashes, etc., but once grief over the loss of a loved one or a job or some other valued "object" enters conscious awareness and is accepted for what it is, the pain can be expressed in tears and in the emotional pain of loss for someone or something that was loved deeply. As a result, physical pain is no longer necessary. Once grief is accepted and expressed as such, it is allowed to evolve from ongoing pain through awareness and tears into something more resembling compassion for oneself and for those we love.

We know the unconscious is there, not only keeping our heart beating and our body functioning, but also storing away every experience we have ever had. The unconscious knows how we have been treated; it knows what we have seen; and, based on our interpretation of these experiences, it reacts accordingly. Gaining an understanding of this process is key to finding the source of chronic pain and providing effective treatment.

For More Information on the Topics Discussed:

American Society of Addiction Medicine (ASAM).

Covington EC, Kotz MM. Psychological issues in the management of pain (Chapter 94). In RK Ries, DA Fiellin, SC Miller, R Saitz, eds. *The ASAM Principles of Addiction Medicine, Fifth Edition.* Philadelphia, PA: Wolters Kluwer; 2014.

In the Literature:

Adler RH, Zlot S, Hurny C, et al. Engel's "Psychogenic pain and the pain-prone patient": A retrospective, controlled clinical study. *Psychosom Med.* 1989;101:87–101.

Darlington ASE, Verhulst FC, De Winter AF, et al. The influence of maternal vulnerability and parenting stress on chronic pain in adolescents in a general population sample: The TRAILS study. *Eur J Pain.* 2012;16:150–159.

Edwards C, Whitfield K, Sudhakar S, et al. Parental substance abuse, reports of chronic pain and coping in adults. *J Natl Med Assn.* 2006;98:420–428.

Engel GL. "Psychogenic" pain and the pain-prone patient. *Am J Med.* 1959;26:899–918.

Gatchel RJ, Peng YB, Peters ML, et al. The biopsychosocial approach to chronic pain: Scientific advances and future directions. *Psychol Bull.* 2007;133:581–624.

References

1. IMS Institute for Healthcare Informatics. *The Use of Medicines in the US: Review of 2010.* Washington, DC: The Institute; April 2011.
2. Avila J, Murray M. Prescription painkiller use at record high for Americans. *ABC News*, 2011 Apr 20: http://abcnews.go.com/US/prescription-painkillers-record-number-americans-pain-medication/story?id=13421828.
3. Wuest J, Ford-Gilboe M, Varcoe C, et al. Abuse-related injury and symptoms of post-traumatic stress disorder as mechanisms of chronic pain in survivors of intimate partner violence. *Pain Med.* 2009;10:739–747.
4. Tietjen GE, Brandes JL, Peterlin L, et al. Childhood maltreatment and migraine (Part III): Association with comorbid pain conditions. *Headache.* 2009;50:42–51.
5. Chapman CR, Tucket RP, Song CW. Pain and stress in a systems perspective: Reciprocal neural, endocrine and immune reactions. *J Pain.* 2008;9:122–145.
6. Garner B, Eftekhar A, Toumazou C. *Neural Control of Immunity.* London, UK: Imperial College London, Centre for Bio-Inspired Technology; 2014.

7. Johnston-Brooks CH, Lewis MA, Evans GW, et al. Chronic stress and illness in children: The role of allostatic load. *Psychosom Med*. 1998;60:597–603.

8. Maes M, Lin A, Delmeire L, et al. Elevated serum interleukin-6 (IL-6) and IL-6 receptor concentrations in posttraumatic stress disorder following accidental man-made traumatic events. *Biol Psychiatry*. 1999:85:833–839.

9. Breuer J, Freud S. *Studies in Hysteria (Nervous and Mental Disease Monograph Series 61)*. New York: Nervous and Mental Disease Publishing (English translation); 1937.

10. Jarvik JG, Hollingworth W, Martin B, et al. Rapid MRI vs. radiographs for patients with low back pain: A randomized controlled trial. *JAMA*. 2003;289(21): 2810.

11. Sivik TM. Personality traits in patients with acute low-back pain: A comparison with chronic low-back pain patients. *Psychother Psychosom*. 1991;56:135–140.

Chapter 4

The Language of Pain and Addiction

MICHAEL M. MILLER, M.D., DFASAM, DLFAPA

Words matter: "She's a real pain" or "I'm addicted to 'The House of Cards.'" Clinicians who work with patients suffering from pain and addiction understand the similarities in the clinical presentations of the two disorders. However, they may not realize that another aspect the disorders have in common is problematic terminology that can be confusing, imprecise, overlapping, and/or stigmatizing.

Such terminology provides inadequate guidance to the clinician on how best to help the patient. Moreover, the terms themselves can generate a subconscious feeling-state in the clinician that may affect his or her empathy, thinking, and interactions with the patient. For example, too many clinicians cringe when they look at their patient list or hear from a member of their team that the patient in the next exam room "has X" or "has Y," because the diagnostic term itself may be laden with meanings and expectations that elicit states of frustration or pessimism about the encounter even before the exam room door is opened.

Many authors have discussed the difference between *pain* and *suffering* [1,2,3]. Others describe the differences between objective pathology and the subjective experience of disease. Distinctions between dependence and abuse are considered essential by some [4] but *passé* by others. Some ask whether a patient has physical or psychological dependence, and debate which is worse (i.e., more disabling, more difficult to repair, and more likely to cause "disease"). They ask whether it matters that a particular patient's addiction involves use of a substance or a particular behavior.

The Language of Pain Medicine

Pain medicine is a specialized area of practice, research, and education, the leaders of which have tried to clarify concepts and terminology in the interest of improving patient care, professional standards, and public policy. Many pain specialists and others have asserted that "pain is what the patient says it is" [5–8] and implored clinicians not to prejudge patients.

Pain has been considered different from nociception, and there are excellent articles on subtypes of pain [9,10]: somatic, neuropathic, phantom, or psychogenic. Pain is a symptom and can be present in many conditions, including major depressive disorder, anxiety disorder, somatoform disorders, and other psychiatric conditions, although no one would assert that pain itself constitutes a mental disorder.

Laypersons and professionals alike allude to differences between "physical pain" and "emotional" or "psychological pain." Most often, they use those terms to describe somatic pain, which results from a problem in some part of the body and is transmitted to the brain via pain pathways in the spinal cord (the spinothalamic tract). Signals transmitted in this manner are collated in the thalamus of the midbrain and transmitted from there to the cerebral cortex, where the organism can become consciously aware that "something hurts."

Thus, pain can be a very useful experience because it signals the presence of a problem somewhere in the body that requires attention. When such signals do not elicit a response (as frequently occurs with neuropathy in a diabetic patient), the source of pain may progress and worsen in severity.

Analgesics such as opioids block the experience of somatic pain. For this reason, they sometimes are referred to as *anti-nociceptive agents* because they block the *perception* of noxious (painful) information. In the case of inflammatory pain (in contrast to visceral pain or musculoskeletal pain), where inflammation is the cause of the pain, an analgesic such as a nonsteroidal anti-inflammatory drug (NSAID) actually blocks the *generation* of the pain.

In contrast, neuropathic pain differs from musculoskeletal or visceral pain in that it does not signal injury to a bone, muscle, or organ in the body, but rather an injury to a nerve cell. This distinction is important in clinical practice because traditional anti-nociceptive agents are not very effective at relieving neuropathic pain [11].

Therefore, distinguishing between somatic (nociceptive) and neuropathic pain is an important component of clinical care [12,13]. Neuropathic pain can result from damage to peripheral nerves (in the limbs, for example) or the spinal cord, as well as damage to nerve structures in the brain (termed "central neuropathic pain," in contrast to "peripheral neuropathic pain").

Because somatic pain is useful in the sense that it allows an organism to adapt to the existence of pain, and because damage to nervous system pathways that usually carry pain information can result in various functional adaptations within the nervous system, it has been suggested [14] that maladaptive pain should be termed "maldynia." This framework, while appealing to some, has not been adopted broadly, and most pain medicine specialists do not embrace it.

There are many other types of pain, as is evident in one of the most respected taxonomies of pain, which has been published by the International

Association for the Study of Pain (IASP) [15]. (See online Appendix A in this book for examples of preferred terminology.) The list includes terms such as *hypoalgesia* (a diminished sensation or appreciation of pain) and *hyperalgesia* (an amplified subjective experience of pain).

Hyperalgesia sometimes is used to describe pain that feels worse because of psychological factors such as anxiety or depression (other psychological states and psychiatric conditions also can contribute to hyperalgesia). A variant is *opioid-induced hyperalgesia*, a syndrome in which an individual experiences pain quite intensely, not because the injury leading to nociceptive or neuropathic pain has become worse, but because feedback loops result in a heightened sensation of pain [16]. This occurs when normal processes of pain information transmission or central nervous system reception are initially blocked, albeit eventually enhanced or upregulated, through the administration of opioid analgesics or via their metabolites.

In the presence of nociceptive blockade, the body attempts to perceive signals by "turning up the gain" on pain areas of the brain so that they become more sensitive. However, in the effort not to miss any important information, the upregulated pain perception systems can experience pain as more intense, even though the actual input is not significantly enhanced.

The patient with opioid-induced hyperalgesia thus perceives everything as more painful because of amplified sensitivity to, or perception of, pain. In such a patient, increasing the use of opioids as an anti-nociceptive agent actually makes the situation worse; in fact, the only way to reduce the patient's subjective discomfort in the presence of opioid-induced hyperalgesia is to reduce or eliminate exposure to the opioid analgesic itself.

Even more terms are included in medical descriptions of pain. There is *paresthesia*, a burning or prickling sensation that can be, but is not always, painful [17]. *Phantom pain* [18] describes a state in which the amputation of all or part of a limb is followed by a subjective sensation that the limb is still in place and painful. Phantom pain is thought to be a manifestation of neuroplasticity [17,18,19] and to represent a central nervous system dysfunction and a neurological condition, but not a psychiatric one.

Psychogenic pain is pain that an individual experiences in the absence of any somatic or neuropathic injury [20]. Psychogenic pain thus can arise in the absence of a specific medical problem, or it can involve a significant amplification of the experience of pain in the presence of an injury. Alternatively, psychogenic pain can constitute a psychiatric illness in itself: a *somatoform disorder*. This is quite different from *hypochondriasis*, which involves excessive fears about having an illness or excessive anxiety about a symptom such as pain. (Note that the *Diagnostic and Statistical Manual of Mental Disorders, 5th Ed.* [DSM-5] [21] features a new set of terms, definitions, and criteria for both somatoform disorders in general and psychogenic pain disorder and hypochondriasis in particular. This and other taxonomies, including the IASP, no longer use the term *psychogenic pain*.)

Although distinctions often are made between physical and psychological pain, it is worth noting that the IASP itself defines pain as "an unpleasant sensory and emotional experience associated with actual or potential tissue damage, or described in terms of such damage. Pain is always subjective" [15]. So whether pain has its origin in a medical/surgical condition or in a psychiatric state or condition, there always is an emotional component to pain, because it feels awful. How much discomfort or misery is experienced by the person in pain is influenced by cultural and sociological variables as well as by an individual's personality variables and expectations (e.g., some individuals are quite distressed by a level of pain that other, more stoic persons withstand without complaint—and, of course, stoicism can be adaptive or maladaptive).

While it is not a true diagnostic category, pain specialists sometimes describe patients as exhibiting *aberrant behaviors* [22,23]. This term is used to characterize the ways in which a patient interacts with his or her caregiver with regard to opioid prescribing, such as by demanding a specific analgesic by brand name and rejecting all other options. Such a patient may share prescribed medications with others or use excessive medications. The medications may be used for an indication other than that for which they were prescribed (for example, to manage anxiety rather than pain). Or the patient may make frequent calls to the physician's office reporting that he or she lost the prescription or their supply of medication.

Physicians who are considering the use of opioid analgesics for pain management typically become uncomfortable when a patient, through their words or actions, manifests such "aberrant behaviors." But one of the biggest challenges in clinical medicine occurs when a physician believes that such aberrant behaviors are pathognomonic for a diagnosis of substance use disorder—which they absolutely are not—or, conversely, believes that aberrant behaviors must be present in order to diagnose a substance use disorder—which also is not the case.

The Language of Addiction Medicine

Like their counterparts in pain medicine, practitioners of addiction medicine—another specialty area of practice, research, and education—have tried to clarify concepts and terminology in an effort to improve patient care, professional standards, and public policy. For example, in the latest edition of the DSM [23], the American Psychiatric Association recommends that the term *abuse* be abandoned in favor of newer, more precise terminology. Similar concerns led the American Society of Addiction Medicine (ASAM), which published its *Definition of Addiction* in 2011 [24], to point out that "abuse" is a stigmatizing and uninformative term. Despite these efforts, "substance abuse" remains the most common term in use today, particularly by federal and state governments and many researchers (also see http://nationalsubstanceabuseindex.org/agencies.htm).

The language of addiction medicine is no less complex than that of pain medicine, and arguably is even more complex because of the emotions attached to the labels applied to patients with substance use disorders, as well as the amount of stigma and discrimination encountered by patients who are labeled "substance abusers" [25]. The problem is that the term "substance abuser" can be used as shorthand for, "This patient is conducting himself or herself in a way that I wish he or she wouldn't." Or the term "substance abuser" might be used to describe a patient with the very discrete syndrome of "substance abuse" as it was defined for 25 years by the American Psychiatric Association (APA) in the DSM [23,26–28]. Or it might be used to describe a person who manifests "substance abuse" in the broad sense of a substance-related disorder of some type.

In the 1980s, the distinction between the minor syndrome of "substance abuse" and the more serious syndrome of "substance dependence" was based on whether or not the patient exhibited physical dependence. However, clinicians and researchers came to understand that the presence of physiological dependence was not the best way to distinguish individuals who have a true substance use disorder from persons who exhibit problematic behaviors with regard to substance use.

As a result, in its 1987 edition [18] of the DSM-III-R, its authors began to reserve the term "substance abuse" for individuals who had experienced repeated problems—at work, in the family, or even with the legal system—related to their use of substances, but who did not meet the criteria for substance dependence. Over time, the presence of substance dependence became an "exclusion criterion" for the condition termed "substance abuse," even if one of the four necessary criteria for substance abuse was present. Thus, a patient could not be assigned a diagnosis of substance abuse if he or she met three or more of the necessary criteria for a diagnosis of substance dependence [29].

With that change, an individual diagnosed with substance abuse could receive behavioral therapy to learn how to use substances responsibly and non-problematically so that he or she no longer met the criteria for substance abuse. However, the majority of experienced clinicians in the area of addiction medicine do not believe that it is responsible clinical practice or even possible to teach someone with substance dependence how to "use drugs responsibly" because of the loss of control over such use evidenced by patients with true substance dependence. Thus, for approximately three decades, clinicians using the DSM-III-R or DSM-IV were careful to make a distinction between "substance dependence" and "substance abuse," because the entire conceptualization of the case and the care plan that flowed from the diagnosis was extremely different for the major syndrome (the one roughly akin to "addiction") and the minor syndrome (unfortunately called "substance abuse"), even while those in general medicine and health policy used the term "substance abuse" to mean something very different from the condition described in the DSM.

In response to this situation, two changes in nosology appeared in the next decade. In 2013, the APA published a major revision of the DSM [23]. In that (fifth) edition, the terms "substance abuse" and "substance dependence" were eliminated—each for very good reasons. As a result, the DSM-5 characterizes substance use conditions as existing on a continuum from mild to moderate to severe, and the criteria for the diagnoses formerly termed "substance abuse" and "substance dependence" were pooled [23]. However, many practitioners of addiction medicine found this terminology challenging because they believe there is a discontinuity between those who use substances problematically and those who have the true brain disease of addiction.

The fifth edition of the DSM also incorporates the concept of *craving* and eliminates the DSM-IV criteria related to legal problems [23]. Prior to the revision, a pain patient could break a law with regard to possession of a controlled substance, or even obtain a prescription through fraudulent means, and have those actions support a diagnosis of substance use disorder. The DSM-5 does not include legal problems among the 11 diagnostic criteria for substance use disorder (SUD), but what remains is a set of criteria by which a non-specialist, when asked to evaluate a pain patient for possible "substance abuse" (in the broad sense), would find: tolerance; a history of episodes of opioid withdrawal; and a patient who spends a significant amount of each day using opioids, recovering from the effects of such use, or even being preoccupied with obtaining adequate supplies of opioid analgesics—and, with those criteria, would reach a diagnosis of opioid dependence.

Physicians who are trained in addiction medicine often are able to make the subtle distinction between a patient who is exposed to high-dose opioids on a regular basis and a patient with a true addiction or who is engaged in real drug misuse. However, in most communities, physicians and other health care professionals have difficulty arranging a consultation with a certified specialist in addiction medicine or addiction psychiatry because of the paucity of such specialist physicians.

Although the DSM contains the most widely accepted diagnostic criteria, the issues cited here led ASAM to adopt its own terminology [32]. (See online Appendix A of this book for examples of ASAM's preferred terms, many of which are quite different than those in the DSM.) The ASAM document is based on the belief that it is not the quantity or frequency of exposure to alcohol, other drugs, or addictive behaviors that determine whether a given individual meets the criteria for addiction; rather, it is the qualitative manner in which the brain of the person with addiction responds to rewards [32].

The ASAM document makes no mention of tolerance or withdrawal, but focuses instead on impairment of control as well as compulsive or impulsive patterns of pathological pursuit of rewards. Thus, the brain disease described in the ASAM Terminology (Box 4.1) is quite different from what the DSM-III-R

BOX 4.1 Excerpt from *ASAM Definition of Addiction (2011)*

"Addiction is a primary, chronic disease of brain reward, motivation, memory and related circuitry. Dysfunction in these circuits leads to characteristic biological, psychological, social and spiritual manifestations. This is reflected in an individual pathologically pursuing reward and/or relief by substance use and other behaviors."

"Addiction is characterized by inability to consistently abstain, impairment in behavioral control, craving, diminished recognition of significant problems with one's behaviors and interpersonal relationships, and a dysfunctional emotional response. Like other chronic diseases, addiction often involves cycles of relapse and remission. Without treatment or engagement in recovery activities, addiction is progressive and can result in disability or premature death."

Excerpted from American Society of Addiction Medicine (ASAM), *Definition of Addiction*. Board of Directors, 19 April 2011: https://www.asam.org/resources/definition-of-addiction

---

termed "substance abuse" [29] or what the DSM-5 refers to as "substance use disorder" [23].

Because the ASAM document is so new, no research has yet been conducted on populations of patients who would meet the ASAM criteria. As a result, the professional literature provides little guidance regarding the epidemiology of differential diagnoses that derive from ASAM's concepts.

Conclusion

A major problem with diagnostic systems in the United States is that there is no broadly accepted term for subsyndromal substance use that has adverse implications for patient health. Especially with respect to alcohol use, an individual can experience problems related to their use of alcoholic beverages—alone or in combination with other substances—and be at statistical risk of developing such problems based on their pattern of use even though they do not (yet) meet the criteria provided in the DSM-III-R, DSM-IV or even the DSM-5. In Europe, there is a diagnostic code for "risky use," and clinicians routinely counsel patients who engage in risky use about the potential for developing medical or other complications. Clearly, in the practice of pain medicine, there could be patients who use opioids in an unhealthy manner but do not meet the criteria for substance use disorder. How to categorize such patients using American diagnostic systems remains a challenge [30,31].

As described, ASAM's terminology incorporates concepts such as unhealthy use, harmful use, and hazardous use [32,33]. There also is the concept of "non-medical use," the occurrence of which is reported annually through the National Survey on Drug Use and Health, sponsored by the National Institute on Drug Abuse (NIDA), part of the National Institutes of Health (NIH) [34]. In this nomenclature, a patient who changes the route of drug administration from oral to intravenous is manifesting "non-medical use" and also "hazardous use," given the risks inherent in injection drug use. Such actions, including obtaining drug supplies from non-medical sources, constitute "non-medical use" and may involve criminal behavior, yet under the DSM-5 they would not be criteria for a diagnosis of substance use disorder.

These issues notwithstanding, what should be of concern to any physician engaged in pain management is that the patient adhere to the treatment plan and does not use prescription medications in an unsafe or unhealthy way. Such a patient may not be diagnosable with a substance use disorder or addiction, and in the United States there may not be a diagnostic code to describe the patient's inappropriate use of medications, but the physician still has a responsibility to monitor treatment compliance and the safe use of any potentially harmful medications that are prescribed, as well as to educate and counsel patients regarding the safe use of prescription medications.

For More Information on the Topics Discussed

American Psychiatric Association (APA):

Diagnostic and Statistical Manual of Mental Disorders, 5th ed. (DSM-5). Arlington, VA: American Psychiatric Publishing; 2013.

American Society of Addiction Medicine (ASAM):

Definition of Addiction. Chevy Chase, MD: The Society; 2011. (Accessed at: http://www.asam.org/for-the-public/definition-of-addiction)

American Society of Addiction Medicine (ASAM). *Terminology Related to the Spectrum of Unhealthy Substance Use.* Chevy Chase, MD: The Society; 2011. (Accessed at: http://www.asam.org/docs/default-source/publicy-policy-statements/1-terminology-spectrum-sud-7-13.pdf?sfvrsn=2)

International Society for the Study of Pain (IASP):

Merskey H, Bogduk N. *Classification of Chronic Pain, 2nd ed.* Seattle, WA: IASP Press; 1994.

Acknowledgment

The author would like to thank pain medicine physicians Bob Wailes, M.D., and Misha Backonja, M.D., for their review of this manuscript.

References

1. Liben S. The difference between pain and suffering. *Canadian Virtual Hospice.* 2014. (Accessed at: https://www.youtube.com/watch?v=rPDLM_XaKds.)
2. Mager D. Pain is inevitable; suffering is optional. *Psychology Today Online.* Posted January 13, 2014. (Accessed at: https://www.psychologytoday.com/blog/some-assembly-required/201401/pain-is-inevitable-suffering-is-optional.)
3. Winterowd C, Beck AT, Gruener D. Theories of pain and treatment approaches to pain management. *Cognitive Therapy with Chronic Pain Patients.* New York: Springer Publishing Company; 2003.
4. White W. Substance abuse versus substance dependence: Implications for management of the DUI offender. *Briefing paper for the Administrative Office of the Illinois Courts and the Illinois Secretary of State.* Springfield, IL: State of Illinois; 2014. (Accessed at: http://www.williamwhitepapers.com/pr/Abuse%26dependencepaperFinal5-30-2007.pdf.)
5. Bernhofer E. Ethics and pain management in hospitalized patients. *OJIN.* 2011;17:1.
6. McCaffery M, Beebe A. *Pain: A Clinical Manual for Nursing Practice.* St. Louis, MO: C.V. Mosby; 1989.
7. Brown EG Jr, Sewell DS, Kirchmeyer K. *Guidelines for Prescribing Controlled Substances for Pain.* Sacramento, CA: Medical Board of California; 2014.
8. Miller LE, Eldredge SA, Dalton ED. "Pain is what the patient says it is": Nurse–patient communication, information seeking, and pain management. *Am J Hospice Palliat Med.* 2016;34(10):966–976. doi:1049909116661815.
9. Vellucci R. Heterogeneity of chronic pain. *Clin Drug Invest.* 2012;32(Suppl 1):3–10. (Accessed at: http://www.ncbi.nlm.nih.gov/pubmed/23389871.)
10. Peyron R. Pathophysiology of chronic pain: Classification of three subtypes of pain. *Rev Prat.* 2013;63(6):773–778. (Accessed at: http://www.ncbi.nlm.nih.gov/pubmed/23923752.)
11. Dworkin RH. Recommendations for the pharmacological management of neuropathic pain: An overview and literature update. *Mayo Clin Proc.* 2010;85(3 Suppl):S3–S14.
12. Bennett M. The LANSS Pain Scale: The Leeds assessment of neuropathic symptoms and signs. *Pain.* 2010;92:147–157.
13. Nicholson B. Differential diagnosis: Nociceptive and neuropathic pain. *Am J Manag Care.* 2006;12(9 Suppl):256–262.
14. Dickinson BD, Head CA, Gitlow S, et al. Maldynia: Pathophysiology and management of neuropathic and maladaptive pain—A report of the AMA Council on Science and Public Health. *Pain Med.* 2010;11(11):1635.

15. Merskey H, Bogduk N. *Classification of Chronic Pain, 2nd ed.* Seattle, WA: IASP Press; 1994.
16. Mitra S. Opioid-induced hyperalgesia: Pathophysiology and clinical implications. *J Opioid Manag.* 2008;4:123–130.
17. Subedi B, Grossberg GT. Phantom limb pain: mechanisms and treatment approaches. *Pain Res Treat.* 2011;864605. https://www.ncbi.nlm.nih.gov/pmc/articles/PMC3198614/
18. Ramachandran VS, Rogers-Ramachandran DC, Stewart M. Perceptual correlates of massive cortical reorganization. *Science.* 1992;258(5085):1159–1160.
19. Knecht S, Henningsen H, Elbert T, et al. Reorganizational and perceptual changes after amputation. *Brain.* 1996;119:1213–1219.
20. National Institute of Neurologic Disorders and Stroke Paresthesia (NINDSP). Information page. (Accessed at: http://www.ninds.nih.gov/disorders/paresthesia/paresthesia.htm.)
21. Nikolajsen L, Jensen TS. Phantom limb pain. *Brit J Anaesth.* 2001;87:107–116.
22. Cleveland Clinic. *Psychogenic Pain.* Cleveland, OH: The Cleveland Clinic; 2014. (Accessed at: http://my.clevelandclinic.org/services/anesthesiology/pain-management/diseases-conditions/hic-psychogenic-pain.)
23. American Psychiatric Association (APA). *Diagnostic and Statistical Manual of Mental Disorders, Fifth ed. (DSM-5).* Arlington, VA: American Psychiatric Publishing; 2013.
24. Chou R, Fanciullo GJ, Fine PG, et al. Opioids for chronic noncancer pain: Prediction and identification of aberrant drug-related behaviors: A review of the evidence for an American Pain Society and American Academy of Pain Medicine clinical practice guideline. *J Pain.* 2009;10:131–146.
25. Michna E, Ross EL, Hynes WL, et al. Predicting aberrant drug behavior in patients treated for chronic pain: Importance of abuse history. *J Pain Symptom Manag.* 2004;28:250–258.
26. American Society of Addiction Medicine (ASAM). *Definition of Addiction.* Chevy Chase, MD: The Society; 2011. (Accessed at: http://www.asam.org/for-the-public/definition-of-addiction.)
27. Rosenblum A, Marsch LA, Joseph H, et al. Opioids and the treatment of chronic pain: Controversies, current status, and future directions. *Exp Clin Psychopharm.* 2008;16:405–416.
28. American Psychiatric Association (APA). *Diagnostic and Statistical Manual of Mental Disorders, 3rd ed. (DSM-III).* Washington, DC: American Psychiatric Publishing; 1980.
29. American Psychiatric Association (APA). *Diagnostic and Statistical Manual of Mental Disorders, 3rd ed., revised (DSM-III-R).* Washington, DC: American Psychiatric Publishing; 1987.
30. American Psychiatric Association (APA). *Diagnostic and Statistical Manual of Mental Disorders, 4th ed. (DSM-IV).* Washington, DC: American Psychiatric Publishing; 1994.
31. Hasin DS, O'Brien CP, Auriacombe M, et al. DSM-5 criteria for substance use disorders: Recommendations and rationale. *Am J Psychiatry.* 2013;170:834–851.

32. American Society of Addiction Medicine (ASAM). *Terminology Related to the Spectrum of Unhealthy Substance Use*. Chevy Chase, MD: The Society; 2011. (Accessed at http://www.asam.org/docs/default-source/publicy-policy-statements/1-terminology-spectrum-sud-7-13.pdf?sfvrsn=2.)

33. Becker WC, Sullivan LE, Tetrault JM, et al. Non-medical use, abuse and dependence on prescription opioids among U.S. adults: Psychiatric, medical and substance use correlates. *Drug Alc Depend*. 2008;94:38–47.

34. National Institute on Drug Abuse (NIDA). *National Survey of Drug Use and Health (NSDUH), 2014*. Bethesda, MD: NIDA, National Institutes of Health; 2015. (Accessed at: http://www.drugabuse.gov/publications/drugfacts/nationwide-trends.)

Chapter 5

Providing Integrated Care
for Pain and Addiction

ALAN A. WARTENBERG, M.D., FACP, FASAM

Over the past several decades, there has been an increased call for "universal precautions" in the evaluation and management of patients with substance use disorders (SUDs) and serious pain issues, particularly chronic pain [1–3]. As with the management of patients with infectious diseases, where clinicians are to assume that all patients could be carriers of serious transmissible agents (HIV, hepatitis B/C, etc.) and take appropriate precautions in every case, clinicians similarly should consider that all presenting patients with pain issues either have, or are at risk for, substance use disorders [3], with the potential for aberrant behaviors and adverse outcomes.

The Rationale for Integrated Care

While there are differences in the levels of risk for misuse of prescription medications between individuals who have active opioid use disorders and those with other substance use disorders, there is a significant overlap [4,5]. This also appears to be the case with patients who have a history of a substance use disorder (including tobacco dependence) that is not currently active [5].

There is concern on the part of many patients and their advocates, as well as practicing physicians, that a history of substance use disorder in patients presenting with pain may result in the dismissal of such patients without adequate evaluation, treatment, and/or referral. On the other hand, successfully integrated treatment of patients with pain and substance use disorder (SUD) or addiction is actually the norm, with the vast majority of patients successfully managed for their pain and addiction problems.

Treating the Pain Patient with a History of Opioid Use Disorder

It is clear that patients with active opioid use disorders are not optimal candidates for opioid-based pain treatment, unless such patients are in active and ongoing treatment for their SUDs. Patients who are actively abusing opioids are at high risk for opioid overdose. They also may be unable to adhere to scheduled visits, medication management, and non-pharmacological therapies, and should be referred to appropriate treatment professionals and/or agencies. Prescribing opioids to such patients may even violate federal and state controlled substance laws and regulations, and state and federal authorities have imposed criminal sanctions on physicians for overdose deaths and other complications attributed to such prescribing [6]. In addition, state boards of medicine have sanctioned physicians (and other prescribers) on similar grounds [7].

While clinicians always should exhaust the possibilities offered by non-pharmacological therapies and non-opioid pharmacotherapies, some patients with a history of, or an active, SUD require even greater efforts to maximize the use of non-opioid approaches, both pharmacological and non-pharmacological. With such patients, if opioids appear to be the only effective therapy, consultation with an addiction specialist is highly recommended so that the physician can make an informed decision regarding such prescribing. Ideally, it is a decision that should be shared with the patient, and with others (including providers of medication-assisted treatment) who are caring for the patient.

Experience shows that many patients receiving opioid agonist therapy (particularly with methadone) are unable to adhere to customary prescribing practices for analgesics and thus have a history of medication misuse. Therefore, ordering a 30-day supply of opioids, benzodiazepines or other medications subject to abuse (which may include certain muscle relaxants and anticonvulsants [8]) may be highly problematic. If opioid analgesics are deemed necessary, the clinician should order the lowest effective dose (which may need to be higher than in opioid-naïve patients) in a smaller quantity than is typically used (for example, involving a once- or twice-weekly medication pick-up). Treatment agreements with such patients must be clear regarding limits on aberrant behaviors, as well as the use of drug testing, pill counts, and other measures to monitor patient progress (see Chapter 9 for further discussion of this point).

It is difficult, or even impossible, to maintain safety in patients who are being prescribed multiple long-acting or extended-release opioids for pain at the same time they are being given other long-acting medications (such as buprenorphine or methadone to treat an SUD). Such prescribing generally should be avoided except in unusual circumstances (such as an acute injury or terminal illness). In such cases, it may be appropriate for the physician who is managing the patient's pain to assume total pharmacological care of the patient, either by prescribing doses of an opioid agonist sufficient to address the patient's pain and SUD, or by titrating other long-acting analgesics upward to "cover" any agonist medication being discontinued (see online Appendix B of this book for more information on these medications).

This advice reflects the disastrous results of multiple prescribers using multiple agents to treat such patients. For example, a 51-year-old man with chronic obstructive pulmonary disease (COPD) who was stable on methadone 120 mg for an SUD was prescribed a fentanyl patch (100 mcg/24h) and MS Contin® 60 mg twice daily (BID) by a pain specialist, in addition to hydromorphone 8 mg four times daily for "breakthrough" pain by his primary care provider. Although each of the care providers was aware of the others' prescribing, there was no effective coordination of care, which culminated in the patient's respiratory failure and death.

It also is important that patients' families and significant others have an opportunity to provide input on a regular basis. In addition, home health care staff, such as a visiting nurse, can be helpful in determining the safety of the patient's environment.

Although methadone and buprenorphine generally are given once a day in formal treatment programs to patients with opioid use disorders, many such programs opt to give medication in divided doses to patients diagnosed with both pain and addiction. This allows one provider to be responsible for the long-acting or extended-release opioid preparations.

Experience shows that pain programs generally are better equipped to provide both non-pharmacological pain management and non-opioid pharmacological treatment, while limiting the use of other opioids to breakthrough pain. If other long-acting or extended-release opioids are needed in addition to methadone or buprenorphine, consideration should be given to gradually weaning the patient from the long-acting opioid while gradually titrating up the other opioid(s) being used for pain. Such patients may remain in a counseling program even when they are not receiving medications for their SUD.

An additional concern in some patients who are in recovery from opioid addiction is that they may refuse to accept opioid therapy out of a fear that such use would constitute a relapse, causing them to "lose" their months (or years) of sobriety. This concern is particularly acute in patients engaged in 12-Step programs. To address their concerns, it may be helpful to meet with them, their family members, and program sponsor(s). Some sponsors form strong and lasting friendships and mentoring relationships with their mentees, and their willingness to engage in frank discussion as to why non-pharmacological treatments may not be sufficient or effective, as well as how opioids can be used safely with appropriate guidelines and precautions, may improve the patient's acceptance of the recommended course of treatment.

Careful documentation by all care providers is critical in treating such patients. For similar reasons, the patient's medical record always should contain documentation of consultations, whether formal or informal (including contacts by telephone and email). More frequent drug monitoring, pill counts, home visits by nurses or health aides, and other interventions also should be considered in the management of these complex patients. As discussed in Chapter 11, such patients (or their family members) should be prescribed naloxone if a risk of overdose is identified.

Treating the Pain Patient with a History of Non-Opioid Substance Use Disorder

The clinician should obtain a thorough history of the patient's past substance use, including use during adolescence and early adult life, a family history of any substance use disorders, and a history of personal and family psychiatric disorders (including any history of traumatic experiences). When interviewing patients, special attention should be given to asking questions such as these in a non-judgmental way (use of written questionnaires that list all drug groups is helpful in this regard).

Testing of urine or saliva should be conducted during a patient's initial visit, as well as before prescribing and (with greater frequency) early in treatment and prior to reducing or increasing drug doses. Other indicators of the need for such testing include patient progress (or lack thereof) and behaviors. Any discordance between the patient's reported use of medications or drugs and confirmed test results should be fully explored and resolved.

Although there are no definitive data on the value of increasing the frequency of screening in patients who have a history of SUDs, this can be a valuable practice for providing a deterrent to relapse and an opportunity for its early detection. For additional information on drug testing, see Chapter 12.

Tobacco

Tobacco use disorder remains the most prevalent SUD in the United States and most developed countries, and is increasing in the developing world. Studies of aberrant behaviors and demographic characteristics of patients that may indicate problematic use of prescription drugs have repeatedly shown that male gender, younger age, and tobacco use are important predictive factors [12–14]. However, there is no suggestion that assisting people in tobacco cessation has a positive effect on the development of non-adherence or aberrant behaviors.

Nevertheless, it is clear that tobacco cessation may favorably influence the underlying pain pathophysiology by allowing better blood flow, as well as reducing the morbidity and mortality associated with tobacco-related disorders.

Health care professionals always should include tobacco use in their patients' problem lists, and should note that patients with other substance use disorders are particularly likely to use tobacco products as well. Pain management specialists and other clinicians should recommend (or refer patients to) the many options available for tobacco cessation, including drug-free counseling; alternative and complementary therapies such as hypnosis, acupuncture, and nicotine replacement therapies; as well as use of bupropion (Zyban®, Wellbutrin®, and generics), and varenicline (Chantix®).

Because tobacco products have a significant influence on a number of p450 hepatic cytochrome enzyme systems involved in metabolic pathways of therapeutic agents, physicians should be aware of the potential influence of both tobacco use and its cessation on medications they prescribe. In addition, patients should be educated about the signs of drug excess or deficiency brought on by tobacco use (as well as its reduction or cessation), and monitoring patients for such changes should be carried out so as to allow appropriate adjustments to drug doses or frequency of dosing.

Alcohol

Beverage or ethyl alcohol is the second most commonly abused drug in the Western world, and it is very prevalent in the developing world as well. Despite this fact, urine drug testing for alcohol metabolites is infrequently conducted, and pain specialists may not be testing for other biological markers of excessive alcohol use [9–11]. Patients with any indicators of active alcohol use disorders or risky drinking should be counseled on the advisability of alcohol abstinence. In fact, many pain specialists require that their patients abstain from even social alcohol use, particularly if it is regular. They do this on the basis of potential additive and/or synergistic effects with a variety of therapeutic agents used in pain management, including opioids, as well as the potential for a significant number of drug–drug interactions. Patients with active alcohol use disorders should be referred to appropriate treatment.

Many patients who present for evaluation and management of chronic pain and who are in short or longer term recovery may not be actively involved in a treatment program. Some may participate in self-help groups and thus may not feel they need any treatment beyond "working their program." Others may not be in treatment and report that they have remained abstinent on their own. Still others may say that they have returned to "social" drinking and are no longer having problems with alcohol.

It is appropriate for a pain provider to insist that patients entering into their treatment—which may well include using medications that will put an individual's continued sobriety at risk—accept all appropriate referrals for consultation. This may include physical or occupational therapy, pain psychology, and addiction treatment. In order to be certain that a patient's recovery is secure and that they are taking appropriate steps to maintain that recovery, it is reasonable for the pain specialist to request a consult. Even individuals with decades of stable sobriety may experience relapse, or relapse triggers, in the face of chronic pain and its treatment.

Many patients with alcohol use disorders can be managed in an outpatient setting, including detoxification and other medical management, which may include anti-craving drugs. Pain specialists should be aware of the utility of various approved pharmacological agents, including naltrexone (ReVia®), extended-release injectable naltrexone (Vivitrol®), acamprosate (Campral®), disulfiram (Antabuse® and generics), and others on the horizon, such as topiramate and gabapentin. Such agents may help prevent relapse in many patients, but prescribing them typically requires consultation with a specialist in addiction medicine or addiction psychiatry [15,16].

Cannabis

Many health care professionals have concerns about the appropriateness and safety of cannabis, whether it is used for pain or for mood alteration. Cannabis remains illegal under federal law, and in most states, physicians' Drug Enforcement Agency (DEA) licenses fall under federal jurisdiction. The federal Department of Veterans Affairs has adopted policies condoning the use of cannabinoids by veterans for either state-certified medical purposes or for their own self-treatment of pain and/or other conditions, particularly in states where marijuana has been decriminalized or legalized for recreational use [17].

These policies indicate that the use of marijuana should be individually judged, and should not preclude appropriate treatment for pain, including use of controlled substances. Therefore, patients undergoing treatment for an SUD should not be discharged from treatment based solely on cannabis use. Such a step should be taken only in cases where it is clear that the patient has a cannabis use disorder or that the cannabis use is destabilizing their other drug use problems.

Benzodiazepines

Benzodiazepines are not benign drugs, even in persons with no history of addiction. However, every case deserves individual consideration. For example, patients with severe anxiety disorders who have not responded to, or cannot tolerate, selective serotonin reuptake inhibitors (SSRIs), serotonin-norepinephrine reuptake inhibitors (SNRIs), and even monoamine oxidase inhibitors (MAOIs), have benefited from the use of benzodiazepines.

It is equally clear that there are many patients who use benzodiazepines problematically and for whom they should not be prescribed. Therefore, the decision about whether to use benzodiazepines should be based on a careful assessment of the patient, including a review of his or her medical record, discussions with clinicians who treated the patient in the past, as well as conversations with family members and others who know the patient well.

Amphetamines, Cocaine, and Other Stimulants

Illicit stimulant use is associated with escalation of use and loss of control more frequently than most substances of abuse. Such loss of control also occurs earlier in the course of a stimulant use disorder than is seen with most drugs. Patients who engage in use of non-prescribed stimulants—particularly methamphetamine and cocaine—should be referred immediately for addiction treatment They should not be treated with controlled substances for pain except in supervised medical or residential settings.

Some patients are diagnosed with attention deficit-hyperactivity disorder (ADHD) or narcolepsy and other disorders that are treated with stimulants on the basis of history alone, often without expert evaluation. Occasionally, stimulants are prescribed in response to complaints of fatigue or sedation in individuals who are using excessive doses of benzodiazepines, opioids, or other central nervous system (CNS) depressants. This can lead to escalating polypharmacy and requires reevaluation by appropriate specialists.

Patients with long histories of ADHD or other disorders for which stimulants may be appropriate, who have demonstrated long-term stability on those agents, can be successfully treated in pain management programs. They should be considered at higher risk than most patients, with monitoring adjusted accordingly.

Other Drugs of Abuse

Pain management physicians rarely see patients whose histories include use of hallucinogenic drugs, and who should be treated as high-risk. Patients who are active users of hallucinogens should be referred for addiction treatment immediately. Standard drug screens rarely test for hallucinogens other than phencyclidine ("angel dust," or PCP), and consideration of specific kits for such agents, or routine use of gas chromatography/mass spectrometry (GC/MS) or liquid chromatography/tandem mass spectrometry (LC/tandem MS) (or other appropriate testing technology) should be employed.

Increased use of synthetic cannabinoids (K2, Spice and many others) has been observed over the past decade, particularly in populations who undergo routine drug testing, such as military personnel, veterans, and persons on probation or parole [18]. While these compounds may produce effects similar to those of marijuana, they also are associated with psychosis, delirium, agitation, seizures, unstable vital signs, and death. Similar risks accompany use of the synthetic stimulants widely known as "bath salts" (and other names such as "plant food"), including methedrone, methylone, and methylenedioxypyrovalerone (MDPV) [19,20]. Patients with histories of using either synthetic cannabinoids or cathinones should be subjected to specialized testing as well.

Barbiturates continue to be used clinically, including phenobarbital and primidone for seizure disorders, but the largest reason for their use is in the treatment of migraine headaches with compounds of butalbital. Like most barbiturates, butalbital tests positive in screening tests. Another atypical sedative is the muscle relaxant carisoprodol (Soma®), in which the active ingredient is the metabolite meprobamate, a barbiturate-like sedative with very high abuse potential. All of these sedatives cause physical dependence in a very short period of time. They also cause respiratory depression and contribute to overdose deaths, and have a withdrawal syndrome that is particularly severe and similar to *delirium tremens*. Thus, in treating patients who have been prescribed barbiturates, communication with other treating providers is essential.

Referral to Treatment

When patients present with active SUDs or in a state of relapse, and when such use may be associated with significant risks of morbidity or mortality if pain management is continued, health care professionals need a good general awareness of the addiction treatment system, both in general and in their particular geographic region. Unfortunately, few physicians who do not regularly work in addiction treatment have a thorough understanding of the organization and processes employed by addiction treatment programs.

Medical detoxification is a critical step in initiating treatment. This may involve management of longer-term post-acute withdrawal syndromes through use of both pharmacological and non-pharmacological modalities. In cases where there are no serious underlying medical issues (such as those seen in elderly or frail patients and those with cardiovascular disorders) and no psychiatric disorders (particularly bipolar and thought disorders), detoxification and its aftermath can be managed in outpatient settings specifically designed for such care. Alternatively, a brief (three- to seven-day) hospitalization can establish stability, followed by a day or evening intensive outpatient treatment program (OTP), generally lasting from two to six weeks. These components of care should be followed up with standard outpatient treatment (involving weekly, biweekly, or bi-monthly visits), and then periodic visits for an indefinite period of time.

In contrast to this recommended progression of care, a worrisome number of patients are dismissed from pain treatment, often with no or very brief medication tapers, and go on to experience severe withdrawal and relapse. Unfortunately, it is all too common for physicians in pain treatment programs to dismiss patients with no more than advice to "get help," without any suggestion as to where appropriate help can be found, or any effort to make a referral, speak with treatment staff, or provide relevant records.

For many such patients, the only available form of treatment available is a publicly funded detoxification program. Most such programs offer minimal services and little physician supervision or skilled nursing care. Most patients in the programs are not seen by a physician and are treated entirely on the basis of standing orders, using one-size-fits-all "cookbook" protocols. Moreover, such detox programs may not provide formal aftercare or outpatient treatment and, even during an inpatient stay, they may offer only minimal access to counseling, assessment, and treatment, with most "groups" consisting of a 12-Step meeting.

This is not a suitable level of care for patients who have complex medical issues, including those who have chronic pain in addition to a substance use disorder. Therefore, clinicians and programs that provide specialized pain treatment should search out hospital-based addiction treatment programs that offer an array of inpatient and outpatient services, or free-standing programs that are directed by certified specialists in addiction medicine or addiction psychiatry and that employ evidence-based techniques and provide appropriate aftercare options.

Pain specialists also should become familiar with alternative approaches to the 12-Step model, such as outpatient counseling delivered by psychiatric social workers, psychologists and certified/licensed alcohol and drug counselors, as well as alternative self-help programs such as Smart Recovery, LifeRing Secular Recovery, Women for Sobriety, and the like [21,22]. Many individuals who do not respond well to 12-Step programs [23] may do well with another form of treatment, and clinicians should be aware of the full array of options for addiction treatment, just as they are aware of options for the management of coronary disease, hypertension, diabetes, or, for that matter, chronic pain.

In fact, there is increasing awareness that 12-Step involvement may be a highly useful adjunct to treatment, but it does not necessarily constitute treatment in and of itself [23,24]. In a study sponsored by Alcoholics Anonymous to assess the efficacy of its own program, researchers found that between 5% and 15% of AA participants achieved long-term sobriety with a 12-Step program alone [25]. For those who fully utilize its program, and whose values align with those of AA, participation can be highly effective. However, as is true with virtually every medical disorder, different individuals respond to different treatment approaches, so that treatments beneficial to some patients may be ineffective or even harmful for others [26].

Conclusion

Health care professionals in the addiction treatment, pain management, and mental health communities are increasingly aware of the need to more fully evaluate patients who present with chronic pain for underlying conditions that complicate pain management and make it more dangerous for patients. It is time for pain treatment professionals and programs to increase their collaboration with addiction treatment specialists and programs. At the very least, pain programs should have strong collaborative relationships with addiction treatment programs, both within their walls and without, and even consider representation of each discipline in the other's treatment team.

Patients who have an active SUD should not be treated for pain without a referral to a comprehensive addiction treatment program that is structured to meet their needs adequately. Patients with histories of such disorders who appear to be in clinical remission also should have an expert evaluation to determine the appropriateness of any pain treatment plan. Those who relapse to opioid or other drug use while undergoing pain treatment should receive a similar referral. Pain specialists should avail themselves of addiction specialists and treatment facilities to meet these patients' complex needs. In fact, it is worthwhile for pain specialists to develop working relationships with carefully vetted practitioners and programs and to maintain regular contact regarding co-managed patients.

When patients are having difficulties and/or are at risk of relapse despite ongoing treatment, it is appropriate to jointly explore the possibility of adding other modalities, such as cognitive behavioral therapy or medication management with anti-craving drugs. If a provider resists use of such treatment, consideration should be given to finding a practitioner or program that promotes evidence-based treatments and referring the patient for such integrated care.

In short, the "failure to thrive" of a patient in pain treatment should lead to a more thorough evaluation, involving a search for missed trauma and other issues, rather than leading to the patient's dismissal from treatment, which leaves the patient without care and often without hope.

For More Information on the Topics Discussed:

American Society of Addiction Medicine (ASAM):

Gallagher RM, Koob G, Popescu A. The pathophysiology of chronic pain and interfaces with addiction (Chapter 93). In RK Ries, DA Fiellin, SC Miller & R Saitz, eds. *The ASAM Principles of Addiction Medicine, Fifth Edition.* Philadelphia, PA: Wolters Kluwer; 2014.

McLellan AT. Moving toward integrated care for substance use disorders: Lessons from history and the rest of health care (Chapter 25). In RK Ries, DA Fiellin, SC Miller & R Saitz, eds. *The ASAM Principles of Addiction Medicine, Fifth Edition*. Philadelphia, PA: Wolters Kluwer; 2014.

Food and Drug Administration (FDA):

Risk Evaluation and Mitigation Strategy (REMS) for Extended-Release and Long-Acting Opioids. Bethesda, MD: FDA, Department of Health and Human Services; 2014. (Access at: http://www.fda.gov/Drugs/DrugSafety/InformationbyDrugClass/ucm163647.htm.)

Substance Abuse and Mental Health Services Administration (SAMHSA):

Kotz MM, Consensus Panel Chair. *Managing Chronic Pain in Adults With or in Recovery From Substance Use Disorders* (Treatment Improvement Protocol [TIP] 54). Rockville, MD: SAMHSA, Department of Health and Human Services; 2012. (Access at: http://store.samhsa.gov/product/TIP-54-Managing-Chronic-Pain-in-Adults-With-or-in-Recovery-From-Substance-Use-Disorders/SMA13-4671.)

References

1. Manchikanti L, Fellow B, Ailinani H, et al. Therapeutic use, abuse, and nonmedical use of opioids: A ten-year perspective. *Pain Physician*. 2010;13:401–435.
2. Office of National Drug Control Policy (ONDCP). *Epidemic: Responding to the Prescription Drug Abuse Crisis*. Washington, DC: ONDCP, Executive Office of the President, The White House; 2015. (Accessed at: www.whitehouse.gov/sites/default/files/ondcp/policy-and-research/rx_abuse_plan.)
3. Gourlay DH, Heit H. Universal precautions: A matter of mutual trust and responsibility. *Pain Med*. 2006;7:210–211.
4. Food and Drug Administration (FDA). *Risk Evaluation and Mitigation Strategy (REMS) for Extended-Release and Long-Acting Opioids*. Bethesda, MD: FDA, Department of Health and Human Services; 2014. (Accessed at: http://www.fda.gov/Drugs/DrugSafety/InformationbyDrugClass/ucm163647.htm.)
5. Okie S. A flood of opioids, a rising tide of deaths. *NEJM*. 2010;363:1981–1985.
6. Johnson SH. Providing relief to those in pain: A retrospective on the scholarship and impact of the Mayday Project. *J Law, Med Ethics*. 2003;31:15–20.
7. Hoffman DE, Tarzian AJ. Oversight of physician opioid prescribing for pain: The role of state medical boards. *J Law, Med Ethics*. 2003;31:21–40.
8. Reeves RR, Burke RS, Kose S. Carisoprodol: Update on abuse. *South Med J*. 2012;105:619–623.
9. Fagan KJ, Irvine KM, McWhinney BC, et al. Diagnostic sensitivity of carbohydrate deficient transferrin in heavy drinkers. *BMC Gastroenterol*. 2014 May 22;14:97. https://www.ncbi.nlm.nih.gov/pmc/articles/PMC4042141/

10. Kissack JC, Bishop J, Roper AL. Ethylglucuronide as a biomarker for ethanol detection. *Pharmacotherapy.* 2008;28:769–781.

11. Aradottir S, Asanovska G, Gjerss S, et al. Phosphatidylethanol (Peth) concentrations in blood are correlated to alcohol intake in alcohol-dependent patients. *Alc Alcoholism.* 2006;41:431–437.

12. Fleming MF, Davis J, Passik SD. Reported lifetime aberrant drug-taking behaviors are predictive of current substance use and mental health problems in primary care patients. *Pain Med.* 2008;9:1098–1106.

13. Liebschutz JM, Saitz R, Weiss RD, et al. Clinical factors associated with prescription drug abuse in urban primary care patients with chronic pain. *J Pain.* 2010;11:1047–1055.

14. Skurtveit S, Furu K, Selmer R, et al. Smoking predicts abuse of opioids. *Ann Epidemiol.* 2010 Dec;20(12):890–897.

15. Swift RM. Drug therapy of alcohol dependence. *NEJM.* 1999;340:1482–1490.

16. Ooteman W, Verheul R, Naasslia M, et al. Patient-treatment matching with anti-craving medications in alcohol-dependent patients: A review of phenotypic, endophenotypic and genetic indicators. *J Subst Use.* 2005;10:75–96.

17. Veterans Health Administration (VHA). *VHA Directive 2010-035.* Washington, DC: VHA, Department of Veterans Affairs; July 22, 2010:1–3.

18. Castaneto MS, Gorelick DA, Desrosiers NA, et al. Synthetic cannabinoids: Epidemiology, pharmacokinetics and clinical implications. *Drug Alcohol Dep.* 2014;144:12–41.

19. Prosser JM, Nelson LS. The toxicology of bath salts: A review of synthetic cathinones. *J Med Toxicol.* 2012;8:33–42.

20. Rosenbaum CD, Carrero SP, Babu K. Here today, gone tomorrow . . . and back again? A review of herbal marijuana alternatives (K2, Spice), synthetic cathinones (bath salts), Kratom, Salvia divinorum, methoxetamine, and piperazines. *J Med Toxicol.* 2012;8:15–32.

21. White W, Kurtz E. *The Varieties of Recovery Experience.* Chicago, IL: Great Lakes Addiction Technology Transfer Center; 2005. (Accessed at: http://www.facesandvoicesofrecovery.org/pdf/White/2005-09_white_kurtz.pdf.)

22. Horvath T. *Sex, Drugs, Gambling and Chocolate: A Workbook for Overcoming Addictions.* Alascadero, CA: Impact Publishers; 2004.

23. Ferri M, Amato L, Davoli M. Alcoholics Anonymous and other 12-step programmes for alcohol dependence. *Cochrane Database Syst Rev.* 2006 Jul 19;(3):CD005032. https://www.ncbi.nlm.nih.gov/pubmed/16856072

24. Dodes L. *Sober Truth: Debunking the Bad Science Behind 12-Step Programs and the Rehab Industry.* Boston, MA: Beacon Press; 2014.

25. Alcoholics Anonymous (AA). *Contemporary Myths and Misinterpretations,* January 1, 2008. (Accessed at: www.AA.org/productsp-48_07survey.pdf.)

26. Glaser G. The irrationality of Alcoholics Anonymous. *Atlantic Monthly.* 2015 Apr;(4):315.

Chapter 6

Ethical Issues in Treating Pain and Addiction

CHRISTOPHER J. SPEVAK, M.D., FASAM

The past decade has seen a serious increase in misuse of prescription opioids, followed by an epidemic of heroin use. The result has been described as a "biopsychosocial catastrophe," involving patients who suffer from pain and addiction and who need treatment for both medical disorders.

A primary goal of this chapter is to help clinicians offer better care to such patients by fostering an enhanced understanding of the ethical issues involved in the treatment of pain and addiction. A secondary goal is to increase clinicians' self-confidence and motivation to deal with such ethical dilemmas, which can provoke clinical uncertainty. Readers are encouraged to consult other chapters of this Handbook, which address a broad spectrum of clinical concerns in addition to the ethical issues discussed here.

An Historical Perspective on Medical Ethics

In order to fully understand the bioethical implications of treating patients diagnosed with pain and addiction, it is first necessary to review some fundamentals of bioethics. The foundation of Western medical ethics dates from the late fifth century BC [1,2]. Versions of the Hippocratic Oath, which emerged nearly a century after the death of Hippocrates, required physicians to swear to various gods that they would uphold certain ethical standards [3]. Today, almost all new physicians take a modern version of the Hippocratic Oath at the time they graduate from medical school.

Over the intervening centuries, and particularly in the past 100 years, medicine has evolved enormously. Modern clinical ethics are said to have emerged in the 1970s, in tandem with the civil rights and women's rights movements. The decade saw a growing recognition that the fundamental rights of patients and research participants were not being respected. For example, patients often were not told about a diagnosis of cancer out of concern that they could not cope with such disturbing news. Anesthetized patients awoke to discover that they had been subjected to surgical procedures to which they had not consented. Individuals were sterilized against their will under state-sponsored eugenics programs. And in the infamous Tuskegee experiment, conducted by the U.S. Public Health Service, treatment was withheld from patients diagnosed with syphilis so that clinicians could observe the progression of the disease.

Paternalism dominated physician–patient relationships. Combined with evolving medical technologies, recognition of such paternalism was a major factor in the birth of the modern bioethics movement. For example, in the 1980s, a Presidential commission called for the creation of an ethics committee at every U.S. hospital. Since that time, ethics committees have been convened in hospitals as well as other institutions and settings, where they address concerns related to genetics, environment, nutrition, and other issues regarding patient care and autonomy [4].

Ethical Theories and Definitions

So what exactly is bioethics? While definitions abound, it is most simply described as the intersection of law, policy, philosophy, anthropology, and medicine with the nature of the patient's personhood and self, in light of health, illness, disease and death. Distinctions have been made between medical ethics, bioethics, and clinical ethics. *Clinical ethics* is defined as the "systematic, critical, reasoned evaluation and justification of right and wrong, good and evil in clinical practice, and the study of the kinds of persons health care professionals ought or ought not to strive to become" [5].

Clinical ethics (unlike *medical ethics*) addresses the needs and rights of all individuals who receive health care. *Bioethics* is even more expansive, covering topics such as environmental issues that affect human health.

It may be presumed that most people are trying to live the most meaningful and good life possible. Morality represents an attempt to do just that, for ourselves and our loved ones, while we remain true to our most deeply held beliefs and help others to clarify and pursue their own chosen good lives. *Moral pluralism* occurs when individuals weigh elements of a good life differently (as when they weigh the relative importance of freedom from pain versus freedom from addiction).

Theoretical Tools

A variety of theoretical tools can be used to guide clinical decision-making when dealing with a patient who presents with both pain and addiction. Two of the most frequently described tools are *deontological theories* and *utilitarianism*.

Originating with the philosopher Immanuel Kant, deontological theories are based on a devotion to duty, with consequences playing no role in determining whether an action is right or wrong. The practical application of deontological theories is evident in situations where there are conflicting obligations and no compromise is possible.

This is in contrast with utilitarianism, in which the consequences of an action are the focus of attention. Under utilitarian theory, the "best overall result is determined from an impersonal perspective that gives equal weight to the interests of each affected party" [6].

Other theories include *consequentialism*, which focuses on outcomes; *existentialism*, which focuses on authenticity; and *virtue*, which focuses on character. More recently, ethicists have examined complex medical issues through the lenses of *rights-based*, *narrative-based*, and *principle-based theories*.

All of these theoretical approaches share key principles that form the framework for moral reasoning [7]. *Beneficence* and *non-maleficence* date back to the Hippocratic Oath. Beneficence is the duty to promote good and to act in the best interest of the patient and society. Non-maleficence prohibits actions that may be harmful to patients. *Autonomy* is the right of an individual to make his or her own decisions regarding health care. *Justice* encompasses the distribution of risks and benefits throughout society.

Several professional societies—including the American Medical Association (AMA), the American Society of Addiction Medicine (ASAM), and the American Academy of Pain Medicine (AAPM)—have developed ethical codes to guide clinicians' decision-making [8,9,10]. Readers are encouraged to explore these resources (see the text box at the end of this chapter).

Ethical Considerations in Delivering Clinical Care

Each of the various ethics frameworks described here has strengths that are especially relevant in different clinical scenarios. For example, the Ethics Work-up published by the Pellegrino Center for Clinical Bioethics [2], which is based on a 10-step process, combines both a substantive and a procedural framework for case analysis, which moves from facts through values to a decision and its justification. The goal is to reach a decision that is the best, most morally acceptable and practically realizable option for the patient. The work-up begins with the following five questions.

What Ethical Issues, Concerns, or Conflicts are Involved?

The process begins by examining the ethical issues, concerns, or conflicts involved in the case. These may involve any of the following:

The *physician–patient relationship* is at the core of recovery and the healing process. Both patients and physicians face challenges on multiple levels. From a patient perspective, physicians may represent the failure of the health care system and society in their quest for recovery and healing.

Patients often find themselves in a "siloed system," with pain treatment in one silo and addiction treatment in another. All too often, the treatment delivered in each silo does not take into account the needs originating in the other silo. Patients may feel marginalized or devalued in both treatment settings. Moreover, many addiction treatment programs are abstinence-based, so patients using opioids for pain or medication-assisted treatment for addiction may feel ostracized.

From the physician's perspective, patients with substance use disorders (SUDs) in a pain clinic may be viewed as drug-seeking or treatment failures. This type of bias often leads to inadequate care.

Informed consent is a crucial part of medical care, and never more so than when treating patients for pain and addiction. As discussed earlier, the era of paternalism ("I am your doctor and I know what is best for you") has been ushered out and replaced by the concept of informed consent. The elements of informed consent include an understanding of the nature of the treatment or procedure and all reasonable alternatives, as well as the risks and benefits of each option. This must be accompanied by an assessment of the patient's competence to understand the information and capacity to make a decision.

The question then becomes, "What type of treatment or procedure requires informed consent?" There is a consensus among bioethicists that all treatment (whether it involves medications, physical or mental health modalities, or procedures) requires informed consent. Such consent should not be confused with the signed document that memorializes the discussion between the physician and patient. The requirement for a signed document may be imposed by a particular program or institution. But even if a signed document is not required, there is an ethical obligation to provide information the patient needs to give a truly informed consent.

The standards for informed consent also vary, with the "reasonable patient" standard employed most often. This standard focuses on what a reasonable patient would need to know in order to make an informed decision.

One area of interest involves the capacity of a patient who is in pain, or taking mind-altering drugs, to make such a decision. Also, evidence shows that an individual's decision-making capacity may fluctuate during the course of an illness, and even according to the time of the day. The physician must be able to evaluate the patient's capacity at the time a decision is made, as well as while treatment continues [11].

Confidentiality is a core principle of bioethics in dealing with a patient to be treated for pain and addiction. As noted earlier, the physician–patient relationship is the foundation of good medical care. Confidentiality is not only required by law, but is at the heart of a strong physician–patient relationship.

Chapter 42 of the Code of Federal Regulations, Part 2, is the legal authority that requires the highest degree of confidentiality in addiction treatment. The standard is higher than that required for psychiatric treatment or general medical care. Here, the guiding principle is that the amount of information disclosed is to be decided by the patient.

Integrated care delivery systems and electronic medical records pose a challenge in this regard, particularly when multiple members of the health care team treat the patient's pain and addiction. All members of the team must be aware that the highest degree of confidentiality and non-disclosure must be observed.

Urine Drug Testing (UDT): UDT has become the standard of care in both pain and addiction treatment (see Chapter 11 of this Handbook). However, such tests raise ethical concerns. While UDT is widely regarded as an essential safety precaution that protects both the patient and society, critics contend that the evidence for random UDT is weak, and add that nonadherence is common. For example, patients may use substances that are not detected by UDT, or adulterate or substitute urine specimens. Moreover, the principle of patient autonomy is put at risk when patients are required to submit to random UDT.

In addition, critics argue that use of UDT stigmatizes patients as drug-seeking and intensifies the mistrust that often accompanies the treatment of pain and addiction.

Opioid Treatment Agreements also have become a standard of care. As with UDT, there is a lack of evidence to support the notion that opioid treatment agreements improve care. From a legal perspective, an argument can be made that such agreements are contracts of adhesion that offer no real option for patients with pain and addiction. Again, the principle of autonomy is at risk.

Treatment Disagreement: Disagreements about various aspects of treatment take many forms, including a patient's unwillingness to participate in the type of care that the physician believes is most appropriate. Because they violate the principle of shared decision-making, treatment disagreements may lead to autonomy challenges.

Abandonment: Even when a patient with pain and/or addiction is nonadherent and causes difficulties in a practice, the treating physician must understand and comply with the legal requirements involved in discharging such a patient from the practice. Although it is tempting to discharge a patient who repeatedly fails urine drug tests or violates opioid treatment agreements, care must be exercised not to abandon the patient. Caution also is required in the more subtle situation in which a patient is functionally discharged because he or she does not receive needed services and is forced to seek care elsewhere.

Pregnancy: The woman who presents for treatment of pain and addiction while pregnant poses a host of ethical challenges involving both mother and fetus. It is well known that opioids, whether prescription or illicit, have teratogenic effects on the fetus. As such, they should be avoided during the first trimester. The question then arises as to what is the optimal treatment for a pregnant woman with co-occurring pain and addiction. The MOTHER study [12] provides guidance in terms of medication-assisted therapy. However, other ethical issues remain.

Pregnant women have concerns about losing their children, or being forced into treatment if a substance use disorder is diagnosed. State requirements that health care providers report such women to child welfare agencies may rest on a patchwork of difficult-to-navigate regulations.

Lesbian, Gay, Bisexual, Transgender (LGBT) issues are a reminder that culturally competent care is essential to good care of the patient with pain and addiction. Evidence shows that lesbian and bisexual women are at three times the lifetime risk of developing SUDs as other women [13,14] see suggested references. Patients coming to treatment are in various stages of "coming out" and therefore must have individualized treatment plans, as addiction is intertwined with sexuality. Clinicians must examine their own views, which may range from anti-LGBT through naïve, tolerant or sensitive, to affirming.

System Constraints also need to be considered. For example, some insurance plans limit access to treatments such as therapy with buprenorphine or other medications. Others limit coverage of certain inpatient or outpatient services. In such a situation, the treating professional and office staff should work with the patient in an effort to gain access to the needed care.

Bias in favor of *abstinence-based treatment programs* is another issue that arises in the treatment of pain and addiction. From an historical and cultural perspective, addiction treatment in the United States has been dominated by abstinence-only approaches. While this situation is changing, it leads to significant ethical issues for both patient and physician. For example, it is not unusual for a patient being treated for pain or addiction with buprenorphine to encounter difficulties in locating an accepting 12-Step program. Other issues that should be considered include end-of-life and research-related issues.

What Are the Facts of the Case?

Facts often drive the decision as to the best course of action. For example, consider the case of a woman who is 10 weeks pregnant, with a history of polysubstance use disorder as well as active opioid use disorder and co-occurring mental health issues. In addition, the woman has an infectious disease related to her intravenous drug use, and tests positive for both hepatitis C and HIV.

In such a case, the goals of treatment and the likelihood of success vary. The facts of the case suggest that initial steps should be focused on minimizing the risk of neonatal abstinence syndrome, as well as any complications of intravenous (IV) drug use, and stabilizing the patient's mental health issues.

In considering the best course of action for a particular patient (based on familial, financial, religious, and cultural dynamics), it is important to recognize that even if there is no clear *best* course of action, some options may be better than others.

What Are the Ethical Arguments For and Against Each Option?

What values or principles are most important? What is the strongest objection to the preferred option, and how could the physician respond to it?

The principle of autonomy dictates that the patient must be at the center of the decision-making process and be informed of the risks and benefits of every treatment option. For each option, ethical considerations include autonomy, beneficence, non-maleficence, and justice.

As an example, while superior outcomes are well documented with medication-assisted therapy, the patient's autonomy is paramount, so a decision in favor of abstinence-based treatment must be respected, even if that requires that the principle of beneficence take second place. In addition, societal consequences must be taken into account, as continued opioid use disorder has significant implications for the public health as well as financial implications for the patient and society as a whole.

Can the Ethically Preferable Option(s) Be Implemented?

If medication-assisted treatment is a preferred option, it is important to consider the limited availability of opioid treatment programs (OTPs), particularly those equipped to treat special populations such as pregnant women. Transportation issues also must be factored in.

Financial, legal, and institutional limitations also must be considered. For example, office-based treatment with buprenorphine may be cost-prohibitive compared with methadone treatment. In addition, the legal implications of office-based treatment of pregnant women must be considered. given that criminal prosecutions as well as loss of custody rights are a possibility in many jurisdictions. Therefore, some pregnant women may wish to avoid medication-assisted therapies, even if they offer an excellent chance of recovery, for fear of the legal difficulties they may trigger.

Conflicts among decision-makers (including the patient, his or her family, and the health care team) may not be resolved. Whatever therapy the patient chooses, it is desirable that every member of the patient's family support the decision, but it is equally important that the treatment team support the patient's decision. The physician needs to be able to provide good care to the patient, even if the patient opts for a treatment the physician regards as less desirable than the recommended option.

Can Any Conflicts Be Resolved?

It is important to consider whether some sort of compromise can be achieved without loss of moral integrity. If compromise is *not* possible, the patient may decide to change physicians, or the physician may transfer care of the patient to another practitioner and withdraw from the case.

Conclusion

Both addiction and pain medicine are beset by bioethical challenges. This chapter began with a brief history of developments in the field of bioethics, followed by a review of key bioethical theories. Readers were asked to consider the steps in a case-based bioethics workup, with the goal of generating interest in the field of bioethics and motivating physicians to apply ethical principles when caring for patients with co-occurring pain and addiction.

For More Information on the Topics Discussed:

American Society of Addiction Medicine (ASAM):

ASAM Public Policy Statement on Principles of Medical Ethics. Chevy Chase, MD: The Society; 2005. (Access at: http://www.asam.org/docs/default-source/public-policy-statements/1prin-of- med-ethics-10-92.pdf?sfvrsn=0.)

Clark HW, Bizzell AC, Campbell A. Ethical issues in addiction practice. In RK Ries, DA Fiellin, SC Miller, R Saitz, eds. *The ASAM Principles of Addiction Medicine, Fifth Edition.* Philadelphia, PA: Wolters Kluwer; 2014.

American Medical Association (AMA):

AMA Code of Medical Ethics. Chicago, IL: The Association, June 2016. (Access at: https://www.ama-assn.org/about-us/code-medical-ethics.)

American Academy of Pain Medicine (AAPM):

AAPM Position Statement on Ethical Practice of Pain Medicine. Chicago, IL: The Academy, March 2011. (Access at: http://www.painmed.org/files/aapm-position-statement-on-ethical-practice-of-pain-medicine.pdf.)

References

1. Department of Veterans Affairs (VA). *VA-DoD Clinical Practice Guidelines: Management of Opioid Therapy for Chronic Pain.* Washington, DC: VA, U.S. Department of Defense; 2017. (Access at: http://www.healthquality.va.gov/guidelines/pain/cot/index.asp.)
2. Pelegrino ED. The metamorphosis of medical ethics. A 30-year retrospective. *JAMA.* 1993;269:1158–1162.
3. Hippocrates. *Decorum* (translator: W Jones). Cambridge, MA: Harvard University Press; 1967:297.
4. Blacksher E. Hearing from pain: Using ethics to reframe, prevent, and resolve the problem of unrelieved pain. *Pain Med.* 2001;2(2):170.
5. Sullmacy D. On the current state of clinical ethics. *Pain Med.* 2001;2(2):98.
6. Beauchamp TL, Childress JF. *Principles of Biomedical Ethics, 4th ed.* New York: Oxford University Press; 1994:11.
7. Novy D. A primer of ethical issues involving opioid therapy for chronic nonmalignant pain in a multidisciplinary setting. *Pain Med.* 2009;10(2):358.
8. American Medical Association (AMA). *AMA Code of Medical Ethics.* Chicago, IL: The Association; June 2016. (Access at: https://www.ama-assn.org/about-us/code-medical-ethics.)
9. American Society of Addiction Medicine (ASAM). *ASAM Statement on Confidentiality of Patient Records and Protections Against Discrimination.* Chevy Chase, MD: The Society; July 1, 2010. (Access at: http://www.asam.org/advocacy/find-a-policy-statement/view-policy-statement/public-policy-statements/2011/12/15/confidentiality-of-patient-records-and-protections-against-discrimination.)
10. American Academy of Pain Medicine (AAPM). *AAPM Position Statement on the Ethical Practice of Pain Medicine.* Chicago, IL: The Academy; March 2011. (Access at:http://www.painmed.org/files/aapm-position-statement-on-ethical-practice-of-pain-medicine.pdf.)
11. Tunzi M. Can the patient decide? Evaluating patient capacity in practice. *Am Fam Physician.* 2001 Jul 15;64(2):299–308. (Access at: http://www.aafp.org/afp/2001/0715/p299.html.)
12. Jones HE, Fischer G, Heil SH, et al. Maternal Opioid Treatment: Human Experimental Research (MOTHER) – Approach, issues, and lessons learned. *Addiction.* 2012 Nov;107(01):28–35.
13. Gonzales G, Henning-Smith C. Health disparities by sexual orientation: Results and implications from the Behavioral Risk Factor Surveillance System. *J Community Health.* 2017 Dec;42(6):1163–1172.
14. Feinstein BA, Dyar C, London B. Are outness and community involvement risk or protective factors for alcohol and drug abuse among sexual minority women? *Arch Sex Behav.* 2017 Jul;46(5):1411–1423.

Chapter 7

Legal Issues in Treating
Pain and Addiction

EDWIN A. SALSITZ, M.D., FACP, DFASAM AND
MARTHA J. WUNSCH, M.D., FAAP, DFASAM

In addition to knowledge about the clinical issues involved in treating pain and addiction, physicians who wish to treat patients for these conditions need to understand applicable federal, state, and local laws and regulations. Key requirements of federal laws and regulations are outlined in this chapter. However, every clinician also needs to know and understand the laws and regulatory requirements in the state in which he or she practices [1,2]. This is important because state laws and licensing board regulations may differ substantially from federal requirements and from one state to another. The Board of Medicine or Board of Pharmacy (or their equivalent) in each state can provide information about the relevant requirements [3].

Federal Laws and Regulations Protecting Confidentiality

Health Insurance Portability and Accountability Act (HIPAA)

Patients expect their caregivers to regard information about them and their treatment as confidential. The medical profession historically attaches a high value to patients' privacy because it is critical that patients give their physicians accurate information. By affording privacy protections to medical information, society assures patients that they can disclose sensitive information to their physicians without worrying about what use others might make of such information [1–3].

The Federal Health Insurance Portability and Accountability Act (Public Law 104-191, known as HIPAA), which was adopted in 1996, established standards for the privacy of "individually identifiable health information." To implement the law, the U.S. Department of Health and Human Services (DHHS) issued a set of regulations governing patients' privacy that apply to a wide range of health care providers. These HIPAA regulations, adopted in 2000, appear in Volume 45 of the Code of Federal Regulations (CFR), Parts 160 and 164.

HIPAA regulations are not as restrictive as the federal confidentiality rules encompassed in 42 CFR (described later), and practitioners who are subject to both sets of rules must follow the more restrictive standards set forth in 42 CFR.

Confidentiality

Confidentiality is especially important when a patient has a substance use disorder (SUD) because of the widespread stigma experienced by such individuals and the very real consequences of such stigma. For example, a patient might fear that his or her relationships with a spouse, parents, children, an employer, or friends would suffer if they learned about his or her problems with alcohol or drugs. If a patient has marital problems, information about an addictive disorder could have an effect on divorce or custody proceedings. A patient whose problem becomes known to an employer could lose an expected promotion or his or her job. Adverse consequences such as these can deter patients from admitting to—or seeking help for—problems with alcohol or other drugs.

In an effort to address these concerns, Congress enacted legislation in the early 1970s to protect information about patients undergoing treatment for SUDs and directed DHHS to issue implementing regulations. The resulting rules are codified at 42 USC §290dd-2. The implementing federal regulations, titled "Confidentiality of Alcohol and Drug Abuse Patient Records," are contained in 42 CFR Part 2 (Volume 42 of the Code of Federal Regulations, Part 2, commonly known as "42 CFR"). These rules permit disclosure of information only in very limited circumstances, such as the following [2]:

1. When a patient signs a consent form that complies with the regulations' requirements;
2. When a disclosure does not identify the patient as an individual with a substance use disorder;
3. When program staff members consult among themselves;
4. When the disclosure is to a "qualified service organization" that provides services to the program;

5. When there is a medical emergency;
6. When the program must report child abuse or neglect;
7. When a patient commits a crime at the program or against program staff;
8. When the information is for research, audit, or evaluation purposes; or
9. When a court issues a special order authorizing disclosure.

In many instances, 42 CFR restricts communications more tightly than either the physician–patient or the attorney–client privilege. For example, the rules of 42 CFR apply regardless of whether the person seeking information already has the information, has other ways to obtain it, has official status, is authorized by state law, or has a subpoena or search warrant. Violations are punishable by a fine of up to $500 for a first offense and up to $5,000 for each subsequent offense [1].

Physicians engaged in general medical practice usually are not subject to the provisions of 42 CFR. However, if a staff member has been designated to provide assessment or treatment of patients with SUDs, and/or the practice benefits from "federal assistance," it must comply with the terms of 42 CFR. Thus, clinicians and their office staffs should handle information about patients' SUDs with great care. Even those who are not *required* to comply with the special provisions of 42 CFR are advised to comply on a voluntary basis (Box 7.1) [1].

State Laws and Regulations Protecting Confidentiality

Many states also have adopted laws and regulations to protect the confidentiality of medical information [2]. Most physicians and patients think of these laws as the "physician–patient privilege." Strictly speaking, the physician–patient privilege is a rule of evidence that governs whether a physician can be compelled to testify in court about a patient. In many states, however, the laws offer wider protections, and some states have special confidentiality laws that explicitly prohibit practitioners from divulging information about patients without their consent [2]. For example, whether a communication (or laboratory test result) is "privileged" or "protected" under state law depends on a number of factors:

- *The type of professional holding the information* and whether he or she is licensed or certified by the state. Most state laws do cover licensed physicians.
- *The context in which the information was communicated.* Some states limit protection to information a patient communicates to a physician in

BOX 7.1 An Early View of the New Federal Rule 42 CFR

A new final rule on 42 CFR Part 2 was issued by the Substance Abuse and Mental Health Services Administration (SAMHSA) in January 2017. Experts who are familiar with the new rule say that it maintains not only the core protections of the rule it replaces, but also the basic requirement that patient must give consent before their information can be disclosed.

In addition, the new rule retains prohibitions on re-disclosure, meaning that when a patient consents to having information released to a particular individual, the individual receiving the information may not re-disclose it to a third party.

Other significant changes in the new rule include the following:

- SAMHSA will allow any lawful holder of patient identifying information to disclose Part 2 patient identifying information to qualified personnel for purposes of conducting scientific research if the researcher meets certain regulatory requirements. SAMHSA also permits data linkages to enable researchers to link to data sets from data repositories holding Part 2 data if certain regulatory requirements are met. These will facilitate much-needed research into substance use disorders.
- SAMHSA will continue to apply Part 2 rules to any program that receives federal assistance and holds itself out as providing substance use disorder diagnosis, treatment, or referral for treatment.
- SAMHSA has added a requirement allowing patients who have agreed to the general disclosure designation the option to receive a list of entities to whom their information has been disclosed, if they request it.
- SAMHSA has made changes to ensure that CMS-regulated entities can perform necessary audit and evaluations activities, including audits of financial and quality assurance functions critical to Accountable Care Organizations and other health care organizations.
- SAMHSA has updated the rule to address both paper and electronic documentation.

SAMHSA will monitor implementation of the final rule and is working to develop additional sub-regulatory guidance and materials on many of the finalized provisions. To read the final rule, go to: https://www.federalregister.gov/documents/2017/01/18/2017-00719/confidentiality-of-substance-use-disorder-patient-records.

Source: Knopf A. Final rule for 42 CFR Part 2 retains core confidentiality protections. *AT Forum*. 2017 Dec/Jan;28:1.

the course of a medical consultation, and do not protect information disclosed to a physician in the presence of a third party, such as a spouse. Other states protect information the patient tells the physician when others are present, as well as information the physician gains during an examination.

- *The circumstances in which "confidential" information will be or was disclosed.* Some states protect medical information only when that information is sought in a court proceeding. If a physician divulges information about a patient in any other setting, the law does not recognize that there has been a violation of the patient's right to privacy. Other states protect medical information in many different contexts.
- *How the right to privacy is enforced.* State legal protection of medical information is useful only when it is backed by enforcement of the law.

States often include requirements such as these in their professional practice acts/licensing laws, which generally prohibit licensed professionals from divulging information about patients. Unauthorized disclosures constitute grounds for disciplinary action, including license revocation. Although enforcement actions remain relatively rare, states do have the right to discipline professionals who violate patients' privacy. Alternatively, they may allow patients to sue the provider for damages [3].

Exceptions

Exceptions to general rules protecting the privacy of information generally include [3]:

- *Consent:* All states permit physicians to disclose information if the patient consents, although states have different requirements for obtaining and documenting such consent. In some states, it must be written; in others, it can be oral. Some states require specific consent forms for disclosures about different diseases.
- *Reporting infectious diseases:* All states require physicians to report certain infectious diseases to public health authorities, although definitions of reportable diseases vary from state to state.
- *Reporting child or elder abuse and neglect:* All states require physicians to report child abuse and neglect to child protective services; however, states' definitions of acts that constitute child abuse vary. Many—but not all—states have similar requirements for the reporting of elder abuse and neglect.
- *Duty to warn:* Most states also require physicians to report credible threats by a patient to harm others.

When Confidentiality Conflicts with Other Principles

Application of the laws may differ depending on whether the physician's obligation is to the patient or another individual or class of individuals. Examples of
such situations include the following cases [1,2].

Employer versus Employee

To whom does a physician owe loyalty when treating a patient who has been
referred by an employer as a condition of retaining a job? Is it to the employer,
who is relying on the physician to help the employee recover and remain (or
return) to work? Or is it to the patient (the employee)? The employer probably
will require reports from the physician on the patient's progress in treatment.
What should the physician do if the employee is not attending or complying with
treatment? This question appears most starkly when the employee is in a safety-
sensitive position and the physician is concerned that his or her behavior poses
an immediate risk to other employees or to the public. To which ethical principle
should the physician adhere: the obligation to safeguard the patient's privacy, or
the obligation to protect those who might be harmed by the patient's actions?

The best way to avoid having to grapple with this problem in an emergency (always a difficult and unpleasant experience) is to create agreed-upon
ground rules before treatment begins. If an employer requires reports, the
physician must have the patient sign a consent form authorizing communication with the employer. The physician and patient must agree on what kinds
of information will be reported, and that agreement should be made part of
the consent form. (Unfortunately, the patient can revoke his or her consent
at any time.) Of course, the employer also must be willing to accept whatever
limitations the agreement places on the kinds of information it will receive.

Reports to employers typically include information about attendance and
progress in treatment. In most cases, it would be inappropriate for a physician
to include detailed clinical information in such reports. However, employers
can require more information when employees in safety-sensitive positions are
in treatment. Employers may want to hear about positive results from a drug
screen test, and the physician may want to be able to report continued drug use
by an employee in a safety-sensitive position.

The physician can discharge his or her duty to the public at large (and to the
employer) without violating the patient's right to privacy if the patient signs
a consent form that documents his or her understanding that certain types of
behavior would be reported to the employer.

Imminent Danger

When a patient presents a danger to self or others, is the treating physician's
obligation to the patient or to society? Most physicians know that society

already has determined that the duty to warn supersedes the duty to protect a patient's privacy. In such cases, the law requires a warning to the potential victim or someone in a position to protect the potential victim.

However, the duty to warn does not completely nullify the patient's right to privacy. The physician can warn others of potential danger without disclosing extraneous information about the patient, including information about his or her use of drugs and alcohol. Physicians who are subject to federal confidentiality rules are required to issue the warning in a way that minimizes harm to the patient's privacy [3,4].

Recordkeeping Requirements

Accurate and up-to-date medical records are the mechanism that protects both the practitioner and the patient. In the event of a legal challenge, detailed medical records documenting what was done, and why, are the foundations of the practitioner's defense [2,3].

Medical Records

Patient medical records should summarize all information relevant to the patient's care so as to facilitate care by another physician if required. The name, telephone number, and address of the patient's pharmacy should be included to facilitate contact as needed. Other documents that should be included in the medical record are [2]:

- Diagnostic assessments, including history, physical examination, laboratory tests ordered and their results;
- Records of past hospitalizations or treatment by other providers, if available;
- The treatment plan;
- Authorization for release of information to other treatment providers;
- Documentation of discussions with and consultation reports from other health care providers;
- A list of all medications prescribed and the patient's response to them, including any adverse events.

Patient History and Physical Examination

The patient history must include information about all medications prescribed or administered, as well as documentation of steps taken to monitor the patient's medication use (such as pill counts, random urine drug screens, and review of the patient's record in the state Prescription Drug Monitoring Program). Pharmacological and non-pharmacological treatments that have been tried and failed also should be documented.

It is wise to obtain the patient's records directly from practitioners who treated the patient in the past. (Caution should be exercised in accepting records supplied by patients, as these occasionally are fraudulent [2].)

The documentation should include information about the patient's personal and family histories of alcoholism, drug use and addiction, as well any personal history of co-occurring psychiatric or medical disorders [2,3].

Prescription Orders

The medical record must include all prescription orders, whether written, e-prescribed, or verbally communicated with confirmation. The record also should include instructions given to the patient as to how the medication should be taken (emphasizing the need to take all medications exactly as prescribed). The prescription order should specify both the milligram dose and the amount of medication to be taken at any given time. (Confusion related to ambiguous orders can lead to adverse outcomes, especially early in treatment [1,3].)

Careful execution of the prescription order can prevent manipulation by the patient or others intent on obtaining opioids for non-medical purposes. For example, federal law requires that prescription orders for controlled substances be signed and dated on the day they are issued. Also under federal law, every prescription order must include at least the following information:

- Name and address of the patient;
- Name, address, and DEA registration number of the prescribing physician. (When buprenorphine is prescribed for the treatment of opioid use disorder, the prescription must contain the prescriber's DEA X Waiver number);
- Signature of the prescribing physician;
- Name and quantity of the drug prescribed;
- Directions for use; and
- Refill information.

In no case is it permissible to post-date a prescription. The prescriber may instruct a patient not to fill a prescription until a specific date, but the prescription order must be dated on the day it is written.

Many states impose additional requirements, which the physician can determine by consulting the medical licensing board for the state in which he or she practices. In addition, there are special federal requirements for drugs in different schedules of the Federal Controlled Substances Act (CSA), particularly drugs in Schedule II, where many opioid analgesics are classified (see online Appendix C at the end of this book).

Special caution is required when paper prescription pads are used because blank pads can be used to forge prescriptions, as can information such as the names of physicians who recently retired, left the state, or died. Therefore, it is a sound practice to lock blank paper prescriptions in a secure place rather than leaving them in examining rooms or carrying them in one's coat pocket.

Physicians should immediately report the theft or loss of prescription forms to the nearest field office of the U.S. Drug Enforcement Administration and to the State Board of Medicine or Pharmacy.

Records of Drugs Dispensed

Under federal law, clinicians who have waivers to prescribe or dispense buprenorphine for the treatment of opioid use disorder may do so in any appropriate practice setting in which they are otherwise credentialed to practice (e.g., an office or hospital). However, it is important to understand that the record-keeping requirements imposed by the U.S. Drug Enforcement Administration (DEA) for such office-based opioid treatment (OBOT) go beyond customary recordkeeping requirements. For example, the DEA requires that clinicians who purchase buprenorphine products to dispense in their practices must document all controlled substances dispensed, including buprenorphine (21 CFR Part 1304.03[b]) [4]. The requirement includes conducting an inventory that accounts for all buprenorphine received and dispensed.

In some cases, patients return to the prescribing physician with their filled prescriptions so that the practitioner or an office staff member can monitor drug administration. While this is acceptable, clinicians are *not* allowed to store or dispense controlled substances obtained through prescriptions filled by patients [4].

In addition, clinicians must keep records of any controlled substances prescribed and dispensed to patients for maintenance or detoxification treatment (21 CFR Part 1304.03[c]) [4]. Many clinicians comply with this requirement by creating a log that identifies the patient (an ID number may be used instead of a name), the name of the drug prescribed or dispensed, its strength and quantity, as well as the date the drug was prescribed or dispensed and the date the supply is expected to be used up. Some clinicians comply with this requirement by keeping a copy of every prescription in the patient record if paper medical records are used. (With electronic medical records and e-prescribing, there is no paper prescription to be tracked.)

Alternatively, the DEA suggests that practitioners keep separate records for controlled substances prescribed and dispensed for opioid maintenance or detoxification treatment, which can simplify record retrieval and review during DEA inspections [5].

Drug Storage

Patients who are prescribed or dispensed any opioid must be cautioned to store the medication properly, preferably in a locked container. They should be advised to store such medications out of the reach of children and pets, in childproof containers, and in locations that are not easily accessible. This warning must be given to all patients, regardless of whether they have children or pets living with them, and should be documented in the medical record [4].

DEA Inspections of DATA-Waivered Physicians

The DEA is responsible for ensuring that practitioners who are registered with DEA pursuant to the Drug Addiction Treatment Act of 2000 (DATA 2000) comply with recordkeeping, security, and other requirements for administering, dispensing, or prescribing controlled substances under the Federal Controlled Substances Act (CSA). As a result, DEA agents conduct regular site inspections of practice facilities. Any clinician who administers, dispenses, or prescribes Schedule III substances, including buprenorphine, also is subject to these routine, random inspections [3].

Required Records

Physicians who prescribe buprenorphine should maintain the records required to be kept on every patient in treatment, with documentation consistent with the recommendations of the DEA [1] and the Federation of State Medical Boards [2].

Records of medications dispensed must be retained for at least two years and made available for inspection by DEA agents and other federal employees authorized by the U.S. Attorney General [4]. The DEA is *not* allowed to review other parts of patient medical records during routine inspections.

Issues When a Practice Closes or Is Shut Down

Whenever a practice closes voluntarily or is shut down involuntarily, numerous logistical, legal, and ethical issues must be addressed. Patients must be notified and offered referral to other providers, medical records must be made available for transfer and storage, and arrangements must be made to ensure continuity of patient care. These matters can be accomplished best when there is sufficient time for providers and staff to make the arrangements, but such tasks must be accomplished regardless of the amount of time available so that patients are not abandoned [4,5].

Closure of a practice poses the risk of involuntary termination of treatment for patients who are dependent on opioids or who have been diagnosed with opioid use disorder and stabilized on prescribed or dispensed medications. In such situations, it is critical to notify patients of the closure and offer prompt, appropriate referrals to other physicians who can provide the needed care [3].

For patients who are taking buprenorphine, the physician must supply sufficient buprenorphine product (or transmit sufficient prescriptions to the patient's pharmacy) to last until the first visit to a new treatment provider. Failure to complete these tasks could cause the patient to experience withdrawal, unintended relapse, overdose, or death, and the physician to be charged with patient abandonment [2].

If a patient will not accept treatment for opioid use disorder in another treatment setting or from another provider, the physician must arrange for or manage withdrawal of the patient from buprenorphine in a manner that minimizes withdrawal discomfort and encourages the patient to seek other forms of effective treatment. In such a situation, the physician must make a good faith effort to ensure that the patient has access to an appropriate level of care after his or her own therapeutic involvement ends [3].

Conclusion

Physicians who prescribe controlled substances for the treatment of pain and/ or opioid use disorder must be aware of federal, state, and local laws and regulations that affect their ability to prescribe or dispense these medications. The 42 CFR sets requirements for the care of patients with SUDs and dictates careful management of these patients to protect confidentiality at a higher level than HIPAA.

Medical records should have adequate documentation to support the care of each patient, to assure a smooth transition to another provider should that become necessary, and to meet DEA requirements should an inspection occur.

Resources to assist health care professionals in understanding and complying with such requirements are available from multiple sources at the federal, state, and local levels.

For More Information on the Topics Discussed:

Federal Laws and Regulations Protecting Confidentiality:

Substance Abuse and Mental Health Services Administration (SAMHSA). *Medical Records Privacy and Confidentiality*. Rockville, MD: SAMHSA,

U.S. Department of Health and Human Services, last updated March 2016. (Access at: https://www.samhsa.gov/laws-regulations-guidelines/medical-records-privacy-confidentiality.)

State Laws and Regulations Protecting Confidentiality:

Federation of State Medical Boards (FSMB). *Model Policy on DATA 2000 and the Treatment of Opioid Addiction in the Medical Office.* Dallas, TX: The Federation; 2013. (Access at: http://www.fsmb.org/Media/Default/PDF/FSMB/Advocacy/2013_model_policy_treatment_opioid_addiction.pdf.)

Federation of State Medical Boards (FSMB):

Contact information for State Medical Boards. (Access at: http://www.fsmb.org/state-medical-boards/contacts.)

Federal Recordkeeping Requirements:

Drug Enforcement Administration (DEA), Diversion Control Division. *Practitioner's Manual, Section IV: Recordkeeping Requirements.* Washington, DC: DEA, U.S. Department of Justice; 2006. (Access at: https://www.deadiversion.usdoj.gov/pubs/manuals/pract/section4.htm.)

National Academy of Sciences:

Improving the Quality of Health Care for Mental and Substance-Use Conditions: Quality Chasm Series, Appendix B: Constraints on Sharing Mental Health and Substance-Use Treatment Information Imposed by Federal and State Medical Records Privacy Laws. Washington, DC: National Academies Press; 2006. (Access at: https://www.ncbi.nlm.nih.gov/books/NBK19829/.)

References

1. Institute for Research, Evaluation and Training in Addictions (IRETA). *Best Practices in the Use of Buprenorphine.* Pittsburgh, PA: Community Care Behavioral Health Organization; 2011.
2. Federation of State Medical Boards (FSMB). *Model Policy on Opioid Addiction Treatment in the Medical Office.* Dallas, TX: The Federation; 2013.
3. Center for Substance Abuse Treatment (CSAT). *Clinical Guidelines for the Use of Buprenorphine in the Treatment of Opioid Addiction.* Treatment Improvement Protocol (TIP) Series 40. DHHS Publication No. (SMA) 04-3939. Rockville, MD: CSAT, Substance Abuse and Mental Health Services Administration; 2004.
4. Salsitz EA, Wunsch MJ, for the Physician Clinical Support System for Buprenorphine (PCSS-B). *PCSS-B Guidance on Drug Enforcement Administration Requirements for Prescribers and Dispensers of Buprenorphine and Buprenorphine/Naloxone.* East Providence, RI: American Academy of Addiction Psychiatry; January 25, 2010.

5. Kraus ML, Alford DP, Kotz MM et al. Statement of the American Society of Addiction Medicine Consensus Panel on the Use of Buprenorphine in Office-Based Treatment of Opioid Addiction. *Addict Med.* 2011 Dec;5(4):254–263.

6. Suzuki J. Logistics of office-based buprenorphine treatment. In JA Renner, Jr., P Levounis, eds. *Handbook of Office-Based Buprenorphine Treatment of Opioid Dependence.* Washington, DC: American Psychiatric Publishing; 2011:24–27.

DIAGNOSING AND TREATING PAIN AND ADDICTION

Common Principles

The chapters in **Section II** examine clinical issues that are relevant to the identification and management of patients who have both pain and addiction.

- In **Chapter 8**, the author reviews the pharmacology of opioids used in the treatment of pain and opioid use disorder, including the pharmacological characteristics that make the use of some opioids riskier than others.
- The authors of **Chapter 9** discuss the reasons opioids are misused and abused, as well as precautions that can be taken by physicians and other health care professionals to maximize benefits while minimizing the risks of opioid use to their patients.
- **Chapter 10** focuses on the process of screening patients for risk of opioid misuse, abuse, or addiction—a step many experts recommend before any opioid is prescribed for pain or addiction.
- The authors of **Chapter 11** discuss on the earliest part of the treatment process, as they review the steps involved in reaching an accurate diagnosis and initiating treatment for pain or addiction.
- In **Chapter 12,** the authors review the importance of monitoring patient compliance with the treatment plan, as well as progress toward treatment goals. The discussion is supported by details on the use of drug testing and other tools to facilitate such monitoring.
- The author of **Chapter 13** discusses steps health care professionals can take to prevent opioid overdose—a rapidly escalating and often fatal problem in the United States—as well as specific methods recommended for reversing overdoses when they occur.

Chapter 8

The Pharmacology of Opioids

CHRISTOPHER CAVACUITI, M.D., CCFP,
M.H.SC., FASAM

Opioids are powerful medications that can provide profound benefits (such as acute pain relief) but also are associated with significant risks (such as overdose, addiction, and death) [1]. In order to help patients make informed decisions about opioid use, it is important that the clinicians who prescribe these medications have the knowledge needed to explain to patients when opioids are likely to help and when they are likely to do harm.

Chemical Classes of Opioids

Opioids can be divided into five chemical classes: phenanthrenes, benzomorphans, phenylpiperidines, diphenylheptanes, and phenylpropanolamines [2,3].

Phenanthrenes

The prototypical class of opioids, encompassing morphine, opium, and codeine, is the phenanthrene class. Phenanthrene opioids can be further subdivided into hydroxylated and dehydroxylated phenanthrenes. Hydrocodone, hydromorphone, oxycodone, and oxymorphone are examples of dehydroxylated phenanthrenes, which are missing a hydroxyl group at the sixth position. Dehydroxylated phenanthrenes are considered to be advantageous due to their better tolerability with respect to decreased gastrointestinal upset and histamine-mediated pruritus. Note that the pruritus that occurs with opioids is not an allergic reaction, though commonly mistaken as such, but a histamine-mediated reaction. Those who are unable to tolerate hydroxylated phenanthrenes may tolerate a dehydroxylated phenanthrene; though if they are unable to handle a dehydroxylated phenanthrene, it is unlikely a hydroxylated phenanthrene will be stomached.

Morphine is metabolized to 3-glucuronide and 6-glucuronide metabolites. The 6-glucuronide metabolite has analgesic activity. although it has a longer half-life than the parent compound. With reduced renal function, the 3-glucoronide metabolite, which lacks analgesic activity, can accumulate, leading to neurotoxicity. Neurotoxicity also may occur in the inpatient setting with high doses of intravenous morphine, >50–100 morphine equivalent daily dose (MEDD). This is the result of the preservatives (parabens, formaldehyde, or bisulfite) found in multi-dose vials of morphine. Preservative-free morphine or hydromorphone are alternatives to avoid this potential adverse event.

Benzomorphans

Benzomorphans have limited utility in pain management. Diphenoxylate and loperamide fall into this category and are not used for the management of pain. Recently, there have been increasing reports of the use of supratherapeutic doses of loperamide, available over the counter, to manage opioid withdrawal symptoms or for purposes of abuse. High doses of loperamide may lead to death as the result of cardiac arrhythmia [3,4].

When combined with other respiratory-depressing medications (such as opioids and benzodiazepines), loperamide and diphenoxylate may cause a patient to succumb to respiratory depression. Pentazocine, another benzomorphan, typically is reserved as a last-line agent for those unable to tolerate alternatives, due to its plateau for analgesic activity, potential for neurotoxicity, and short-acting nature.

Phenylpiperidines

Fentanyl, sufentanil, and remifentanil belong to the phenylpiperidine class of opioids. Sufentanil and remifentanil are phenylpiperidines that have no role in the primary care setting; their use should be limited to skilled anesthesiologists because of the risks they pose. Interestingly, the least and most tolerated opioids fall into the phenylpiperidine class. If a patient is experiencing opioid-induced pruritus, a switch to fentanyl may alleviate this adverse event because fentanyl has less histamine reactivity.

Increasing reports of fentanyl-related deaths are attributed to illicit formulations of fentanyl combined with other illicit substances, such as cocaine or heroin, rather than prescribed fentanyl [5].

Fentanyl patches are reserved for use in patients who require around-the-clock opioids and who are opioid-tolerant. Dosing of the fentanyl patch is determined by the patient's previous opioid dose, taking into account individual factors [5]. According to the package insert, there is some interpatient variability in the fentanyl patch dosing interval, with some patients not achieving adequate analgesia with q72h dosing; such patients may benefit from q48h dosing, which allows the levels to remain in therapeutic range while avoiding toxicity.

Some patients experience application site reactions to the adhesive in the fentanyl patches. This is easily treated with triamcinolone aerosol spray applied to the application area (wait for the spray to dissipate before placing a patch). Another frequent complaint is patch displacement, which can be prevented by placing an occlusive dressing atop the fentanyl patch.

Transmucosal immediate-release fentanyl (TIRF) products are available in multiple formulations. These medications are indicated for the management of breakthrough cancer pain, generally in patients over 18 years of age who are receiving and tolerant to opioid medications. Life-threatening respiratory depression may occur with TIRFs if they are used in patients who are not opioid-tolerant. A risk evaluation and mitigation strategy (REMS) program is available for TIRFs and must be completed prior to prescribing them [6].

Diphenylheptanes

Examples of the diphenylheptane class of opioids include propoxyphene and methadone. Although propoxyphene is no longer available, patients' previous response to and tolerance of diphenylheptanes may indicate that they are good candidates for a trial of methadone.

Methadone, a racemic mixture, is a unique medication because of its long and variable half-life (15–60h), its propensity for multiple drug–drug interactions (attributable to interactions with cytochrome p-450 enzymes and p-glycoprotein), and its association with cardiac arrhythmias arising from prolongation of the QTc interval. (A more detailed review of methadone appears elsewhere in this chapter.)

Phenylpropylamines

The final class of opioids is the phenylpropylamines, which include tapentadol and tramadol. Further discussion of these medications is found in Chapter 14 of this Handbook.

Pharmacodynamics of Opioids

The pharmacology of opioids and other drugs often is described in terms of *pharmacodynamics*, which is the study of what a drug does to the human body. Understanding the activity of a particular opioid at the opioid receptor is a key factor in using these medications as safely as possible.

Although opioid activity can be measured in many different ways, clinicians generally are interested in how the drugs are synthesized—that is, the observable physiological and clinically relevant responses that occur when an opioid is administered (see Table 8.1).

Opioid Antagonists

At one end of the mu-opioid agonist/antagonist spectrum are the opioid antagonists. Clinically useful opioid antagonists tend to have a high level of affinity for opioid receptors, but no intrinsic opioid receptor activity. The high affinity

TABLE 8.1 Classifying Opioids by the Manner in Which They Are Synthesized

Opioid Subtype	Description	Examples
Endogenous opioids	Opioid peptides that are produced by the body	Endorphins, enkephalins, dynorphins, endomorphins
Exogenous non-synthetic opioid agonists	Natural opioids derived from *Papaver somniferum* (the opium poppy)	Codeine, morphine, thebaine, diacetylmorphine (morphine diacetate, heroin)
Exogenous semi-synthetic opioid agonists	Natural opioids that have been chemically altered in a laboratory	Oxycodone, hydrocodone, hydromorphone
Exogenous synthetic opioid agonists	Opioids that are synthesized entirely in a laboratory	Buprenorphine, fentanyl, methadone

of these compounds means that opioid antagonists can "out-compete" other opioids at the opioid receptor. However, their lack of intrinsic activity at the opioid receptor means that they produce no opioid effect.

If an opioid antagonist is administered to an individual who is opioid-dependent, it will precipitate acute opioid withdrawal. Such antagonist properties often are clinically useful. For example, naloxone (which is a short-acting opioid antagonist) can be very useful in reversing opioid overdose, while naltrexone (a longer-acting opioid antagonist) appears to be helpful in reducing relapse risk in individuals who are trying to achieve and maintain opioid abstinence.

It should be noted that safety concerns with oral naltrexone persist, especially with regard to patients who have difficulty complying with the prescribed naltrexone regimen. Such individuals are at risk of overdose due to loss of tolerance. However, newer (intra-muscular/depot) formulations of naltrexone appear to reduce the safety concerns associated with rapid changes in opioid tolerance that occur with abrupt cessation of oral naltrexone.

Opioid Partial Agonists

The next group of compounds along the "agonist/antagonist potency spectrum" are the partial agonists. Clinically useful opioid partial agonists (such as buprenorphine) have enough intrinsic activity at the opioid receptor to relieve withdrawal and pain, but ideally, not enough to cause intoxication, overdose, or death. It is estimated that in physically dependent opioid users, 50–60% of mu opioid receptors must be occupied with buprenorphine before any significant relief of pain or withdrawal occurs, and that optimal relief of these symptoms often requires that 80–90% of mu receptors be occupied by buprenorphine.

Unlike full agonists, the relatively weak agonist effect of partial agonists such as buprenorphine means that even 99–100% receptor occupation by buprenorphine typically does not lead to intoxication and overdose or death among opioid-experienced individuals, whereas 99–100% mu receptor occupation with a full agonist would almost certainly lead to overdose and death.

Opioid Low-Potency Full Agonists

The next-strongest group of opioid compounds are the weaker or "lower potency" full agonists. These weaker opioids generally are considered to be safer and to have a lower addictive potential than the "high potency" agonists. The World Health Organization (WHO)'s Analgesic Ladder classifies these lower potency agonists as Step 2 medications.

It is important to recognize that the physiological effects of an opioid are determined as much by the drug's dose as by its potency. Thus a large dose of a "low-potency" full agonist is much the same in terms of mu opioid effect as a small dose of a "high-potency" full agonist.

Opioid High-Potency Full Agonists

The strongest opioid compounds are the group of "high-potency" agonists (such as heroin, oxycodone, fentanyl, morphine, and hydromorphone). These are the compounds with the greatest ability to provide analgesia. However, they also are the group with the greatest addiction liability and the highest risk of causing overdose and death. These are the medications generally listed as "Step 3" (the highest step) medications in the WHO Analgesic Ladder. Most are listed in Schedule II of the Federal Uniform Controlled Substances Act (CSA). (See Table 8.2.)

TABLE 8.2 Common Physiological Effects Associated with Various Opioid Receptor Subtypes

Opioid Receptor Subtype	Endogenous Ligand	Physiological Effects
Mu (μ)	Beta-endorphins	Analgesia (major effect) Euphoria Tolerance Withdrawal Respiratory depression QT prolongation Constipation Miosis Sedation Hypogonadism (suppressed secretion of Gonadotropin-releasing hormone [GNRH])
Delta (δ)	Enkephalins	Analgesia (minor effect) Convulsant effects Antidepressant effect
Kappa (κ)	Dynorphins	Analgesia (minor effect) Dissociative/hallucinogenic effects Diuresis Dysphoria

Pharmacokinetics of Opioids

Another common way to classify opioids is by examining their *pharmacody-namic* properties to understand what the body does to the drug (Table 8.2). From a practical perspective, exactly the same dose of a particular opioid can potentially have a very different effect on different individuals (or even at different times on the same individual), depending on the route of administration.

The effect of any opioid depends to a considerable degree on whether or not it is injected (which provides a very fast onset and short duration of action) or administered orally (which yields a slower onset and longer duration of action). Another important factor is whether the drug formulation is altered (as by embedding the active ingredient in a matrix of insoluble substances) so that intestinal absorption is further delayed (resulting in even slower onset and longer duration of action).

Short-Acting Opioids

Short-acting opioids (SAOs), because of their fast onset of action, rapidly flood the brain with high levels of opioids. This can be very useful in achieving acute pain relief, when the goal is to increase opioid levels quickly. For this reason, opioids with a rapid onset of action are the drugs of choice in situations in which pain is acute and severe. Opioids with a rapid onset of action also are the drugs of choice among individuals with opioid use disorder whose intent is to achieve a strong state of opioid-induced euphoria as quickly as possible.

Flooding the brain with high doses of potent opioids not only leads to more intense and rapid analgesia and euphoria, it also leads to much more intense and rapid neuroadaptation (which is the brain's way of trying to compensate for these high opioid levels, or homeostasis). The neuroadaptive changes that occur with chronic opioid use generally are commensurate with the potency and rapidity of the opioid effect. The stronger the opioid and the more rapidly it enters the brain, the greater the neuroadaptive response. This neuroadaptive response is what leads to tolerance and withdrawal, which occur much earlier in the course of treatment with SAOs than with longer-acting opioids.

Longer-Acting Opioids

Longer-acting opioids (LAOs) typically are used to treat chronic rather than acute pain. As noted earlier, many LAOs are derived by combining SAOs with an insoluble substance matrix that delays intestinal absorption. While the euphoric/reinforcing effects of LAOs are somewhat weaker than for SAOs, clinicians should not assume that LAOs are therefore safer or less addictive than

SAOs. LAOs can be quite addictive and their use is associated with high levels of tolerance and withdrawal.

Moreover, individuals with opioid use disorder often go to great lengths to overcome these matrices so that they can convert LAOs back into their SAO form. Methods employed range from peeling off the chemical wraps (hence the street name "peelers" for MS Contin® and OxyContin®), to squeezing out the gel in fentanyl patches and injecting it in an effort to attain the intense euphoria of the SAO product. Various Internet sites feature methods that can be used to convert LAOs back to their SAO form.

Another potential safety risk with LAOs is dose accumulation. With LAOs (and even more so with very long-acting opioids [VLAOs]), it is important that clinicians remember the pharmacology adage: "It takes five half-lives to achieve steady state." This means that in LAOs (which have a half-life of roughly 12 hours), clinically significant dose accumulation occurs over the first 60 hours. Individuals who are impatient to achieve their desired opioid effect (because of addiction or uncontrolled pain) may not be willing to wait for 60 hours to experience the full steady-state of their dose and may not be aware of how much dosage accumulation is occurring at the point LAOs are altered.

The prolonged dose-accumulation period for LAOs and VLAOs means that it is very important that patients be educated in the fact that any change in an LAO regimen can take two to three days to take effect and that the dose-titration phase of opioid treatment is a time of increased risk of accidental overdose.

Very Long-Acting Opioids (VLAOs)

The two most well-known and clinically relevant VLAOs are methadone and buprenorphine. Everything said about LAOs also applies to these drugs.

Affinity for the Opioid Receptor

The *affinity* of opioids for the opioid receptor is an important (and clinically relevant) property. Opioids interact with mu, delta, and kappa receptors, which are responsible for opioids' analgesic effects as well as adverse events (see online Appendix B, Table B-1) [3]. Mu-opioid receptors are the prototypical receptors involved with analgesia, respiratory depression, and euphoria. With kappa-opioid receptors—depending on the receptor subtype involved—dysphoria or analgesia may occur [7].

Not only do opioids act on different types of receptors, but they can affect those receptors in different ways; for example, as an agonist, partial agonist, antagonist, or agonist/antagonist (see online Appendix B, Figure B-1). Pure opioid agonists wrap around the receptor tightly. With increasing doses of an opioid agonist, analgesia and respiratory depression both increase. Partial agonists result in receptor activation, but to a lesser extent than do full opioid agonists. As the dose of a partial agonist increases, the activity eventually plateaus.

Buprenorphine and—to a lesser extent—methadone also have high affinity for the opioid receptor. This is clinically useful because other(higher potency, lower affinity) opioids cannot out-compete buprenorphine and methadone for the opioid receptor. Clinically, what this means is that individuals who are on medication-assisted therapy (MAT) with methadone or buprenorphine find high-potency opioids much less euphoric and reinforcing because the high affinity of methadone and buprenorphine makes it relatively difficult for other opioids to bind to the mu receptor.

Buprenorphine and other partial agonists are safer options for patients who have respiratory problems because there is a limit to the amount of carbon dioxide that can accumulate and/or a limit to their ability to cause respiratory depression.

Agonists/antagonists include pentazocine, which acts as an agonist at some opioid receptors and an antagonist at others. Naloxone is an opioid antagonist because it occupies the receptor but does not lead to receptor activity [3].

The effect of every opioid differs according to whether it is injected (causing a very fast onset and short duration of action) or given orally (with a slower onset and longer duration of action), or whether the drug formulation is altered (as by embedding the active ingredient in a matrix of insoluble substances) so that intestinal absorption is even further delayed. (See Table 8.3.)

Opioid Metabolism and Drug Interactions

Opioids undergo two primary metabolic pathways: Phase 1 metabolism through the cytochrome (CYP) P450 enzyme system, and Phase 2 by glucuronidation

TABLE 8.3 Opioid Activity: Least Active to Most Active

Opioid Antagonists (LEAST ACTIVE)	Partial Agonists	Low-Potency Full Agonists	High-Potency Full Agonists (MOST ACTIVE)
Naloxone Naltrexone	Buprenorphine	Codeine Hydrocodone Tramadol Methadone	Fentanyl Oxycodone Hydromorphine

via uridine diphosphate glucuronosyltransferase 2B7 (UGT2B7). In some cases, both pathways may be involved [3].

Opioids that undergo Phase 1 metabolism primarily involve CYP3A4 and CYP2D6 enzymes. The CYP3A4 enzyme metabolizes the majority of drugs, while CYP2D6 is involved to a lesser degree. As a result, opioids metabolized through CYP3A4 pose a higher risk of drug–drug interactions, while CYP2D6 metabolism poses only an intermediate risk [8].

On the other hand, opioids such as hydromorphone, levorphanol, morphine, oxymorphone, and tapentadol, which undergo Phase 2 conjugation by glucuronidation via UGT2B7, exhibit very little to no involvement with the CYP system and pose a very low risk of causing drug interactions [8].

Patients also should be monitored for rug interactions involving p-glycoprotein (P-gp) drug transporters. For example, patients being treated for hepatitis C may be susceptible to a significant risk of drug interaction associated with P-gp inhibitors such as telaprevir or boceprevir when they are used at the same time as methadone or morphine. In situations such as this, levorphanol or tapentadol may be better options because both avoid the CYP450 system and have not been shown to be problematic with P-gp [9].

In general, clinical effects of drug inhibition include higher concentrations of opioids, potentially prolonging analgesic effects as well as the risk of opioid-related adverse effects, including opioid-induced respiratory depression (OIRD). Conversely, drug inhibition may reduce analgesic efficacy as well as possibly inducing symptoms of opioid withdrawal. If and when drug interactions occur, the clinical effects of inhibitors may emerge within hours to days, while the effects of inducers may not occur for weeks. Inability to recognize significant drug interactions may increase the risk for opioid-related adverse events, including overdose and death.

Pharmacokinetic and Pharmacogenetic Variability

Genetic susceptibility to opioid analgesics can be multifaceted, encompassing multiple genes [10]. Research shows that several genes can alter the perception of pain, affect analgesic activity, and increase the risk of toxicity when polymorphisms occur.

Although CYP2D6 exhibits lesser impact on drug metabolism and drug interactions than does CYP3A4, it is susceptible to genetic variability that may significantly affect the metabolism of codeine, hydrocodone, oxycodone, and tramadol. CYP2D6 functional variants consist of four phenotypes: poor metabolizers (PM), intermediate metabolizers (IM), extensive metabolizers (EM), and ultra-rapid metabolizers (UM) [11]. These traits may vary by ethnicity [12].

Adverse Effects of Opioids

Adverse effects of opioids are summarized in online Appendix B, Table B-1. With the exception of constipation, tolerance to many side effects typically develops with continued use. Opioid-induced constipation (OIC) occurs because opioid receptors are located throughout the gastrointestinal tract and, when activated, they interfere with normal functioning. The standard regimen to prevent OIC is the use of stool softeners and stimulant laxatives. Bulk laxatives should be avoided because they may make the condition worse. A relatively new class of medications, peripherally acting mu receptor opioid antagonists (PAMORAs), are another option for management of OIC.

Respiratory depression is a significant concern with the use of opioids (see online Appendix B, Figure B-2) (Box 8.1). In addition, opioids are implicated with sleep-disordered breathing. The risk of overdose and death increases with the opioid dose. or if the opioid is used in combination with other CNS depressants such as alcohol, benzodiazepines, and/or sedative/hypnotics (Table 8.1) [3].

The profound alterations in brain neuroanatomy that occur with longer-term opioid use can lead to numerous unintended negative consequences, including opioid-induced hyperalgesia and opioid use disorder, tolerance, and withdrawal [12]. All too often, individuals who suffer from these unintended consequences are blamed by society and the medical system [13]. (Also see Chapters 14 and 19 of this Handbook.)

Conclusion

Different opioids have very different pharmacological properties. A detailed understanding of these differences is necessary in order to use opioids safely

---

BOX 8.1 Related Figures and Tables in Online Appendix B of This Handbook

Online Appendix Figure B-1. Opioid Receptor Affinity and Activity
Online Appendix Figure B-2. Relationship of Opioid Dose to Respiratory Depression
Online Appendix Table B-1. Opioid Metabolism and Detection Times
Online Appendix Table B-2. Opioid Pharmacogenetics in Pain Management
Online Appendix Table B-3. Opioid-Related Adverse Effects
Online Appendix Table B-4. Comparison of Oral Drug Formulations That Deter or Prevent Misuse and Abuse

and effectively. Opioids are powerful medications that offer profound benefits (such as pain relief), but they also are associated with significant risks (such as addiction, overdose, and death). In order to help patients make fully informed decisions about opioid use, it is important that the clinicians who treat them possess the expertise necessary to identify when opioids are most likely to help and when they are more likely to harm.

Understanding the pharmacology of opioids and how these drugs "rewire" brain neurocircuitry can be an important step in destigmatizing those individuals who suffer from problems associated with opioid use [14].

For More Information on the Topics Discussed:

American Society of Addiction Medicine:

Borg L, Buonora M, Butelman ER, et al. The pharmacology of opioids (Chapter 9). In RK Ries, DA Fiellin, SC Miller, R Saitz, eds. *The ASAM Principles of Addiction Medicine, Fifth Edition.* Philadelphia, PA: Wolters Kluwer; 2014.

Substance Abuse and Mental Health Services Administration (SAMHSA):

The Facts About Buprenorphine (patient education brochure) SMA09-4442. Rockville, MD: SAMHSA, Department of Health and Human Services, rev. 2011. (Access at: http://store.samhsa.gov/shin/content/SMA09-4442/SMA09-4442.pdf.)

Medication-Assisted Treatment: Methadone (for clinicians). Rockville, MD: SAMHSA, Department of Health and Human Services, 2015. (Access at: https://www.samhsa.gov/medication-assisted-treatment/treatment/methadone.)

Acknowledgment

The author acknowledges with gratitude the valuable input to this chapter by the following individuals: Abigail Brooks, Pharm.D., Thien C. Pham, Pharm.D., Courtney Kominek, Pharm.D., BCPS, CPE, and Jeffrey Fudin, Pharm.D., DAIPM, FCCP, FASHP.

References

1. Juurlink DN, Dhalla IA. Dependence and addiction during chronic opioid therapy. *J Med Toxicol.* 2012;8(4):393–399.

2. Fudin J. Chemical Classes of Opioids. 2016. http://paindr.com/wp-content/uploads/2016/11/Opioid-Structural-Classes_edited-November-2016.pdf

3. Brooks A, Pham TC, Kominek C, et al. Personal communication, May 27, 2017.

4. Food and Drug Administration (FDA). *Loperamide (Imodium): Drug Safety Communication*: Serious heart problems with high doses from abuse and misuse. (Accessed at: http://www.fda.gov/Safety/MedWatch/SafetyInformation/SafetyAlertsforHumanMedicalProducts/ucm505303.htm.)

5. Centers for Disease Control and Prevention (CDC). *Fentanyl Overdose Data.* Atlanta, GA: CDC. No date. (Accessed at: http://www.cdc.gov/drugoverdose/data/fentanyl.html.)

6. TIRF REMS. (Accessed at: https://http://www.tirfremsaccess.com/TirfUI/rems/home.action.)

7. Smith HS. Opioid metabolism. *Mayo Clin Proc.* 2009 Jul;84(7):613–624.

8. Fudin J, Fontenelle DV, Fudin HR, et al. Potential P-glycoprotein pharmacokinetic interaction of telaprevir with morphine or methadone. *J Pain Palliat Care Pharmacother.* 2013 Aug;27(3):261–267.

9. Pham TC, Fudin J, Raffa RB. Is levorphanol a better option than methadone? *Pain Med.* 2015 Sep;16(9):1673–1679.

10. Kapur BM, Lala PK, Shaw JL. Pharmacogenetics of chronic pain management. *Clin Biochem.* 2014 Sep;47(13–14):1169–1187.

11. Janicki PK in Deer, TR et al. (Eds.). *Pharmacogenomics of Pain Management. Comprehensive Treatment of Chronic Pain by Medical, Interventional, and Integrative Approaches.* Chicago, IL: American Academy of Pain Medicine; 2013:22–33.

12. Vallejo R, Barkin RL, Wang VC. Pharmacology of opioids in the treatment of chronic pain syndromes. *Pain Physician.* 2011 Jul–Aug;14(4):E343–E360.

13. Fishbain DA, Cole B, Lewis J, et al. What percentage of chronic nonmalignant pain patients exposed to chronic opioid analgesic therapy develop abuse/addiction and/or aberrant drug-related behaviors? A structured evidence-based review. *Pain Med.* 2008;9(4):444–459.

14. Earnshaw V, Smith L, Copenhaver M. Drug addiction stigma in the context of methadone maintenance therapy: An investigation into understudied sources of stigma. *Int J Ment Health Addict.* 2013;11(1):110–122.

Chapter 9

Understanding and Preventing Opioid Misuse and Abuse

ROBERT L. DUPONT, M.D., THEODORE V. PARRAN, JR., M.D., AND BONNIE B. WILFORD, M.S.

Opioids have a central role in relieving human suffering today, as they have for thousands of years. They also cause great harm. This duality has provoked confusion and concern on the part of policymakers and the public. Opioids confront physicians and other health care professionals with the dilemma of how to balance their patients' need for the treatment of pain or addiction with the risk that prescribed opioids will be misused by the patients to whom they are prescribed, or given or sold to others. This duality constitutes a major quality-assurance and risk-management issue for all health care professionals.

In recent years, the significance of the problem has increased exponentially as the use of opioids to treat non-cancer pain has become widespread, leading to growing reports of opioid misuse, addiction, overdose, and death [1,2,3,4,5,6]. (See Table 9.1 for descriptions of appropriate and inappropriate opioid use.)

Given the need to balance such risks and benefits, how do physicians decide who should receive an opioid prescription? Are opioids more likely to be prescribed to and misused by some patients than by others? How can physicians organize their practices so as to afford protection to themselves and their patients as they pursue the optimal management of pain or addiction? [1] This chapter will explore strategies for addressing the dilemma.

TABLE 9.1 Terms Used to Characterize Prescription Opioid Use, Misuse, and Abuse

Characterization	Definition	Clinical Examples	Intervention Strategies
Appropriate Use	Use of an opioid as prescribed for a defined condition, with no signs of misuse or abuse.	A 10-day course of post-operative opioid analgesics, taken as prescribed.	Explain to the patient that the prescribed opioids will be used only for a limited time. Assist with safe and comfortable withdrawal when use ends.
Misuse or Inappropriate Use	Use of an opioid for a reason other than that for which it was prescribed or in a dose different than prescribed, but without a pattern of ongoing misuse leading to disability or dysfunction.	— A single episode of opioids use twice as often as prescribed. — Use of a "leftover" prescribed opioid for a new clinical problem without consulting a physician.	Educate the patient about proper use of the opioid and the risks associated with misuse.
Prescription Opioid Abuse	Use of an opioid (whether prescribed or not) outside the normally accepted standards of use, resulting in disability and/or dysfunction.	— Continued misuse despite interventions. — Use of a prescribed drug for "recreational" purposes unrelated to any medical condition.	— Express concerns in an empathetic way. — Discontinue the medication that is being abused. — Consult with an expert (e.g., an addiction or pain specialist).
Catastrophic Use	Use of a controlled substance in ways that involve illegal activity or that place the patient at imminent risk of harm, as from opioid overdose.	— Altering or forging a prescription to obtain more opioid than prescribed. — Selling a prescribed medication. — Overdosing on an opioid.	— Immediately stop prescribing all opioids and other controlled drugs. — Consult with or refer the patient to a specialist in addiction medicine. — Notify legal authorities if indicated.

Source: Adapted from Isaacson HJ, Hooper JA, Alford DP, et al. Prescription drug abuse: What primary care physicians need to know. *Postgrad Med.* 2005.

Factors That Contribute
to Opioid Abuse

Three major influences help shape the current situation: *drug factors, physician factors,* and *patient factors* [1,7–10].

Drug Factors

Over the course of human history, virtually all substance abuse and addiction has involved the use of substances that produce brain reward by way of an acute surge of dopamine from the mid-brain to the forebrain (an important concept that has replaced the older notions of "euphoria producing" or "mind-altering" substances) [2,7,11–16]. Historically, in clinical practice, confusion has arisen between the term "addiction" or the *Diagnostic and Statistical Manual 5* (DSM-5) term "substance use disorder moderate or severe," and the term "physical dependence," which is associated with withdrawal symptoms when an opioid is abruptly discontinued. Many non-addicting substances—including antihypertensive and anti-epilepsy agents—produce withdrawal symptoms when they are abruptly discontinued. On the other hand, many addicting substances do not produce prominent withdrawal symptoms on abrupt discontinuation, including cannabis and central nervous system (CNS) stimulants. Patients can be addicted to a substance with or without physical dependence, and patients can be physically dependent on a substance with or without addiction.

The four major classes of brain-rewarding substances are:

- *Stimulants*, such as cocaine, methamphetamine, nicotine, caffeine, and certain prescribed stimulant medications.
- *Sedative-hypnotics*, including alcohol, benzodiazepines, barbiturates, and other hypnotics.
- *Opioids*, including illicit drugs such as heroin and prescription analgesics.
- *"Other drugs,"* including the psychedelics, dissociative anesthetics, cannabinoids, and hallucinogens.

As mentioned earlier, the drugs in each of these classes either directly or indirectly produce an *acute release of dopamine* from the mid-brain (ventral tegmental area [VTA] and nucleus accumbens) to the forebrain. It is this characteristic dopamine surge that makes certain drugs rewarding to the brain, and hence liable to "social use," abuse, and even addiction in susceptible patients [6,7].

The individual characteristics of the dopamine surge produced by various controlled drugs and various routes of administration render them more or less likely to be abused—that is, more or less rewarding to the brain. Drugs with a more rapid onset of action are more likely to be sought for purposes of abuse than those with a slower onset, with a corresponding increase in their "street" or market value. The variability of each substance in terms of the rapidity and intensity of brain reward is reflected in the placement of each controlled drug in one of five progressively more restrictive schedules of the Federal Controlled Substances Act (CSA) [1,7,17,18].

Physician Factors

Physicians report a lack of training in the appropriate prescribing of controlled drugs, specifically in the areas of differential diagnosis and management of acute chronic and malignant pain, anxiety and depression, insomnia, and addiction [7,10]. It is in these areas of clinical practice that physicians commonly confront dilemmas about prescribing controlled drugs, yet it is precisely in these areas where most physicians report suboptimal education and clinical preparation. The resulting problems have been classified by the American Medical Association as the "4 D's"—Dated, Deceived (or Duped), Disabled, and Dishonest physicians [8]. To these, many experts add a fifth "D"—the Defiant practitioner—and a sixth: the Distracted practitioner [11,12].

- *Dated physicians* are those whose knowledge of one or another aspect of patient care is out of date. Therefore, they are likely to prescribe the wrong drug or dose to the wrong patient, or to prescribe a controlled drug when one is not required [8].
- *Deceived or Duped physicians* are those who are misled by patients about the presence of symptoms or conditions that would indicate the need for a controlled drug [8]. Virtually any physician can be deceived by so-called professional patients, who often employ very sophisticated ruses.
- *Disabled physicians*—that is, those with psychiatric or medical disorders (including addiction)—have been characterized as more lax in their prescribing to others [8], although there is good evidence that this is not the case [13].
- *Dishonest physicians* typically prescribe large amounts of controlled drugs for other than legitimate medical purposes and generally for money. Fortunately, this group is an exceedingly small part of the overall physician population [8].
- *Defiant physicians* have come to believe that they have greater expertise in a specific area of practice than everyone else, and practice in ways that are not supported by the evidence base. When such practices involve prescribing controlled drugs, the result can be a marked surge in illicit local availability of such drugs [12,13].
- *Distracted physicians* are practitioners who are so overwhelmed by patient care duties or the related paperwork that they lose track of their controlled drug prescribing, or refills, or the monitoring strategies necessary when prescribing controlled drugs.

Some experts have described two additional physician factors that appear to facilitate inappropriate prescribing: *pathological enabling* and *confrontation phobia* [11]. One of the most ennobling characteristics of the medical profession is the willingness of physicians to do whatever is necessary to help patients achieve an improved quality of life; however, this quality of "enabling" can become detrimental when the physician accedes to patients' nonmedical drug-seeking behavior. The situation worsens if the physician is reluctant to confront such a patient about his or her inappropriate behavior.

It is widely recognized that as long as patients need and physicians prescribe controlled drugs, some proportion will be used non-medically or diverted to intentional abuse; however, certain physician practice characteristics heavily influence the *proportion* of controlled drugs that are available for diversion or abuse. Fortunately, each of the risky prescribing behaviors described here is readily corrected.

Practices that *increase the risk of diversion* include [1–3]:

1. Willingness to prescribe relatively potent controlled drugs at the patient's first visit.
2. Willingness to initiate a controlled drug prescribing regimen without obtaining a complete patient history, especially the history of prior substance abuse and other data (including screens for a personal or family history of substance use disorders).
3. Failure to order periodic toxicology screens for patients to whom controlled drugs are prescribed on a continuing basis.
4. Lack of collaboration with colleagues (e.g., physicians who treated a patient in the past, other physicians currently treating the patient, pharmacists, and other expert consultants, including specialists in pain and addiction).
5. Continued prescribing despite evidence of out-of-control behavior by a patient (e.g., alteration or forgery of prescription orders; reports of selling, bingeing, or overdose; use of an opioid in combination with alcohol and other drugs; multi-sourcing; unplanned escalation in dose; multiple requests for early refills, and/or threatening behavior).
6. A tendency to underemphasize the aspects of a treatment plan that do not involve pharmacotherapy.
7. Willingness to concomitantly prescribe multiple controlled drugs, from the same and different classes, over long periods of time.

Patient Factors

Addiction is defined as a chronic disorder, with clear physical, psychological, and genetic components. It is characterized by the intermittent, repetitive *loss of control* over the use of one or more brain-rewarding substances, resulting in repeated *adverse consequences* in the patient's life.

As it relates to the use of prescribed opioids, addiction can be conceptualized as a brain reward in susceptible individuals, characterized by a persistent craving for more of the drug, continued escalation in use despite adverse consequences, increasingly global dysfunction in the patient's life, and a willingness to cause stress in other meaningful relationships in pursuit of the pathological relationship with the opioid drug. Another behavior that is a hallmark of addiction is *dishonesty*, typically including dishonesty with the prescribing physician, as well as *craving* for the substance when it is not present. Addiction-prone individuals have been described as having "high-risk brains" when it comes to the use of brain-rewarding substances of all types.

When applied to opioid use, addiction pathology typically results in rapid escalation in dose, patient reports that the medicine is "ineffective," requests for early visits and refills, reports of "lost" prescriptions and medicines, and a developing sense of tension in the physician–patient relationship [1–3,18–20].

When a patient who is addicted to opioids or other controlled drugs loses control of his or her drug use, the supply runs short. Such a patient has relatively few options: (1) pressure the physician for more medication, (2) pressure the pharmacist for early refills, or (3) seek additional sources of supply (as from family members, "doctor shopping," or purchases from illicit sources).

In contrast, the patient who is not at risk for addiction will not experience brain reward when using controlled drugs as prescribed and thus will not misuse these medications. Such patients—who clearly constitute the vast majority to whom controlled drugs are prescribed—tend to remain stable on low doses of medication for extended periods of time, and to report that the prescribed medication is effective. Indeed, the chief clinical challenge often is to ensure that such patients take the prescribed medications as often and in the dose prescribed. Inappropriate fears of addiction on the part of patients (or their caretakers) where there is no history of such addiction is a common reason for underuse of prescribed opioids and other controlled drugs by patients with non-addictive "low-risk" brains [1,18].

It is important for physicians to be able to clearly distinguish between typical medical use of opioids and other controlled drugs and typical nonmedical use. The former does not involve the brain reward associated with addiction, while the latter does. Typical medical use is oral and at routine doses, while typical nonmedical use involves excessive doses, often by routes of administration other than oral, and at times and in ways that are more similar to an alcoholic binge than to the use of a vitamin tablet. This distinction needs to be explained to patients who are prescribed opioids so that they (and their family members) are reassured and so that those who do not use the prescribed drug appropriately can recognize the pathological nature of their behavior.

Factors that are helpful in distinguishing medical from non-medical use are described in Table 9.2.

The level of risk for abuse of or addiction to opioids varies from one individual to the next, but a history of illicit substance use and a willingness to use

TABLE 9.2 Characteristics That Help Distinguish Medical from Nonmedical Use of Opioids

Characteristic	Medical Use	Nonmedical Use
Intent	Used to treat a diagnosed illness	Used to party or to "treat" distressing effects of alcohol or other drug abuse
Effect	Improves the user's quality of life	Worsens the user's quality of life
Pattern	Stable and medically justified	Unstable; usually involving escalating or high doses
Control	Quantity and frequency of use is shared honestly with the physician	Self-controlled
Legality	Legal	Illegal

controlled substances at doses and by routes of administration that are not prescribed all are associated with a markedly elevated level of risk. The single strongest risk factor for future misuse, abuse, or addiction to a prescribed controlled drug is a current or past history of abuse of any substance.

Patient behaviors that suggest loss of control include [1,2,21]:

- *Early requests for refills* (the patient who makes an urgent, unscheduled visit late in the day, or who claims he/she "took too many," "lost the prescription," "washed it with the laundry," "the dog ate it," "left it in . . . ," "the pharmacist shorted the count," "spilled it in the toilet," or had his/her supply lost, stolen, etc.).
- *Multi-sourcing* (recruiting surrogates to obtain the medication, visiting multiple physicians, purchasing drugs over the Internet or from illicit drug dealers, etc.).
- *Intoxicated behavior* (slurred speech or disinhibited calls to the office, presenting to pharmacies under the influence, emergency department visits for repeated falls or other traumatic injuries, accidental overdoses, etc.).
- *Pressuring behaviors* (begging or pleading, being excessively complimentary, breaching boundaries, vague or even clear threats to harm self or others, and the like) [1,19].

If the physician fails to respond firmly to these out-of-control behaviors—such as by stopping prescribing of the controlled drug—the patient's out-of-control addictive behavior is likely to progress to increasingly aberrant levels, with escalating adverse consequences. Such adverse consequences commonly include domestic problems such as violence and divorce, arrests and incarceration, hospitalization, accidental overdose, suicide attempts, and even death. It is for these reasons that it is critically important for physicians who are prescribing opioids and other controlled drugs to closely monitor their patients for aberrant behaviors, so as to avoid doing harm while trying to help the patient achieve improved comfort and function [1].

Strategies to Reduce the Risk of Opioid Abuse

The same three factors—physician factors, patient factors, and drug factors—that contribute to abuse of prescription drugs also contribute to its mitigation and management. By developing strategies to address each of these three factors, physicians can make substantial progress in achieving an appropriate balance in prescribing [7].

Physician Factors

It is widely recognized that some level of prescription drug diversion and abuse is unavoidable. However, specific physician practice behaviors can *minimize* the risk that controlled drugs will be diverted or abused, while providing appropriate therapy to low-risk patients [1]. Basic principles for all physicians to consider when prescribing controlled drugs—and especially when prescribing opioids on a long-term basis—include the following:

1. Develop skills to efficiently and effectively screen for a history of substance abuse or addiction in patients with "high-risk brains," and perform this screening *before as well as after* initiating therapy with an opioid or other controlled drug [2,14,15].
2. Avoid prescribing opioids or other controlled drugs to patients with "high-risk brains," especially on a long-term basis. High-risk drugs combined with high-risk brains are likely to result in high-risk behavior, with attendant harm to the patient, family, community, and even the prescriber.
3. Become knowledgeable about the differential diagnosis and management of acute versus chronic versus malignant pain.

4. Rigorously employ a process of informed consent and treatment agreements when prescribing opioids or any other controlled drugs, and carefully inform patients of their ethical and legal obligations. Document this conversation in an informed consent form specifically designed for long-term management of patients who are prescribed opioids or other controlled drugs.

5. Adopt a policy of refusing requests for early refills (see the discussion later in the chapter).

6. Collaborate with pharmacy colleagues by writing complete and clear prescription orders, as well as responding promptly and completely to their questions or requests for verification.

7. Never commit to long-term prescribing of opioids in the presence of diagnostic uncertainty or discomfort about the indication.

8. Stay in your area of expertise, both in terms of the conditions you treat as well as in the medications and doses you prescribe. Saying "I am so sorry, but no," early in the course of treatment is much better than having to do so later on.

9. Always stop or revise the therapeutic regimen if a patient demonstrates any concerning or out-of-control behaviors.

10. Do not prescribe controlled drugs to yourself, family, or close friends or colleagues—sufficient therapeutic distance is essential to effective patient monitoring.

11. Never prescribe a controlled drug unless there is a medical record to document the presence of a physician–patient relationship and a legitimate medical purpose for the prescription.

12. Perform periodic toxicology testing when prescribing a controlled drug over the long term. Such testing is useful in establishing compliance and in detecting the use of other, non-prescribed controlled substances. Drug test monitoring is especially helpful because a high percentage of patients who abuse opioids and other controlled drug prescriptions also abuse multiple licit and illicit drugs, many of which are readily identified on routine urine testing. (See Chapter 11 of this Handbook for a discussion of urine drug testing.) [1,5,7]

13. Follow a thorough, carefully structured monitoring strategy once prescribing is initiated.

14. Regularly check your state's (and neighboring states') Prescription Drug Monitoring Program (PDMP) and the patient's local pharmacy printout. This helps avoid patient multi-sourcing and helps ensure the patient's adherence to all of the prescribed medications—non-controlled drugs as well as the controlled ones.

Remember that one of the basic principles of medicine is "First, do no harm, then comfort always and cure sometimes." If, in the process of attempting to provide comfort to a patient by prescribing an opioid or other controlled drug, evidence suggests that harm is being done (such as through diversion or abuse), it is ethically mandatory to reassess the entire clinical situation and to change treatment strategies as quickly as possible [5,7].

Identification of a patient who is abusing prescribed opioids or other controlled drugs presents a major therapeutic opportunity. Every physician needs to have a plan for working with patients who are misusing or addicted to alcohol and other drugs, including opioids. Physicians must be proficient in putting this plan into action. Such a plan typically involves ending the use of all controlled drugs, working with the patient and the patient's family, referral to an addiction expert for assessment, (perhaps) placement in a formal addiction treatment program, long-term participation in a 12-Step mutual help program such as Alcoholics Anonymous or Narcotics Anonymous, and follow-up of any medical or psychiatric sequelae.

If opioids are involved, the patient should be offered medical withdrawal options, referral for office-based opioid treatment (buprenorphine) or a clinic-based opioid maintenance (methadone) program, as well as an "overdose plan" to share with friends, partners, and/or caregivers. Such a plan would contain information on the signs of overdose and how to administer naloxone or otherwise provide emergency care (such as by calling 911) [22]. (Additional information on opioid overdose is found in Chapter 13 of this Handbook.)

Patient Factors

Patients share with physicians a responsibility for safe and appropriate use of prescription medications, including opioids (see Table 9.3). Some patients fail to fulfill this responsibility because of lack of information or failure to appreciate the resulting risks. In response, multiple federal agencies and private-sector organizations have launched public education campaigns that involve public service announcements for television and radio, as well as distribution of print messages about the dangers of misusing or abusing opioids and other prescription medications. Nevertheless, there is no substitute for physician advice at the time an opioid or other drug is prescribed. This is the "teachable moment" when the physician should explain that it is illegal to sell, give away, or otherwise share their medication with others, including family members.

The patient's obligation also extends to keeping the medication in a locked cabinet or otherwise restricting access to it, and to safely disposing of any unused supply.

Drug Factors

Among emerging solutions that focus on the drugs themselves are state programs to monitor drug distribution through PDMPs, which are helpful in

TABLE 9.3 Physicians' and Patients' Shared Responsibility for Safe and Appropriate Use of Opioids

Responsibilities of the Physician	Responsibilities of the Patient
To have the patient's well-being as his or her primary concern.	To seek medical attention for conditions that a physician can cure or ameliorate.
To formulate a working diagnosis of the patient's problems based on the patient's history and findings of the physical examination.	To be truthful in reporting historical information and to cooperate with the physical examination.
To order appropriate laboratory tests (or consultations with specialists) to clarify the diagnosis.	To obtain the laboratory tests or consultations requested by the physician.
To prescribe appropriate therapy. (This assumes that the physician is acting within his or her scope of expertise.)	To comply with the physician's instructions. (This includes taking medications as prescribed.)
To monitor the effects of treatment, including the side effects or toxicity of any drugs prescribed.	To report symptoms accurately.
To continue to follow the patient until the condition is relieved or the patient's care is assumed by another physician.	To follow through with appointments until discharged by the physician.

Source: Wesson DR, Smith DE. Prescription drug abuse. Patient, physician, and cultural responsibilities. *West J Med.* 1990;152(5):613–616.

identifying "doctor shopping" and other methods of multi-sourcing. Accessing other programs that address Internet sales of controlled drugs (many of which are substandard or counterfeit) also are important steps.

Changes in drug formulation also hold the promise of significantly reducing tampering and abuse. On the horizon are novel compounds that will depend on enzymatic action in the body to convert to, and deliver, their medicinal properties. In theory, such novel delivery systems will prevent the extraction of the active ingredient from the bonded adjuvant [20]. However, "abuse-resistant" is not synonymous with *abuse-proof*, so the physician still must use care in prescribing, and the patient must exhibit responsibility in using these drugs.

Special Precautions with New Patients

Many experts recommend that additional precautions be taken with new patients, particularly those to whom the physician considers prescribing opioid analgesics and other medications with a significant potential for abuse [21]. Recommended precautions include the following:

- *Obtaining Identification.* The patient's identity should be verified by asking for proper identification.
- *Consulting Past Providers.* In addition to the patient history and examination, the physician should determine who has been caring for the patient in the past, what medications have been prescribed and for what indications, and which other substances (including alcohol, illicit drugs and over-the-counter [OTC] products) the patient has been using. With the patient's consent, a good-faith effort must be made to obtain medical records from health care professionals who have treated the patient in the past.
- *Limiting Prescriptions.* In non-emergency situations, the physician should prescribe only enough of an opioid to meet the patient's needs until the next appointment. The patient should be directed to *return to the office* for additional prescriptions, as telephone orders do not allow the physician to reassess the patient's continued need for the medication.

In emergency situations, the physician should prescribe the smallest possible quantity of medication (for example, no more than a one- to three-day supply of an opioid analgesic) and arrange with the patient for a return visit the next day [1,6,7,26].

Policies on Replacing "Lost" Prescriptions and Requests for Early Refills

Treatment agreements generally state that ". . . lost medications will not be replaced regardless of the reasons for such loss" [22]. However, several guidelines advise that actual decisions be individualized by the prescribing physician, based on multiple sources of information (including in-person evaluation of the patient), using strategies to reorient patients into more complete adherence to the treatment regimen [6,7,23–26].

Adherence can be a complex process, and patients frequently experience setbacks, especially early in the treatment process. A high index of suspicion is warranted when patients claim to lose prescriptions or report that they have been stolen. However, on rare occasions, patients do experience extenuating circumstances (such as a documented assault, hurricane-related evacuations, or vomiting due to a gastrointestinal disorder), and a patient may actually lose his or her prescription or medication. Physicians need to establish clear policies on how such requests will be evaluated, so that staff and patients know what to expect [22].

Most physicians experienced in treating patients with substance use disorders view requests for replacement prescriptions as a reason for great concern (i.e., a "red flag") that may signal that the patient is taking more medication than prescribed, or not taking the medication and diverting it for profit instead. Other red flags include inconsistent toxicology screens, inability to consistently keep appointments, requests for early refills, a sudden request for a dose increase in a previously stable patient, purported intolerance or allergy to naloxone, lost prescriptions, use of multiple prescribers, prescription forgery, ongoing close ties to those who illegally sell opioids, and close acquaintances or relatives who are addicted to opioids but not in treatment [1,6,23].

A patient who has a good track record of adherence to appointments and following up referrals would be treated differently from someone who never has stabilized in treatment. Egregious behaviors such as selling prescribed medications may result in immediate discontinuation of controlled drug prescribing, or even dismissal from the practice. Threatening behavior on the part of the patient is typically best handled by ending the physician–patient relationship [6,23].

In considering requests for replacing "lost or stolen" prescriptions, physicians and other team members should [6]:

- First, consider the relative frequency of early refill requests involving prescriptions for controlled drug prescriptions compared to those for non-controlled drugs. Many clinicians have virtually never been asked for an early refill for a non-controlled drug, while requests for early refills involving controlled drugs are not uncommon. That is why most informed consent forms or patient–prescriber agreements (PPA) explicitly state that lost or stolen controlled drug prescriptions will not be replaced on a routine basis.
- Meet promptly with the patient for evaluation, with special emphasis on detecting the presence of signs or symptoms of withdrawal.
- Use motivational interviewing techniques to encourage the patient to be more forthcoming regarding the reasons for requesting an early refill.
- Check available state prescription drug monitoring programs for any evidence that the patient has filled prescriptions from multiple prescribers.
- Perform a urine drug screen or other biological monitoring to determine the patient's current status.

If the patient demonstrates withdrawal symptoms, it is incumbent on the prescriber to treat these symptoms or refer the patient for urgent treatment. Doing otherwise can be considered a form of patient abandonment.

If the prescriber decides to provide an early refill, it should be used as an opportunity for patient education and to reinforce the informed consent form or PPA.

Prescribers should avoid any pattern or formula for providing refills of controlled drugs (the "one, two, or three strikes" approach).

Repeated reports of lost prescriptions must be regarded as an indicator of substance use disorder, out-of-control behavior, or drug diversion, especially when corroborated by information from urine drug tests or PDMPs. Patients who demonstrate any of these behaviors should not continue to receive prescriptions for controlled drugs. In many cases, such patients should be referred to inpatient or outpatient medical withdrawal services [23].

Conclusion

Abuse of prescription opioids and other controlled substances is disconcerting in a way that is different than abuse of illegal opioids such as heroin. Prescription opioids are socially sanctioned to relieve the pain of surgery, medical illness, or substance use disorders (as in office-based opioid agonist treatment), and few persons would want their access to opioid medications unduly restricted. The misuse and abuse of opioid medications thus perverts the intended medical order: instead of being agents that ameliorate disease, the medications themselves—and the physicians who prescribe them—become agents of another disease—substance use disorder or addiction. In this increasingly common situation, health care professionals and pharmaceutical manufacturers become facilitators of illness rather than of health [27].

The history of controlled drug prescribing leads to the recognition of physician factors, patient factors, and drug factors that can raise or reduce the risk that such valuable medications will be subjected to diversion and abuse. Educational and practice management strategies can mitigate and manage such risks. Adopting approaches like those outlined in this chapter can help physicians address the prescription drug abuse problem, while still providing appropriate treatment to those without problematic responses to controlled drugs, and thus contribute to an overall improvement in the quality of care for all patients [1,7].

For More Information on the Topics Discussed:

American Society of Addiction Medicine (ASAM):

Wunsch MJ, Gonzalez PK, Hopper JA, McMasters MG, Boyd CJ. Nonmedical use, misuse, and abuse of prescription medications (Chapter 34). In RK Ries, DA Fiellin, SC Miller, R Saitz, eds. *The ASAM*

Principles of Addiction Medicine, fifth Edition. Philadelphia, PA: Wolters Kluwer; 2014.

Finch JW, Parran TV Jr., Wilford BB, et al. Clinical, ethical and legal considerations in prescribing drugs with abuse potential (Chapter 111). In RK Ries, DA Fiellin, SC Miller, R Saitz, eds. *The ASAM Principles of Addiction Medicine, fifth Edition.* Philadelphia, PA: Wolters Kluwer; 2014.

Federation of State Medical Boards (FSMB):

[updated version available]

Guidelines for the Chronic Use of Opioid Analgesics. Washington, DC: The Federation, May 2017.

Fishman S. Responsible Opioid Prescribing. Dallas, TX: The Federation; 2013. This 150-page book by pain expert Scott Fishman, M.D., translates the FSMB's model policy on pain management into practical guidelines for office-based practice.

References

1. Parran TV, Wilford BB, DuPont RL. Clinical issues in prescribing controlled drugs. *Up-to-Date* online medical education service. 2010, http://cursoenarm.net/UPTODATE/contents/mobipreview.htm?21/41/22175?source=HISTORY
2. Dart RC, Surratt HL, Cicero TJ, et al. Trends in opioid analgesic abuse and mortality in the United States. *NEJM.* 2015 Jan 15;372(3):241–248.
3. Portenoy RK. Opioid therapy for chronic non-malignant pain: A review of critical issues. *J Pain Symptom Manag.* 1996;11:203–217.
4. Federation of State Medical Boards (FSMB). *Guidelines for the Chronic Use of Opioid Analgesics.* Washington, DC: The Federation, May 2017.
5. Finch JW, Parran TV, Wilford BB, et al. Clinical, legal and ethical considerations in prescribing drugs with abuse potential (Chapter 109). In Ries RK, Alford DP, Saitz R, Miller S, eds. *Principles of Addiction Medicine, Fifth Edition.* Philadelphia, PA: Lippincott, Williams & Wilkins; 2014.
6. Substance Abuse and Mental Health Services Administration (SAMHSA). *Training Curriculum for Courses on Office-Based Opioid Treatment with Buprenorphine.* Rockville, MD: SAMHSA, U.S. Department of Health and Human Services; 2014.
7. Longo LP, Parran TV, Johnson B, et al. Addiction, Part II. Identification and management of the drug-seeking patient. *Am Fam Physician.* 2000;61:2401–2408.
8. American Medical Association (AMA). Drug abuse related to prescribing practices (Report of the Council on Scientific Affairs). *JAMA.* 1982;247:864–866. [Updated 1992, 2002, 2012.]
9. Federation of State Medical Boards (FSMB). *Model Policy on Opioid Addiction Treatment in the Medical Office.* Dallas, TX: The Federation; 2013.

10. Parran TV. Prescription drug abuse: A question of balance. *Med Clin North Am.* 1997;81(4):967–978.
11. Longo LP, Parran TV, Johnson B, et al. Addiction, Part II. Identification and management of the drug-seeking patient. *Am Fam Physician.* 2000;61:2401–2408.
12. Isaacson JH, Hopper JA, Alford DP, et al. Prescription drug use and abuse. Risk factors, red flags, and prevention strategies. *Postgrad Med.* 2005;118:19.
13. Parran T, Grey S, Adelman C. The role of disabled physicians in the diversion of controlled Drugs. *J Addict Dis.* 2000;19(3):35–42.
14. Michna E, Ross EL, Hynes WL, et al. Predicting aberrant drug behavior in patients treated for chronic pain: Importance of abuse history. *J Pain Symptom Manag.* 2004 Sep;228(3):250–258.
15. Reed MC, Engles-Horton LL et al. Use of opioid medications for chronic non-cancer pain in primary care. *J Gen Intern Med.* 2002;17:173–179.
16. Volkow ND, Fowler JS, Wang GJ. The addicted human brain viewed in the light of imaging studies: Brain circuits and treatment strategies. *Neuropharmacology.* 2004;47(Suppl 1):3.
17. Zacny J, Bigelow G, Compton P, et al. College on Problems of Drug Dependence Taskforce on Prescription Opioid Non-Medical Use and Abuse: Position statement. *Drug Alc Depend.* 2003;69:215–232.
18. DuPont RL. *The Selfish Brain—Learning from Addiction.* Center City, MN: Hazelden; 2003.
19. Council of State Governments (CSG). Drug abuse in America—Prescription drug diversion. *Trends Alert.* Lexington, KY: The Council; April 2004.
20. Coleman JJ, Bensinger PB, Gold MS, et al. Can drug design inhibit abuse? *J Psychoact Drug.* 2005;37(4):343–362.
21. Czechowicz D, ed. *Prescription Drug Abuse and Addiction* (NIDA Research Report Series, 7/2001; NIH Publication # 01-4881). Rockville, MD: NIDA, National Institutes of Health; 2001.
22. Center for Substance Abuse Treatment (CSAT). *Clinical Guidelines for the Use of Buprenorphine in the Treatment of Opioid Addiction.* Treatment Improvement Protocol (TIP) Series 40. DHHS Publication No. (SMA) 04-3939. Rockville, MD: CSAT, Substance Abuse and Mental Health Services Administration; 2004.
23. Michna E, Ross EL, Hynes WL, et al. Predicting aberrant drug behavior in patients treated for chronic pain: Importance of abuse history. *J Pain Symptom Manag.* 2004;28:250.
24. Veterans Health Administration (VHA), Department of Veteran Affairs. *VHA/DoD Clinical Practice Guidelines for Management of Substance Use Disorders (SUD), Version 2.0.* Washington, DC: VHA, Department of Veterans Affairs; 2009.
25. Institute for Research, Education and Training in Addiction (IRETA). *Best Practices in the Use of Buprenorphine. Final Expert Panel Report.* Pittsburgh, PA: IRETA, Community Care Behavioral Health Organizations; October 18, 2011.
26. Substance Abuse and Mental Health Services Administration (SAMHSA). *Opioid Overdose Prevention Toolkit.* Rockville, MD: SAMHSA, U.S. Department of Health and Human Services; 2016.
27. Cheatle MD. Prescription opioid misuse, abuse, morbidity, and mortality: Balancing effective pain management and safety. *Pain Med.* 2015 Oct;16(Suppl 1):S3–S8.

Chapter 10

Screening Patients for Opioid Risk

JEFFREY FUDIN, PHARM.D., DAIPM, FCCP,
FASHP, JACQUELINE CLEARY, PHARM.D., BCACP,
COURTNEY KOMINEK, PHARM.D., BCPS, CPE,
ABIGAIL BROOKS, PHARM.D., BCPS, AND
THIEN C. PHAM, PHARM.D.

Screening tools are available to aid in assessing patients and formulating treatment plans, as well as to assess patients' response to treatment. Tools are categorized as either *risk stratification tools* or *opioid misuse tools*, each of which will be described in this chapter. That discussion is followed by a description of how to assess a patient's level of risk for opioid overdose.

Risk Stratification Tools

Risk stratification tools include the Opioid Risk Tool (ORT), the Diagnosis Intractability Risk Efficacy (DIRE) score, the Prescription Drug Use Questionnaire (PDUQ), and the Screener and Opioid Assessment for Patients with Pain–Revised (SOAPP-R).

Opioid Risk Tool

The ORT is an office-based brief screening tool that is designed to predict which patients who are prescribed opioids are likely to develop aberrant drug use behaviors [1]. The tool is divided into five main items, which include family history of substance use disorder (SUD), personal history of SUD, age, and history of preadolescent sexual abuse and/or mental disorder (if any). Items are assigned specific point values, which may vary depending on whether the patient is male or female.

Total scores determine the patient's risk category, with 0–3 points, 4–7 points, and ≥8 points classified as low, medium, or high risk, respectively. In a validation study, the ORT demonstrated sensitivity and specificity in identifying patients at risk for aberrant behavior [1].

Diagnosis, Intractability, Risk, Efficacy Scale

Another tool for risk stratification is the DIRE. This tool was developed to help primary care physicians forecast analgesic efficacy and patient compliance with long-term opioid therapy for chronic non-cancer pain [2].

The DIRE score is composed of ratings of four factors: diagnosis, intractability, risk (further broken down into psychological, chemical health, reliability, and social support), and efficacy. A total score of 7–13 predicts that a patient is not a suitable candidate for opioid therapy, while a score of 14–21 suggests that a patient is a good candidate for treatment with opioids. A retrospective review found the DIRE to be a valid and reliable tool [2].

Prescription Drug Use Questionnaire

The PDUQ was constructed to help clinicians identify chronic pain patients who have a co-occurring SUD [3]. The instrument collects information on five domains, including characteristics of the pain condition, opioid use patterns, social/family factors, familial/personal history of SUD, and psychiatric history. This information is collected in a 42-item clinician-led interview [3].

The tool was validated in a study that compared PDUQ results to clinician assessments [4]. Patients who scored >15 met the criteria for SUD, while those who scored >25 met the criteria for substance dependence.

Screener and Opioid Assessment for Patients with Pain–Revised

The SOAPP-R is useful in determining the intensity of monitoring that a patient on chronic opioid therapy may require. The tool is composed of a 24-item patient questionnaire (this has been revised upward from the original tool, which contained 14 items) [5].

Each answer to an item is rated. A total of ≥18 is considered a positive screen. Patients who score ≥22 are considered to be at high risk, while those scoring 10–21 are rated as being at moderate risk, and a score of <9 signifies low risk for opioid misuse. Clinicians can use the scores in deciding whether treatment settings and plans should be altered to reflect the patient's level of risk.

The SOAPP-R has been validated in 500 chronic pain patients [6].

Table 10.1 compares the risk stratification tools discussed previously on a number of important factors.

Opioid Misuse Screening Tools

Opioid misuse screening tools include the Addiction Behaviors Checklist (ABC), the Current Opioid Misuse Measure (COMM), and the Pain Assessment and Documentation Tool (PADT).

Addiction Behaviors Checklist

When using opioid analgesics to treat patients for chronic pain, the ABC is useful in monitoring patients for behaviors suggestive of SUDs, as defined in a consensus statement published jointly by the American Academy of Pain Medicine (AAPM), the American Pain Society (APS), and the American Society of Addiction Medicine (ASAM) [7].

Information for the ABC is collected through patient interviews, information in the patient's chart, and observations of the patient in the clinic setting. The instrument includes 20 items, which address behaviors suggestive of the development of an SUD since the last office visit, and behaviors evidenced during the current visit.

A score of 3 or more indicates a potential for opioid misuse. The ABC has been validated in a Veterans Affairs health care setting [7].

Current Opioid Misuse Measure

The COMM was developed to help clinicians assess the severity of current opioid misuse [8]. In that respect, it is different from other tools that aim to *predict* medication misuse at some point in the future [9].

For the COMM, patients rate the frequencies of 17 thoughts or behaviors that may have occurred in the preceding 30 days on a scale of 0 = *never*, to 4 = *very often*. The sum of the items determines the final score, with a score of ≥9 indicating opioid misuse (although this cut-off may overestimate the severity of opioid misuse) [10]. The COMM has been validated in two separate studies of pain management and primary care patients [9,10].

Pain Assessment and Documentation Tool

The PADT, which is in the form of a brief note for the patient's chart, addresses four domains: analgesia, aberrancy, activities of daily living, and adverse effects

TABLE 10.1 Comparison of Screening Tools for Risk Stratification

Risk Tool	Indication	Question Format	Scoring	Advantages	Disadvantages
DIRE*	Risk of opioid abuse and suitability of candidate for long-term opioid therapy	7 via patient interview	Numerical score; simple to interpret	2 minutes to complete; Correlates well with patient's compliance and efficacy of long-term opioids therapy	Prospective validation needed
ORT*	Categorizes patients as low, medium, high risk	5	Numerical score; simple to interpret	<1 minute to complete; Simple scoring; High sensitivity and specificity for stratifying patients; Validated	1 question based on patient's knowledge of family history of substance abuse
PDUQ*	Assess for presence of addiction in chronic pain patients	42 items via patient interview	Numerical score; simple to interpret	3 items correctly predicted addiction or no addiction in 92% of patients	20 minutes to administer
SOAPP-R*	Primary care	24	Numerical score; simple to interpret	5 minutes to complete; Cross-validated; Easy to interpret results	–

* DIRE, Diagnosis, Intractability, Risk, Efficacy Score; ORT, Opioid Risk Tool; PDUQ, Prescription Drug Use Questionnaire; SOAPP-R, Screener and Opioid Assessment for Patients with Pain–Revised

Source: Revised and reprinted with permission from *paindr.com*. (Accessed May 5, 2015, at: http://paindr.com/wp-content/uploads/2012/05/Risk-stratification-tools-summarized_tables.pdf.)

Reference: Compton P, Darakjian J, Miotto K. Screening for addiction in patients with chronic pain and "problematic" substance use: Evaluation of a pilot assessment tool. *J Pain Symptom Manag.* 1998;16(6):355–363.

TABLE 10.2 Comparison of Tools for Assessment of Opioid Misuse

Tool	Indication	Question Format	Scoring	Advantages	Disadvantages
ABC	Ongoing assessment of patients on COT	20	≥3 indicates possible inappropriate opioid	· Concise · Easy to score · Studied at VA	· Need validation outside VA
COMM	Assess aberrant medications-related behaviors in chronic pain	17	Numerical	· 10 minutes to complete · Useful for adherence assessment	· Unknown reliability long-term
PADT	Streamline assessment of chronic pain outcomes using the 4 A's	N/A	N/A	· 5 minutes to complete · Documents progress · Complements other tools listed	· Not intended to predict drug-seeking behavior or positive/negative outcomes

ABC, Addiction Behaviors Checklist; COMM, Current Opioid Misuses Measure; PADT, Pain Assessment and Documentation Tool; COT, Chronic Opioid Therapy

Source: Revised and reprinted with permission from *paindr.com*. (Accessed May 5, 2015, at: http://paindr.com/wp-content/uploads/2012/05/Risk-strat-ification-tools-summarized_tables.pdf.)

[11]. It is intended as a tool to provide consistent documentation of progress in pain management. It is not designed to replace other pain assessment tools, but rather to augment them. In studies, clinicians typically needed 10–20 minutes to complete the PADT [11].

Table 10.2 compares the opioid misuse assessment tools discussed previously.

Assessing Overdose Risk

Given that overdose is a possibility for any patient who is prescribed opioids or who engages in nonmedical use, determining which patients should have direct access to naloxone is crucial [12]. Indeed, naloxone is the standard of care for opioid and heroin overdose [13].

As an opioid receptor antagonist, naloxone works by reversing the respiratory depressant effects of opioids [14]. The American Medical Association (AMA) recently released a policy statement advising that all at-risk patients who are being prescribed chronic opioid therapy also should be prescribed naloxone [15]. In addition, the Centers for Disease Control and Prevention (CDC) Guideline for Prescribing Opioids for Chronic Pain recommends prescribing naloxone as a risk-mitigation tool for patients whose risk factors increase possible overdose, including (but not limited to) those who have a history of overdose, patients who are prescribed more than 50 milligrams of morphine equivalents (MME), and those who are concurrently prescribed opioids and a benzodiazepine [16].

Clinicians also must select the formulation of naloxone based on the desired route of administration. To assist in this task, Zedler et al. developed the Risk Index for Overdose or Severe Opioid-induced Respiratory Depression (RIOSORD), a risk-stratification tool that has been validated in a veteran population of almost 2 million patients [17] (Table 10.3).

The RIOSORD score reflects factors related to overdose risk, such as the patient's history of psychiatric disorder, the presence of pulmonary or liver disease, use of an extended-release opioid, concurrent use of an antidepressant or benzodiazepine, the morphine equivalents consumed per day, and recent hospitalizations or emergency department visits. To elicit this information, the RIOSORD contains 17 questions, with a maximum score of 115. Each variable described above contributes a certain number of points to the overall score [18].

Subsequently, Zedler and colleagues developed a similar and overlapping schematic in a retrospective case-control study of 18,365,497 patients in the general medical population, using opioid claims data from integrated commercial health plans in the United States [19].

According to the Zedler team, chronic pain patients for whom risk factors have been identified are excellent candidates for an in-home naloxone overdose kit (Table 10.4).

TABLE 10.3 Scoring the RIOSORD Tool

Question	Points for a "Yes" Response
In the past 6 months, has the patient had a health care visit (outpatient, inpatient, or ED) involving any of the following health conditions?	
Opioid dependence?	15
Chronic hepatitis or cirrhosis?	9
Bipolar disorder or schizophrenia?	7
Chronic pulmonary disease? (e.g., emphysema, chronic bronchitis, asthma, pneumoconiosis, asbestosis)?	5
Chronic kidney disease with clinically significant renal impairment?	5
An active traumatic brain injury, excluding burns (e.g., fracture, dislocation, contusion, laceration, wound)?	4
Sleep apnea?	3
Does the patient consume:	
An extended-release or long-acting (ER/LA) opioid formulation of any prescribed opioid?	9
Methadone? (also check ER/LA- 9 points)	9
Oxycodone? (if ER/LA formulation, also check ER/LA- 9 points)	3
A prescription antidepressant?	7
A prescription benzodiazepine?	4
Is the patient's current maximum prescribed opioid dose:	
≥100 mg morphine equivalents per day?	16
50 – <100 mg morphine equivalents per day?	9
20 – <50 mg morphine equivalents per day?	5

TABLE 10.3 Continued

Question	Points for a "Yes" Response
In the past 6 months, has the patient:	
Had one or more emergency department (ED) visits?	11
Been hospitalized for one or more days?	8
Total point score (maximum 115)	

Source: Adapted from Zedler B, Saunders W, Joyce A, et al. Validation of a screening questionnaire for serious prescription opioid-induced respiratory depression or overdose. Presented at the 2015 American Academy of Pain Medicine 31st Annual Meeting. National Harbor, MD. LB010. 2015.

TABLE 10.4 Risk Classes and Predicted Probabilities

Risk Class	Risk Index Score (Points)	Observed Incidence
1	0–24	0.03
2	25–32	0.14
3	33–37	0.23
4	38–42	0.37
5	43–46	0.51
6	47–49	0.56
7	50–54	0.60
8	55–59	0.79
9	60–66	0.75
10	≥67	0.86

Source: Adapted with permission from Zedler B, Saunders W, Joyce A, Vick C, Murrelle L. Validation of a screening questionnaire for serious prescription opioid-induced respiratory depression or overdose. Presented at the 2015 American Academy of Pain Medicine 31st Annual Meeting. National Harbor, MD. LB010. 2015.

At present, legislation defining which patients can be prescribed naloxone by their physician, pharmacist or other clinician varies from state to state.

Naloxone is a life-saving medication to which patients should have access to help reduce the risk of a fatal overdose [15].

Conclusion

When carefully selected and correctly used, screening tools can enhance patient safety and mitigate the risks associated with opioid therapy. Therefore, they are useful in monitoring patients who require long-term use of opioids for pain or addiction. Such screening tools should be used to assess the risk of opioid misuse or abuse, as well as the risk of opioid-induced respiratory depression. Risk assessment should include comorbid conditions, stratified risk assessment, and urine monitoring [20].

However, it is important to remember that, although these tools are useful, they are not a substitute for good clinical judgment throughout the course of opioid therapy.

For More Information on the Topics Discussed:

American Society of Addiction Medicine (ASAM):

Bradley KA, Williams EC. Implementation of screening and brief intervention in clinical settings using quality improvement principles (Chapter 18–Sidebar). In RK Ries, DA Fiellin, SC Miller, R Saitz, eds. *The ASAM Principles of Addiction Medicine, Fifth Edition.* Philadelphia, PA: Wolters Kluwer; 2014.

Zgierska A, Fleming MF. Screening and brief intervention (Chapter 18). In RK Ries, DA Fiellin, SC Miller, R Saitz, eds. *The ASAM Principles of Addiction Medicine, Fifth Edition.* Philadelphia, PA: Wolters Kluwer; 2014.

Centers for Disease Control and Prevention (CDC):

Dowell D, Haegerich TM, Chou R. CDC Guideline for prescribing opioids for chronic pain—United States, 2016. *MMWR Rec Rep.* 2016;65(No. RR-1):1–49.

References

1. Webster LR, Webster RM. Predicting aberrant behaviors in opioid-treated patients: Preliminary validation of the Opioid Risk Tool. *Pain Med.* 2005;6(6):432–442.

2. Belgrade MJ, Schamber CD, Lindgren BR. The DIRE score: Predicting outcomes of opioid prescribing for chronic pain. *J Pain*. 2006;7(9):671–681.
3. Compton PA, Wu SM, Schieffer B, et al. Introduction of a self-report version of the Prescription Drug Use Questionnaire and relationship to medication agreement noncompliance. *J Pain Symptom Manag*. 2008 Oct;36(4):383–395.
4. Banta-Green CJ, Merrill JO, Doyle SR, et al. Measurement of opioid problems among chronic pain patients in a general medical population. *Drug Alc Depend*. 2009 Sep 1;104(1–2):43–49.
5. Compton P, Darakjian J, Miotto K. Screening for addiction in patients with chronic pain and "problematic" substance use: Evaluation of a pilot assessment tool. *J Pain Symptom Manag*. 1998 Dec;16(6):355–363.
6. Butler SF, Fernandez K, Benoit C, et al. Validation of the revised Screener and Opioid Assessment for Patients with Pain (SOAPP-R). *J Pain*. 2008;9(4):360–372.
7. Wu SM, Compton P, Bolus R, et al. The Addiction Behaviors Checklist: Validation of a new clinician-based measure of inappropriate opioid use in chronic pain. *J Pain Symptom Manag*. 2006 Oct;32(4):342–351.
8. Butler SF, Budman SH, Fernandez KC, et al. Development and validation of the Current Opioid Misuse Measure. *J Pain*. 2007 Jul;130(1–2):144–156.
9. Butler SF, Budman SH, Fanciullo GJ, et al. Cross validation of the Current Opioid Misuse Measure to monitor chronic pain patients on opioid therapy. *Clin J Pain*. 2010 Nov–Dec;26(9):770–776.
10. Meltzer EC, Rybin D, Saitz R, et al. Identifying prescription opioid use disorder in primary care: Diagnostic characteristics of the Current Opioid Misuse Measure (COMM). *J Pain*. 2011;152(2):397–402.
11. Chou R, Turner JA, Devine EB, et al. The effectiveness and risks of long-term opioid therapy for chronic pain: A systematic review for a National Institutes of Health Pathways to Prevention Workshop. *Ann Intern Med*. 2015 Feb 17;162(4):276–286.
12. Department of Health and Human Services (DHHS). Opioid abuse in the United States and Department of Health and Human Services actions to address opioid-drug-related overdoses and deaths. *J Pain Palliat Care Pharmacother*. 2015 Jun 5;29(2):133–139.
13. Robinson A, Wermeling DP. Intranasal naloxone administration for treatment of opioid overdose. *Am J Health-Syst Pharm*. 2014 Dec 15;71(24):2129–2135.
14. Dowell D, Haegerich TM, Chou R. CDC Guideline for prescribing opioids for chronic pain—United States, 2016. *MMWR Rec Rep*. 2016;65(No. RR-1):1–49.
15. Harris PA. It's about saving lives: Increasing access to naloxone. *AMA Wire*, 2015. (Accessed at: http://www.ama-assn.org/ama/ama-wire/post/its-savint-lives-increasing-access-naloxone.)
16. Zedler B, Xie L, Wang L, et al. Development of a risk index for serious prescription opioid-induced respiratory depression or overdose in Veterans' Health Administration patients. *Pain Med*. 2015;16(8):1566–1579.
17. Zedler B, Saunders W, Joyce A, et al. Validation of a screening questionnaire for serious prescription opioid-induced respiratory depression or overdose.

Presented at the 2015 American Academy of Pain Medicine 31st Annual Meeting. National Harbor, MD. 2015.

18. Zedler B, Saunders W, Joyce A, Vick C, Murrelle L. Validation of a screening risk index for serious prescription opioid-induced respiratory depression or overdose in a U.S. commercial health plan claims database. *Pain Med.* 2017 Mar 6. doi:10.1093/pm/pnx009. [Epub ahead of print]

19. Canadian Agency for Drugs and Technologies in Health. *Education and Assessment for Overdose Prevention: A Review of the Clinical Evidence and Guidelines—Rapid Response Report: Summary with Critical Appraisal.* Ottawa, Ontario: The Agency; 2015 Sep 24.

20. Gourlay DL, Heit HA, Almahrezi A. Universal precautions in pain medicine: A rational approach to the treatment of chronic pain. *Pain Med.* 2005;6(2):107–112.

Chapter 11

Diagnosing Patients
and Initiating Treatment

THEODORE V. PARRAN, JR., M.D., JOHN A.
HOPPER, M.D., AND BONNIE B. WILFORD, M.S.

Any patient identified as potentially suffering from chronic pain and/or addiction must undergo a thorough evaluation so that the clinician can reach an accurate diagnosis and compile information needed to formulate an appropriate treatment plan [1]. Such an evaluation should be designed to:

- Collect information about the patient's past and present use of alcohol, tobacco, and other substances.
- Identify comorbid medical and psychiatric conditions and disorders.
- Screen for communicable diseases and address them as needed.
- Assess the patient's level of pain.
- Reach a diagnosis of (or eliminate) opioid use disorder, including the duration, pattern, and severity of opioid misuse; the patient's level of tolerance; results of previous attempts to discontinue opioid use; past experience with agonist therapies; the nature and severity of previous episodes of withdrawal; and the time of last opioid use and current withdrawal status.
- Evaluate the patient's readiness to participate in treatment.
- Assess the patient's access to social supports, family, friends, employment, housing, financial resources, and assistance with legal problems.

Patients also should be evaluated for a broad array of psychosocial issues (also see Chapters 3 and 24 of this Handbook) to help determine how best to meet all of their health care needs.

Approach to the Patient

The clinician's approach and attitude are extremely important in obtaining an accurate history, developing a therapeutic alliance, and engaging the patient in treatment. Patients often are reluctant to disclose their alcohol or drug use and associated problems. Many report discomfort, shame, fear, distrust, hopelessness, and the desire to continue using drugs as reasons they do not discuss addiction openly with their physicians [2–4]. When one study asked patients what one single thing their physician could do to help them engage in treatment for opioid dependence, the most frequent answer was "don't judge me" [5–8].

The clinician's personal beliefs about drug use, individuals who have substance use disorders, sexual behavior, lifestyle differences, and other emotionally laden issues must be set aside or dealt with openly and therapeutically [9]. Physicians, other clinical staff, and community pharmacists may need to adjust their personal and professional attitudes to best serve patients who are being treated for pain and addiction [10].

Clinicians are more likely to elicit useful information if they approach the patient in a respectful, matter-of-fact manner, similar to the approach they would employ when inquiring about any other medical illness or problem. Desirable communication skills include friendliness, empathy, and respect. Techniques such as Motivational Interviewing can be helpful in establishing a therapeutic alliance [6,7].

A successful approach is best achieved by a clinician who can:

- Express empathy through reflective listening.
- Communicate respect for and acceptance of the patient and his/her feelings.
- Establish a nonjudgmental, collaborative relationship.
- Be a supportive and knowledgeable consultant.
- Compliment rather than denigrate.
- Listen rather than tell.
- Gently persuade, with the understanding that change is up to the patient.
- Tactfully point out discrepancies between the patient's goals or values and current behavior.
- Avoid arguments and direct confrontation, which can degenerate into a power struggle.
- Adjust to, rather than oppose, resistance on the part of the patient.
- Focus on the patient's strengths to support the hope and optimism needed to make change [8].

Sources of Information

The patient's history (including any history of substance use or abuse) and physical examination are key sources of information, without which it is difficult to reach an accurate diagnosis. Used appropriately, screening tools and laboratory tests also provide useful information.

Patient History

A thorough patient history is essential in arriving at an accurate diagnosis and developing a safe and appropriate treatment plan [11]. Ideally, the history should include the nature of the patient's problem(s), any underlying or co-occurring diseases or conditions, the effect of opioid use on the patient's physical and psychological functioning, and the results of any past treatment for pain or substance use disorder.

It is essential to ascertain whether the patient is currently taking (or recently took) methadone or any other long-acting opioid, because those agents have variable half-lives and may greatly increase the risk of overdose [12,13]. In addition, patients who engage in abuse of, or who are dependent on, sedative-hypnotics may be at risk of overdose or death from the combination of sedative-hypnotics and opioids [9].

In-depth interviews, combined with the use of standardized assessment instruments, are effective means of gathering this information from the patient. All patients should be asked whether they: (1) use substances before operating a motor vehicle, (2) ride with intoxicated drivers, (3) engage in sexual activity without contraception or use of condoms, and (4) have sex while intoxicated [14].

Other historical information that is helpful for logistical and administrative purposes includes employment status, insurance benefits, and legal status and/or pending criminal charges.

Information from family members and significant others can provide useful additional perspectives on the patient's status [3], as does contact with or records from clinicians who have treated the patient in the past.

Screening Tools

Appropriate use of screening tools allows the clinician to: (1) make a diagnosis of pain or substance use disorder with appropriate differential, (2) complete a psychological assessment, including the risk that initiating pain treatment will trigger a substance use disorder or relapse to such a disorder in a patient who is in recovery, and (3) periodically review the patient's diagnosis and any co-occurring disorders [5].

Physical Examination

The physical examination should focus on physical findings related to pain and addiction and their complications. For example, examination of skin injection sites can provide useful information about the duration of injection drug use. Although many sites can be used, the cubital fossa and groin are the most common injection sites. Recent injection marks are small and red, and sometimes are inflamed or surrounded by slight bruising. Older injection sites typically are not inflamed, but sometimes show pigmentation changes (either lighter or darker), and the skin may have an atrophied or sunken appearance. A combination of recent and old injection sites suggests that an opioid-dependent patient may have a long-standing disorder and current neuroadaptation [15].

Individuals who have engaged in alcohol, tobacco, and other drug abuse should have the cervical, axillary, supraclavicular, and inguinal lymph node regions examined for lymphadenopathy. Also, tuberculosis, chancroid, syphilis, and HIV are more common in persons with addictive disorders who present with lymphadenopathy [14].

A thorough neurological examination and evaluation of mental status is another important component of the physical examination. In addition, all women of childbearing age should have a pregnancy test [12].

Laboratory Tests

As a rule, a urine drug screen and other laboratory tests are useful in identifying or confirming recent opioid use and to screen for unreported use of other drugs. Ideally, urine drug screens should include all opioids commonly prescribed and/or misused in the local community, as well as illicit drugs that are available locally [2].

Other useful tests include those of liver enzymes, serum bilirubin, and for hepatitis and HIV, particularly in patients who have engaged in injection drug use (in the latter group, serum creatinine levels should be tested for the presence of silent renal disease [3,4].

Other Sources of Information

It also is advisable to access the patient's prescription drug use history through the state's Prescription Drug Monitoring Program (PDMP), to confirm compliance in taking prescribed medications and to detect any unreported use of other prescription medications.

Reaching a Diagnosis

In order to be diagnosed with substance use disorder, the patient must meet criteria set forth in standardized sources, the most widely recognized of which are the *International Classification of Diseases, 10th edition* (ICD-10) [16], and the *Diagnostic and Statistical Manual of Mental Disorders, 5th edition* (DSM-5) [17].

International Classification of Diseases, 10th Edition (ICD-10)

The ICD-10 [16] defines opioid dependence as "a cluster of physiological, behavioral, and cognitive phenomena in which the use of opioids takes on a much higher priority for a given individual than other behaviors that once had greater value." In order to establish a clear diagnosis of opioid dependence, the ICD requires that three or more of the following symptoms must have been experienced or exhibited at some time during the preceding year:

- A strong desire or compulsion to take opioids;
- Difficulty in controlling opioid-use behaviors in terms of the onset, cessation, or intensity of use;
- The presence of a physiological withdrawal state when opioid use has stopped or been reduced, as evidenced by one of the following: (a) the characteristic withdrawal syndrome, or (b) use of opioids (or closely related substances) with the intention of relieving or avoiding withdrawal symptoms;
- Evidence of tolerance, such that larger doses of opioids are required to achieve effects originally produced by smaller doses;
- Progressive neglect of alternative sources of pleasure or interests in favor of opioid use;
- Increased amounts of time spent in obtaining opioids or recovering from their effects; and
- Persistent opioid use despite clear evidence of overtly harmful consequences [16].

Diagnostic and Statistical Manual of Mental Disorders, 5th Edition (DSM-5)

For diagnostic and reimbursement purposes, it also is important to document how many of the 11 criteria in the American Psychiatric Association's DSM-5 category of "substance use and addictive disorders" [17] have been identified in or by the patient. Finally, it is essential to verify or exclude the presence of physiological dependence before deciding on the mode of treatment [18,19].

Formulating a Treatment Plan

No single treatment is appropriate for all persons at all times. Therefore, treatment should be guided by an individualized plan that is developed in consultation with the patient. Such a plan should be based on a comprehensive biopsychosocial assessment of the patient. Treatment options include [9,24]:

- Medication tapering and no other treatment;
- Medication tapering followed by antagonist therapy;
- Counseling and/or peer support without medication-assisted therapy;
- Referral to short- or long-term residential treatment;
- Referral to an opioid treatment program (OTP) for maintenance treatment with either buprenorphine or methadone; or
- Treatment with buprenorphine or naltrexone in a medical office setting.

The treatment plan should list problems (such as obstacles to recovery, deficits in the patient's knowledge or skills, or patient dysfunction or loss), as well as strengths (such as a patient's readiness to change, positive social support system, or strong connection to a source of spiritual support), treatment priorities (such as obstacles to treatment and risks, identified within the list of problems and arranged according to severity) and goals (a statement to guide realistic, achievable, short-term resolution or reduction of the problems), methods or strategies (the treatment services to be provided, the site of those services, the staff responsible for delivering treatment), and a timetable for follow-through with the treatment plan that promotes accountability.

Finally, the plan should be written to facilitate measurement of progress [9,25]. Both the plan and the steps taken to implement it should be documented in the patient's medical record [23].

Before proceeding with treatment, it is helpful to consider each of the items listed in the Treatment Checklist, Box 11.1.

Selecting an Appropriate Medication

Whenever a medication is to be used, the treatment plan should give attention to steps that will promote patient adherence to the instructions for use [9]. Depending on the needs of the patient, these might include: (a) a description of specific strategies for remembering to take medications; (b) use of blistercard

BOX 11.1 Treatment Planning Checklist

1. Does the patient understand the risks and benefits of the proposed treatment?
2. Did the patient agree to treatment after a review of all relevant options?
3. What is the patient's level of motivation?
4. Can the patient be expected to adhere to the treatment plan?
5. Is the patient willing and able to follow safety precautions?
6. Can the necessary treatment resources be provided, either in the physician's office or another accessible location?
7. Is the patient currently dependent on or abusing alcohol or using tobacco?
8. Is the patient currently dependent on opioids, benzodiazepines, barbiturates, or other sedative/hypnotics (all of which increase the risk of overdose)?
9. Does the patient have a history of multiple previous treatments or relapses, or is the patient at high risk for relapse non-medical drug use?
10. Has the patient had prior adverse reactions to any medications involved in the treatment plan?
11. Is the patient taking other medications that may interact with any proposed pharmacotherapies?
12. Is the patient pregnant or of childbearing age?
13. Does the patient have medical problems that are contraindications to proposed pharmacotherapies? Are there physical illnesses that complicate treatment?
14. Is the patient psychiatrically stable? Is the patient actively suicidal or homicidal; has he or she recently attempted suicide or homicide? Does the patient exhibit emotional, behavioral, or cognitive conditions that will complicate treatment?
15. Are the patient's psychosocial circumstances sufficient to support recovery?

Source: Center for Substance Abuse Treatment (CSAT). *Clinical Guidelines for the Use of Buprenorphine in the Treatment of Opioid Addiction.* (Treatment Improvement Protocol [TIP] Series 40. DHHS Publication No. [SMA] 04-3939. Rockville, MD: CSAT, Substance Abuse and Mental Health Services Administration; 2004.

packs or pill boxes; (c) a schedule for monitoring medication adherence that reflects the patient's history of adherence to other medication regimens; and (d) steps to involve the patient's family members in assisting with and monitoring adherence [12].

Additional safeguards are recommended before deciding to prescribe an opioid analgesic. For example, even when sound medical indications have been established, physicians typically consider three additional factors before deciding to prescribe [9,22]:

- The *severity of symptoms,* in terms of the patient's ability to accommodate them. Relief of symptoms is a legitimate goal of medical practice, but using opioid analgesics requires caution.
- The patient's *reliability in taking medications,* noted through observation and careful history-taking. The physician should assess a patient's history of and risk factors for drug abuse before prescribing any psychoactive drug and weigh the benefits against the risks. The likely development of physical dependence in patients on long-term opioid therapy should be monitored through periodic check-ups.
- The *dependence-producing potential of the medication.* The physician should consider whether a product with less potential for abuse, or even a non-drug therapy, would provide equivalent benefits. Patients should be warned about possible adverse effects caused by interactions between opioids and other medications or illicit substances, including alcohol.

As in the treatment of any medical disorder, physicians who choose to offer medication-assisted therapy for pain or addiction need to understand the nature of the underlying disorder, the specific actions of each of the available medications (as well as any associated contraindications or cautions), and the importance of careful patient selection and monitoring [15].

Educating the Patient and Obtaining Informed Consent

Discussing the diagnosis with the patient and explaining the recommended treatment options is an essential step. For example, exploring the patient's expectations of treatment for his or her pain or addiction is an important way to avoid unrealistic hopes and expectations [1,2]. A patient who fully understands what treatment can and cannot do ultimately may experience a more successful outcome [3].

Because opioids can contribute to fatal overdoses in individuals who have lost their tolerance to opioids or in those who are opioid-naïve (such as a child or other family member), proper and secure storage of the medication must be discussed. Especially if there are young people in the patient's home, the subject of safe storage and use should be revisited periodically throughout the course of treatment, with the discussions documented in the patient record [19,21].

Patients should give their informed consent to treatment in a written agreement that is signed by both the patient and the physician. Issues should be thoroughly discussed in terms of potential risks and benefits as part of the informed consent process. With the patient's consent, this conversation could include family members, significant other(s), or a guardian [9]. Patients and family members often are ambivalent about treatment, and their concerns may influence subsequent treatment choices. (Also see Chapter 7 of this Handbook.)

A written *informed consent document*, discussed with and signed by the patient, can be helpful in reinforcing this information and establishing a set of "ground rules" [11].

Creating a Treatment Agreement

Beyond the general provisions of the informed consent document, a *treatment agreement* should be used to describe the goals of treatment and what is expected of the patient in terms of cooperation and involvement in the treatment process, as well as what the patient can expect from the provider [4]. (Although the term is widely used, it is best not to label this a treatment "contract" because of the legal connotation.) Many clinicians use the term "Patient–Prescriber Agreement" (PPA) to denote the collaborative and patient-centered nature of the treatment agreement.

The treatment agreement also should describe the conditions under which treatment will be discontinued [11]. It should address contingencies for failure to improve or problems with treatment adherence; for example, these might include referral to a more structured treatment environment (such as an opioid treatment program). It also is important for patients to agree to the goal of abstinence from all illicit drugs and nonmedical use of prescription drugs [7].

Initiating Treatment

When an appropriate medication has been selected, the *dose, schedule,* and *formulation* should be determined. These choices often are just as important in optimizing pharmacotherapy as the choice of medication itself. Decisions involve:

1. Dose (based not only on the age and weight of the patient, but also on severity of the disorder, possible loading-dose requirement, and the presence of potentially interacting drugs);

2. Timing of administration (such as a bedtime dose to minimize problems associated with sedative or respiratory depressant effects);
3. Route of administration (chosen to improve compliance/adherence as well as to attain peak drug concentrations rapidly); and
4. Formulation (e.g., selecting a patch in preference to a tablet, or an extended-release product rather than an immediate-release formulation).

At the time a drug is prescribed, the patient should be informed that it is illegal to sell, give away, or otherwise share their medication with others, including family members. The patient's obligation extends to keeping the medication in a locked cabinet or otherwise restricting access to it, as well as safely disposing of any unused supply. (Helpful information on disposal options from the U.S. Food and Drug Administration [FDA] can be accessed at: http://www.fda.gov/ForConsumers/ConsumerUpdates/ucm101653.htm.)

Integrate Pharmacological and Nonpharmacological Therapies

Some patients may respond to psychosocial interventions and others to medication therapy alone, but most patients need both. The different approaches—medications, professional counseling, and mutual help groups—are complementary. They share the same goals while addressing different aspects of the patient's problem: neurobiological, psychological, and social. Offering the full range of effective treatments also maximizes patient choice and outcomes, as no single approach is universally successful [22]. Many studies show that the combination of pharmacological and nonpharmacological interventions may be more effective than either approach used alone [26].

Encourage Participation in Mutual-Help Programs

The support of a mutual-help group can be critical to the patient's well-being. The oldest, best-known, and most accessible mutual-help program for persons with opioid use disorders is offered by Narcotics Anonymous (NA). Patients may resist attending NA meetings and may fear that disclosure of medication use will make them unwelcome [9]. Although some NA members may have negative attitudes toward medication, the organization itself supports appropriate medication use. Providers should encourage patients to try different group meetings until they find one that is a "good fit." Lists of local meetings to give to patients can be obtained from http://www.na.org.

Other mutual-help groups, while not as universally available as NA, have a strong presence in many communities. Contact information for a number of groups that may be helpful to patients and their families is provided in online Appendix E of this volume.

Special Considerations

Some patients present with specific conditions or at life stages that require special consideration in formulating a treatment plan. The most frequently seen special populations of these are discussed in Chapters 24 to 31 of this Handbook.

Conclusion

Identification of a patient who is abusing a prescribed opioid or other controlled drug presents a major therapeutic opportunity. The physician should have a plan for managing such situations, which typically involves working with the patient and the patient's family, referral to an addiction expert for assessment and placement in a formal addiction treatment program, long-term participation in a 12-Step mutual-help program such as Narcotics Anonymous, and follow-up of any associated medical or psychiatric comorbidities [9].

In all cases, patients should be given the benefit of the physician's concern and attention. It is important to remember that patients who are unable to maintain controlled use of controlled substances often have very real medical problems that demand and deserve the same high-quality medical care offered to any patient [19,23].

For More Information on the Topics Discussed:

American Society of Addiction Medicine (ASAM):

Parran TV Jr., McCormick RA, Delos Reyes CM. Assessment (Chapter 20). In RK Ries, DA Fiellin, SC Miller, R Saitz, eds. *The ASAM Principles of Addiction Medicine, fifth Edition*. Philadelphia, PA: Wolters Kluwer; 2014.

Warner E, Lorch E. Laboratory diagnosis (Chapter 19). In RK Ries, DA Fiellin, SC Miller, R Saitz, eds. *The ASAM Principles of Addiction Medicine, fifth Edition*. Philadelphia, PA: Wolters Kluwer; 2014.

Medscape.com:

www.medscape.com. Two course modules sponsored by the National Institute on Drug Abuse (NIDA) and posted on MedScape can be accessed at http://www.medscape.org/viewarticle/770687 and http://www.med-scape.org/viewarticle/770440. Continuing Medical Education (CME) credits are available.

OpiodPrescribing.com:

www.opioidprescribing.com. Sponsored by the Boston University School of Medicine, with support from the federal Substance Abuse and Mental Health Services Administration (SAMHSA), this site presents course modules on various aspects of prescribing opioids for chronic pain. To view the list of courses and to register, go to http://www.opioidprescrib-ing.com/overview. CME credits are available at no charge.

Prescriber's Clinical Support System for Opioids:

www.pcss-o.org. Sponsored by the American Academy of Addiction Psychiatry in collaboration with other specialty societies and with support from SAMHSA, the Prescriber's Clinical Support System for Opioids (PCSS-0) offers multiple resources—including live and recorded webinars—related to opioid prescribing and the diagnosis and manage-ment of opioid use disorders.

Informed Consent:

Sample informed consent documents can be accessed at the PCSS-B web-site (www.pcssb.org) and in SAMHSA's TIP 40 (CSAT, 2004).

References

1. Levounis P. Patient assessment. In Renner JA, Levounis P, eds. *Handbook of Office-Based Buprenorphine Treatment of Opioid Dependence.* Washington DC: American Psychiatric Publishing; 2011.
2. Gourlay DL, Heit HA, Caplan YH. *Urine Drug Testing in Clinical Practice: The Art and Science of Patient Care.* Sacramento, CA: California Society of Family Physicians; 2010.
3. Substance Abuse and Mental Health Services Administration (SAMHSA). *Brief Guide to the Clinical Use of Extended-Release Injectable Naltrexone in the Treatment of Opioid Use Disorders.* Rockville, MD: SAMHSA, U.S. Department of Health and Human Services; 2014.
4. Saitz R. Medical and surgical complications of addiction. In RK Ries, DA Fiellin, SC Miller, R Saitz, eds. *Principles of Addiction Medicine, Fourth Edition.* Philadelphia, PA: Lippincott, Williams & Wilkins; 2009.
5. Wilford BB. *Briefing Paper on Screening and Brief Intervention.* (Prepared for the Third National Leadership Conference on Medical Education in Substance Abuse, Jan. 16, 2008.) Washington, DC: Office of National Drug Control Policy, Executive Office of the President, The White House; 2008.

6. Carpenter KM, Jiang H, Sullivan MA, et al. Betting on change: Modeling transitional probabilities to guide therapy development for opioid dependence. *Psychol Addict Behav*. 2009 Mar;23(1):47–55.

7. Fitzgerald J, McCarty D. Understanding attitudes toward use of medication in substance abuse treatment: A multilevel approach. *Psychol Serv*. 2009;6(1):74–84.

8. Miller NS, Sheppard LM. The role of the physician in addiction prevention and treatment. *Psychiatr Clin North Am*. 1999 Jun;22(2):489–505.

9. Center for Substance Abuse Treatment (CSAT). *Clinical Guidelines for the Use of Buprenorphine in the Treatment of Opioid Addiction*. Treatment Improvement Protocol (TIP) Series 40. DHHS Publication No. (SMA) 04-3939. Rockville, MD: CSAT, Substance Abuse and Mental Health Services Administration; 2004.

10. Rieckmann T, Daley M, Fuller B, et al. Client and counselor attitudes toward the use of medications for treatment of opioid dependence. *J Sub Abuse Treat*. 2007 Mar;32(2):207–215.

11. Federation of State Medical Boards (FSMB). *Model Policy on Opioid Addiction Treatment in the Medical Office*. Dallas, TX: The Federation; 2013.

12. Kraus ML, Alford DP, Kotz MM, et al. Statement of the American Society of Addiction Medicine Consensus Panel on the use of buprenorphine in office-based treatment of opioid addiction. *J Addict Med*. 2011 Dec;5(4):254–263.

13. Breen CL, Harris SJ, Lintzeris N, et al. Cessation of methadone maintenance treatment using buprenorphine: Transfer from methadone to buprenorphine and subsequent buprenorphine reductions. *Drug Alcohol Depend*. 2003 Jul 20;71(1):49–55.

14. Center on Addiction and Substance Abuse (CASA). *Missed Opportunity: National Survey of Primary Care Physicians and Patients on Substance Abuse*. New York: The Center; April 2000.

15. World Health Organization (WHO). *Guidelines for the Psychosocially Assisted Pharmacological Treatment of Opioid Dependence*. Geneva, Switzerland: WHO; 2009.

16. World Health Organization (WHO). The ICD-10 *Classification of Mental and Behavioural Disorders: Clinical Descriptions and Diagnostic Guidelines*. Geneva, Switzerland: WHO; 1992.

17. Hasin D, Hatzenbuehler M, Keyes K, et al. Substance use disorders: Diagnostic and Statistical Manual of Mental Disorders, Fourth edition (DSM-IV) and International Classification of Diseases, Tenth edition (ICD-10). *Addiction*. 2006 Sep 2;101:59–75.

18. American Psychiatric Association (APA). *Diagnostic and Statistical Manual of Mental Disorders, 5th Edition (DSM-5)*. Washington, DC: American Psychiatric Publishing; 2013.

19. Substance Abuse and Mental Health Services Administration (SAMHSA). *Opioid Overdose Toolkit*. Rockville, MD: SAMHSA, U.S. Department of Health and Human Services; 2014.

20. Isaacson JH, Hopper JA, Alford DP, Parran T. Prescription drug use and abuse. Risk factors, red flags, and prevention strategies. *Postgrad Med*. 2005;118:19.

21. Lingford-Hughes AR, Welch S, Peters L, et al., for the British Association for Psychopharmacology (BAP) Expert Reviewers Group. BAP Updated Guidelines: Evidence-Based Guidelines for the Pharmacological Management of Substance Abuse, Harmful Use, Addiction and Comorbidity: Recommendations from BAP. *J Psychopharm.* 2012 July;26(7):899–952.

22. Fiellin DA, for the Physician Clinical Support System for Buprenorphine (PCSS-B). *PCSS-B Guidance on Treatment of Acute Pain in Patients Receiving Buprenorphine/Naloxone.* East Providence, RI: American Academy of Addiction Psychiatry; Nov. 10, 2005.

23. Finch JW, Parran TV, Wilford BB, Wyatt SA. Clinical, legal and ethical considerations in prescribing drugs with abuse potential (Chapter 111). In RK Ries, DA Fiellin, R Saitz, S Miller, eds. *The ASAM Principles of Addiction Medicine, Fifth Edition.* Philadelphia, PA: Lippincott, Williams & Wilkins; 2014.

24. National Institute on Drug Abuse (NIDA). *Principles of Drug Addiction Treatment, Third Edition.* (NIH Publication No. 12–4180.) Rockville, MD: NIDA, National Institutes of Health; 2012.

25. American Society of Addiction Medicine (ASAM). *Public Policy Statement on Office-Based Opioid Agonist Treatment (OBOT).* Chevy Chase, MD: ASAM; 2010.

26. Fishman MJ, Mee-Lee D, Shulman GD, Wilford BB et al., eds. *Supplement to the ASAM Patient Placement Criteria on Pharmacotherapies for the Management of Alcohol Use Disorders.* Philadelphia, PA: Lippincott, Williams & Wilkins, Inc.; 2010.

Chapter 12

Drug Testing and Other Tools for Patient Monitoring

LOUIS E. BAXTER, SR., M.D., DFASAM

The issues of pain and addiction, which often are intertwined in patient care, need to be dissected, evaluated, and identified in order to achieve the best possible treatment outcomes for patients and providers.

Patients who are being treated for pain run the risk of developing physical dependence, substance misuse, or addiction, while patients who are being treated for pain and who have a history of substance use disorder (SUD) are at risk of reactivating that disorder if they are not properly treated and monitored for drug efficacy and safety, adherence to the treatment plan, and the development of tolerance or other complications [1,2].

Drug Testing as a Tool for Patient Monitoring

Drug testing and toxicology are very important tools to help navigate the confluence of pain and addiction. This chapter will describe how drug testing can be employed as a useful tool for the delivery of safe and effective care. First, let us review some definitions:

- *Toxicology* is a branch of biology, chemistry, and medicine that is concerned with the study of adverse effects of chemicals on living organisms [1].
- *Drug testing* is the means by which chemicals, drugs, and other substances are identified (many of these substances are

particularly relevant to the care of patients undergoing treatment for pain and addiction). Many drug testing modalities can be employed, with selection of the appropriate modality representing the key to success.

Although virtually any body fluid or tissue can be assayed for drugs of abuse, those used most frequently are urine, blood, oral fluid, sweat and hair, because testing these modalities is noninvasive [2]. It is vitally important that the correct modality be selected in order to obtain the most clinically relevant information to answer the patient care questions at hand.

Hair Testing

Hair testing is best used to test for drugs of abuse for forensic or research purposes. Hair samples are easily collected and are not easily substituted or adulterated (both of which are problems with unobserved urine specimens). However, hair testing presents its own problems. For example, drug deposition into hair is related to melanin content, so highly pigmented hair acquires a greater concentration of drug. On the other hand, cosmetic procedures and ultraviolet light can lead to artificially reduced drug concentrations. Environmental contamination also is a problem in hair testing and can render interpretation problematic [3].

For these reasons, a hair test is helpful in looking back at drug use over time, but not helpful in examining acute or recent use, as it cannot detect the presence of drugs until at least one to two weeks following the time use occurred [4].

Blood Testing

Blood testing is more useful than urine testing for detection of recently ingested drugs and alcohol. Most compounds are detected in the blood only a few hours before redistribution, metabolism, and elimination occur.

Obtaining blood by venipuncture requires training. It is much more invasive than urine collection and carries the risk of infection. Many injection-drug-using patients have very poor venous access due to previous intravenous injections and sclerosis of their veins. Exposure of personnel administering the test to infectious disease transmission also is a legitimate concern that must be considered.

Testing Oral Fluids

Oral fluids are a mixture of saliva, fluid from gingival crevices, and remnants of food and drink. Concentrations of drugs in oral fluid approximates concentrations found in blood, but only for short periods of time. Differences in collection techniques can affect the drug concentrations. Also, it has been shown than contamination of oral fluids can occur as the result of recent smoking or ingesting of drugs [5].

Sweat Testing

Testing sweat (perspiration) can be useful in identifying drugs and alcohol that were administered through the use of patches. This modality allows detection of drugs that were excreted over an extended period of time. The problem is that the quantity of sweat collected is so small that it is difficult to measure drug levels, because it is not possible to measure the total amount of sweat not captured by the patch [6].

Urine Testing

Urine testing is preferred and is the most widely used modality. It is easily collected and non-invasive, and yields large quantities of fluid for testing. Urine can be used to detect drug or alcohol use within hours of such use and for as long as three days after use. In some chronic drug users, such use can be detected for weeks after the most recent use (see Table 12.1).

Technology exists (involving gas or liquid chromatography–mass spectrometry) that allows the quantification of drugs and their metabolites, and also detects drugs and metabolites and specifically identifies them at very low concentrations—even below the usual cutoff levels established by the drug-testing industry [7].

In pain management settings, point-of-care testing (POCT) is sufficient because positive test results do not result in dire consequences, but rather lead to modification of the treatment plan.

Suggested urine drug panels for evaluation of pain and addiction patients should include: amphetamines, cocaine, hydrocodone, hydromorphone, morphine, oxycodone, fentanyl, methadone, oxymorphone, heroin, tetrahydrocannabinol (THC), and buprenorphine. In addition, the panel should test for the presence of sedative-hypnotics in all age groups, and stimulants in young adults.

NOTE: *Whenever a concern is raised about a POCT test result, a sample should be sent for more definitive laboratory testing and confirmation.*

Interpreting Test Results

Urine test results in pain management and addiction treatment are indispensable in clarifying and expanding diagnoses, assessing treatment efficacy, and assuring that the treatment plan is efficacious for the patient. It is important

TABLE 12.1 Urine Drug Testing in Pain Management: Detection Times Vary for Different Opioid and Sedative Drugs*

Substance	Lower Limit for Screening Purposes	Duration of Detection
Barbiturates	200 ng/mL	Up to 24 hours with short-acting formulations; up to 30 days with long-acting formulations
Benzodiazepines	NA	Up to 24 hours with short-acting formulations (e.g., triazolam); up to 12 days with intermediate-acting formulations (e.g., alprazolam); up to 8 days with long-acting formulations (e.g., diazepam)
Buprenorphine	0.5 ng/mL	Up to 4 days after use
Codeine	300 ng/mL	Up to 2 days after use
Heroin	10 ng/mL	Up to 3 days after use
Hydrocodone	100 ng/mL	Up to 2 days after use
Hydromorphone	300 ng/mL	Up to 2 days after use
Methadone	300 ng/mL	Up to 3 days after single use; up to 11 days with maintenance dosing
Morphine	300 ng/mL	Up to 2 days after use
Oxycodone	100 ng/mL	Up to 1.5 days after use (immediate-release formulation) or up to 3 days after use (extended-release formulation)
Oxymorphone	100 ng/mL	Up to 2.5 days after use (immediate-release formulation) or up to 4 days after use (extended-release formulation)
Propoxyphene	NA	Up to 2 days after use

TABLE 12.1 Continued

Substance	Lower Limit for Screening Purposes	Duration of Detection
Other opiates	50 ng/mL	Up to 2 days after a single use

*Higher doses and some pathologies may extend the window of detection.

Sources: Excerpted from Heit HA, Gourlay DL. Urine drug testing in pain medicine. *J Pain Symptom Manag.* 2004;27(3):260–267; DuPont RL, Goldberger BA, Ferguson JL. The science and clinical uses of drug testing (112). In RK Ries, DA Fiellin, SC Miller, R Saitz, eds. *The ASAM Principles of Addiction Medicine, Fifth Edition.* Philadelphia, PA: Wolters Kluwer; 2014; and Substance Abuse and Mental Health Services Administration (SAMHSA). *Clinical Drug Testing in Primary Care.* Technical Assistance Publication (TAP) 32. HHS Publication No. (SMA) 12-4668. Rockville, MD: SAMHSA; 2012.

that such tests be interpreted by experts—preferably a certified Medical Review Officer (MRO).

Inaccurate interpretations can foil a brilliant treatment plan and leave the patient inadequately diagnosed and inappropriately treated. The MRO can verify that the chain of custody and the appropriate collection processes and testing standards have been followed, and that the test result was not a false positive screening result or the result of a legitimately prescribed medication.

Confusion regarding positive drug test results arises from the assumption that most drug users who are undergoing pain treatment use drugs infrequently. Moreover, many such individuals either deny or minimize their drug use, leading to the assumption that their actual use is occasional.

To the contrary, most positive drug tests are the result of regular drug use, as shown in a study that found 55% of positive test results were attributable to daily or near-daily use. Only 7% of urine-positive drug test results were from individuals who used drugs only a few times a year [8]. *Positive urine drug test results require further evaluation of the donors.* Multiple test results that are positive for drugs that were not prescribed warrant evaluation by an addiction specialist.

False negative and false positive results can occur (See Table 12.2, below). In fact, POCT testing by immunoassay returns false results (positive and negative) in nearly half of all cases, depending on the drug class. It should be noted that the absence of a prescribed drug, in and of itself, does not indicate diversion, hoarding, or bingeing. It may be that the POCT immunoassay is falsely negative because it did not detect the drug, or that the drug was present at a level below the reportable cutoff limit [9].

TABLE 12.2 Compounds and Medications That Can Cause False Positive Results on Urine Immunoassay Tests

False Positive for:	Substance(s) Causing the False Positive
Barbiturates (short-acting)	Phenytoin
Benzodiazepines	Oxaproxin, sertraline
Methadone	Quetiapine
Morphine	Amitriptyline, codeine, dextromethorphan, heroin, poppy seeds, pyrilamine, quinine water
Other opiates	Gatifloxacin, levofloxacin, ofloxacin, papaverine, poppy seeds, rifampicin

Sources: Excerpted from DuPont RL, Goldberger BA, Ferguson JL. The science and clinical uses of drug testing (112). In RK Ries, DA Fiellin, SC Miller, R Saitz, eds. *The ASAM Principles of Addiction Medicine, Fifth Edition.* Philadelphia, PA: Wolters Kluwer; 2014; Heit HA, Gourlay DL. Urine drug testing in pain medicine. *J Pain Symptom Manag.* 2004;27(3):260–267; and Substance Abuse and Mental Health Services Administration (SAMHSA). *Clinical Drug Testing in Primary Care.* Technical Assistance Publication (TAP) 32. HHS Publication No. (SMA) 12-4668. Rockville, MD: SAMHSA; 2012.

A false positive occurs when a test result is positive for a drug that is not present when subjected to confirmation testing. *Cross-reactivity* with foods, over-the-counter (OTC) medications, and prescribed medications may be the cause of such problems (see Table 12.2) [10,11].

Laboratory errors or test insensitivity also are possible problem areas. Laboratory errors can occur when the forensic chain of custody is not documented or maintained. Such problems sometimes occur at testing laboratories and can be discovered by speaking with the lab's Certifying Scientist.

Frequency of Testing

There is not yet consensus as to the optimal frequency of urine testing in pain patients. Nevertheless, as a valuable tool, it appears that it would be prudent to obtain a urine sample at the beginning of a patient's engagement in treatment and then periodically as clinical concerns arise or as part of routine assessment.

Limitations of Drug Testing

Drug testing is not a treatment for pain or addiction, but a tool to facilitate and evaluate the effectiveness of a treatment plan for a particular patient. Test results merely reflect the presence or absence of a drug or its metabolites at a specific point in time, *if* the assay is sensitive to that particular drug, *if* the drug has been used recently, and *if* its level is detected above the established cutoff level. If the test panel does not include a specific drug or class of drug, it will not detect the drug.

Drug tests cannot detect the exact dose or time of the most recent use of any drug, licit or illicit. Individuals metabolize drugs at different rates, and different amounts have different effects on different people. The presence or absence of a drug, by itself, does not confirm the presence of an SUD or a drug-free existence. Neither does a positive or negative drug test determine wellness or illness. Finally, drug testing cannot reveal whether a patient is using more or less medication than prescribed.

Even within these limitations, however, drug testing is far more accurate in detecting recent drug use than patients' self-reports. Modern laboratory-based testing for drugs of abuse meets the highest standards of analytical technology to produce reliably accurate findings and test results [11,13].

Other Methods of Patient Monitoring

Other sources and types of information that are useful in patient monitoring include the following [14,15]:

- Laboratory tests, such as the serum aspartate aminotransferase (AST), gamma-glutamyl ttransferase (GGT), carbohydrate-deficient transferrin (CDT), ethyl glucuronide (EtG), and urine drug screens (see Chapter 11 of this Handbook);
- The patient's record of keeping (or failing to keep) appointments for office visits, following up on referrals, or attending mutual support groups;
- Information on the patient's use of prescribed opioids or other medications, as documented in the state's Prescription Drug Monitoring Program (PDMP);
- Reports from family members (obtained with a signed release from the patient);
- Periodic status reports from professionals who are providing psychosocial therapies and other forms of support.

Patient self-reports can be useful indicators of treatment progress. The physician should ask about the frequency and intensity of symptoms such as pain or craving, especially during stressful periods such as holidays, celebrations, and major life changes. The patient should be asked to assign a rating between 1 and 10 (with 1 indicating *no symptoms* and 10 the *most intense symptoms* the patient can imagine), as well as how he or she felt over the preceding week.

In addition, the patient may be asked whether any episodes have caused particular problems. Identifying such patterns over time can be useful. Both the clinician and the patient can see that the patient's symptoms may fluctuate throughout the day and over longer periods, indicating the need to continue, adjust, supplement, or discontinue use of a particular therapy [16].

In patient monitoring, subjective symptoms are as important as objective clinical signs (such as body weight, pulse rate, temperature, blood pressure, and levels of drug metabolites in the bloodstream). With this information, the clinician can modify the treatment plan as needed, decide whether to continue pharmacotherapy or other forms of treatment, and address any co-occurring medical, psychiatric, and substance use issues [14].

Asking the patient to keep a log of signs and symptoms gives him or her a sense of participation in the treatment program and facilitates the physician's review of therapeutic progress and adverse events [15].

If the physician becomes concerned about a patient's behavior or clinical progress (or lack thereof), it usually is advisable to seek a consultation with an expert in the primary disorder for which the patient is being treated *as well as* an expert in addiction [13].

Conclusion

The optimal frequency of urine testing in pain management is yet to be determined. Nevertheless, it appears reasonable to conduct a urine assay at the beginning of engagement in treatment and then periodically as clinical concerns may arise, or as part of a pain program management policy and protocol. Because both chronic pain and addiction are chronic medical conditions, the frequency of testing should mirror the standard of frequency for other chronic medical disorders such as diabetes (A1C testing for diabetes is recommended to be performed on a quarterly basis) [17].

Finally, whenever an unexpected test result or other information is obtained, it is appropriate to refer the patient to an addiction specialist for a comprehensive assessment and evaluation. Identifying substance use disorders early and providing treatment promptly can only improve patient outcomes in the management of pain and addiction.

For More Information on the Topics Discussed:

American Society of Addiction Medicine (ASAM):

Parran TV Jr., McCormick RA, Delos Reyes CM. Assessment (Chapter 20). In RK Ries, DA Fiellin, SC Miller, R Saitz, eds. *The ASAM Principles of Addiction Medicine, Fifth Edition.* Philadelphia, PA: Wolters Kluwer; 2014.

Medscape.com:

www.medscape.com. Two course modules sponsored by the National Institute on Drug Abuse (NIDA) and posted on MedScape can be accessed at http://www.medscape.org/viewarticle/770687 and http://www.medscape.org/viewarticle/770440. Continuing medical education (CME) credits are available.

OpiodPrescribing.com:

www.opioidprescribing.com. Sponsored by the Boston University School of Medicine, with support from the federal Substance Abuse and Mental Health Services Administration (SAMHSA), this site presents course modules on various aspects of prescribing opioids for chronic pain. To view the list of courses and to register, go to http://www.opioidprescribing.com/overview. CME credits are available at no charge.

Prescriber's Clinical Support System for Opioids:

www.pcss-o.org. Sponsored by the American Academy of Addiction Psychiatry in collaboration with other specialty societies and with support from SAMHSA, the Prescriber's Clinical Support System for Opioids (PCSS-0) offers multiple resources—including live and recorded webinars—related to opioid prescribing and the diagnosis and management of opioid use disorders.

References

1. Heit HA, Gourlay DL. Using urine drug testing to support healthy boundaries in clinical care. *J Opioid Manag.* 2015 Jan–Feb;11(1):7–12.
2. Gareri J, Klein J, Koren G. Drug of abuse testing in meconium. *Clin Chima Acta* 2006;366:101–111.
3. Pragst F, Balikova MA. State of the art in hair analysis for detection of drug and alcohol abuse. *Clin Chim Acta* 2006;370:17–49.
4. Spiehler V. Hair analysis by immunologic methods from beginning to 2000. *Forensic Sci Int* 2000;107:249–259.
5. Crouch DJ. Oral fluid collection: The neglected variable in oral fluid testing. *Forensic Sci Int* 2005;150:165–173.

6. Kidwell DA, Holland JC, Arthanaselis S. Testing for drugs of abuse in saliva and sweat. *J Chromatogr B Biomed Sci Appl.* 1998;713:111–135.

7. Federal Register. *Notices,* Vol. 69, No. 71, 2004 April 3.

8. DuPont RL, Griffin DW, Siskin BR. Random drug tests at work: The probability of identifying frequent and infrequent users of illicit drugs. *J Addict Dis.* 1995;14:1–17.

9. Manchikanti L, Molia Y, Wargo BW, et al. Comparative evaluation of the accuracy of immunoassay with liquid chromatography tandem mass spectrometry of urine testing opiates and illicit drugs in chronic paint patients. *Pain Physician.* 2011;14:175–187.

10. Hammey-Stabler CA, Webster LR. *A Clinical Guide to Urine Drug Testing.* Stamford, CT: PharmaCom Group Ltd; 2008.

11. DuPont RL, Selvaka CS. Test to identify recent drug use. *American Psychiatric Press Textbook of Substance Abuse Treatment, 4th Edition.* Washington DC: American Psychiatric Press; 2007.

12. American Diabetes Association (ADA). Standards of Medical Care in Diabetes – 2014. *Diabetes Care.* 2014;37(Suppl 1):S14–S80.

13. Federation of State Medical Boards of the United States (FSMB). *Model Policy Guidelines for Opioid Addiction Treatment in the Medical Office.* Dallas, TX: The Federation; 2013.

14. Center for Substance Abuse Treatment (CSAT). *Clinical Guidelines for the Use of Buprenorphine in the Treatment of Opioid Addiction.* (Treatment Improvement Protocol [TIP] Series 40.) DHHS Publication No. [SMA] 04-3939. Rockville, MD: CSAT, Substance Abuse and Mental Health Services Administration; 2004.

15. Finch JW, Parran TV, Wilford BB, et al. Clinical, legal and ethical considerations in prescribing drugs with abuse potential (Chapter 111). In RK Ries, DA Fiellin, R Saitz, S Miller, eds. *The ASAM Principles of Addiction Medicine, Fifth Edition.* Philadelphia, PA: Lippincott, Williams & Wilkins; 2014.

16. National Institute on Drug Abuse (NIDA). *Principles of Drug Addiction Treatment, Third Edition.* (NIH Publication No. 12–4180.) Rockville, MD: NIDA, National Institutes of Health; 2012.

17. Fishman MJ, Mee-Lee D, Shulman GD, et al., eds. *Supplement to the ASAM Patient Placement Criteria on Pharmacotherapies for the Management of Alcohol Use Disorders.* Philadelphia, PA: Lippincott, Williams & Wilkins; 2010.

Chapter 13

Opioid Overdose Education, Prevention, and Management

BERND WOLLSCHLAEGER, M.D.

The United States is experiencing an epidemic of drug overdose (poisoning) deaths. Since 2000, the overall rate of overdose deaths has increased by 137%. This represents an increase of 6.5% in total overdose deaths in a single year. Moreover, 61% of the 47,000 overdose deaths in 2014 involved a prescription opioid or heroin—a 200% increase since the year 2000 [1,2].

Physicians and other health care professionals can make a major contribution toward reducing the toll of opioid overdose through the care they take in prescribing opioid analgesics and monitoring patient response, as well as their ability to identify and effectively address opioid overdose. Accordingly, this chapter provides a brief review of education, prevention and treatment approaches that are readily deployed in clinical practice.

Incidence and Prevalence of Opioid Overdose

Over the past two decades, the amount of opioid analgesics prescribed in the United States has quadrupled [3], yet there has not been a comparable increase in the number of Americans who report severe pain [4,5]. What has changed is the way many health care professionals prescribe opioid analgesics. In 2012, health care providers wrote 259 million prescriptions for opioid analgesics, enough for every American adult to receive a prescription [4]. Subsequently, nearly 2 million Americans aged 12 or older either abused or were dependent on opioids in 2013 [4]. As a result, the number of deaths associated with opioids nearly tripled between 1999 and 2014, when more than 28,000 persons in the United States died of opioid overdose [5,6]. Deaths from opioid overdoses among women increased by more than 400% between 1999 and 2010 [7], while overdoses among men increased by 237% in the same period (Figure 13.1) [8,9].

Most of those who died from prescription opioid overdose between 1999 and 2013 were between the ages of 25 and 54. In fact, this cohort experienced a higher rate of opioid overdose than any other age group. However, the overdose rate for adults aged 55–64 increased more than sevenfold during the same time period [2].

In a review of data on prescriptions dispensed over a five-year period, researchers from the Centers for Disease Control and Prevention (CDC) and the

Drug overdose death rates, United States, 2014*

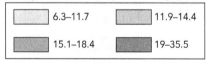

Drug overdose deaths per 100,000 population

	6.3–11.7		11.9–14.4
	15.1–18.4		19–35.5

*Age-adjusted death rate per 100,000 population

Figure 13.1 *Drug Overdose Death Rates, United States, 2014*

Source: CDC National Vital Statistics System, 2015.

U.S. Food and Drug Administration (FDA) found that practitioners in nine medical specialty groups accounted for 70.5% of all prescriptions written and 84.3% of opioid prescriptions. Orthopedic surgeons and dentists prescribed opioids at a higher rate than did primary care physicians. Physicians in other specialties, such as emergency medicine, initially had large increases in opioid prescribing, but in the years since 2010, emergency medicine experienced the greatest decline in opioid prescribing (–5.7%), followed by dentistry (–5.7%) and surgery (–3.9%) [3].

Data from the National Survey on Drug Use and Health [6] and the National Vital Statistics System [9] provide evidence that the dramatic increase in deaths caused by opioid overdose has been propelled in part by widespread use of heroin, often adulterated with illicitly manufactured versions of drugs such as fentanyl and carfentanyl. (According to data from the National Forensic Laboratory Information System, the number of fentanyl seizures was seven times higher in 2012 than in2014, with 4,585 fentanyl confiscations in 2014 alone [10].) Overall use of heroin in the United States increased by 63% from 2002 through 2013 [6,9], while the number of deaths associated with heroin overdose nearly quadrupled [6,9].

The increase in heroin-related deaths occurred across a broad range of demographic groups, including men and women, most age groups, and all income levels [9,11].

Assessing Patients' Risk of Opioid Overdose

Patient-centered opioid overdose prevention involves the use of risk stratification tools to identify patients who are at elevated risk of opioid abuse. This requires use of a structured approach in order to obtain a complete and comprehensive assessment of the patient, with particular attention to his or her risk for opioid abuse [12].

An essential step in appropriate prescribing is to compile a complete history of the patient's past use of drugs (either illicit drugs or prescribed medications with abuse potential). Obtaining such a history involves asking very specific questions. For example [1]:

- In the past six months, have you taken any medications to help you calm down, keep from getting nervous or upset, raise your spirits, make you feel better, and the like?
- Have you been taking any medications to help you sleep? Have you been using alcohol for this purpose?
- Have you ever taken a medication to help you with a drug or alcohol problem?
- Have you ever taken a medication for a nervous stomach?
- Have you taken a medication to give you more energy or to cut down on your appetite?

The patient history also should include questions about use of alcohol and over-the-counter (OTC) preparations. For example, the ingredients in many common cold preparations include alcohol and other central nervous system (CNS) depressants, so these products should not be used in combination with opioid analgesics.

Use of screening tools like those discussed in Chapter 8 of this Handbook also can be helpful. Positive answers to any of the history questions or screens warrant further investigation.

State Prescription Drug Monitoring Programs (PDMPs) have emerged as a key strategy for detecting the misuse and abuse of prescription opioids and thus preventing opioid overdoses and deaths. Specifically, prescribers can check their state's PDMP database to determine whether a patient is filling the prescriptions provided and/or or obtaining prescriptions for the same or similar drugs from other physicians [1].

PDMPs differ from one state to another in terms of the exact information collected, how soon that information is available to physicians, and who may access the data. Therefore, information about the program in a particular state is best obtained directly from the state's PDMP or Board of Medicine or Pharmacy [1].

Overdose Education and Prevention

Information for Patients and Caregivers

It is vital to inform patients about the risks and benefits of any medication prescribed, as well as the ethical and legal obligations such therapy imposes on both the physician and the patient [1,13].

Such informed consent can serve multiple purposes: (1) it provides the patient with information about the risks and benefits of opioid therapy; (2) it encourages adherence to the treatment plan; (3) it limits the potential for inadvertent drug misuse; and (4) it improves the efficacy of the treatment program.

Patient education and written informed consent should specifically address the potential for physical dependence and cognitive impairment as side effects of opioid analgesics. Other issues that should be addressed in the informed consent or treatment agreement include the following [1,13]:

- The patient is instructed to stop taking all other pain medications, unless explicitly told to continue by the physician. Such a statement reinforces the need to adhere to a treatment regimen overseen by a single clinician.
- The patient agrees to obtain prescriptions from only one physician and, if possible, to cash them at one designated pharmacy.

- The patient agrees to take the medication only as prescribed. (For some patients, it may be possible to offer latitude to adjust the dose as symptoms dictate.)
- The agreement makes it clear that the patient is responsible for safeguarding the written prescription and the supply of medications, as well as for arranging refills during regular office hours. This responsibility includes planning ahead so as not to run out of medication during weekends or vacation periods.
- The agreement specifies the consequences for failing to adhere to the treatment plan, which may include weaning and discontinuation of opioid therapy if the patient's actions compromise his or her safety.

In addition, some physicians provide patients with a laminated card that identifies the individual as a patient of their practice. This is helpful to other physicians who may see the patient and in the event the patient is seen in an emergency department [1].

Encouraging Public Awareness

Creating public awareness about opioid overdose provides the foundation for a continuous and extensive education and training program on how to manage and treat overdose victims [1]. Physicians should be reminded of studies showing that more than 90% of patients who overdosed continued to receive prescriptions for opioid analgesics [14].

The Opioid Overdose Toolkit published by the Substance Abuse and Mental Health Services Administration (SAMHSA) [1] is an essential resource for the education and training of naloxone prescribers and first responders. The Toolkit also contains step-by-step guidance for family members and patients on how to prevent and manage opioid overdose.

Overdose Management

Opioid overdose occurs when a patient accidentally or intentionally misuses a prescription opioid, a combination of various opioids, a combination of opioids with benzodiazepines or alcohol, or an illicit opioid such as heroin. It also can occur when a patient attempts to take an opioid as directed but misunderstands the directions for its use. Less common causes include instances in which the prescriber miscalculated the opioid dose or the pharmacist made an error in dispensing the prescribed drug.

Multiple cases of fatal opioid overdose have been associated with the use of fentanyl-laced heroin (often involving illicitly manufactured fentanyl or carfentanyl), which potentiates the effects of the heroin. In 2014, law enforcement officials cited heroin laced with fentanyl as the drug suspected in at least 50 fatal opioid overdoses in Pennsylvania, Maryland, and Michigan [14].

Clinical Presentation

Physical signs of *opioid intoxication* include slurred speech, abnormal behavior, lack of coordination, constricted pupils, and constipation. Other effects include euphoria followed by apathy and impaired judgment. Although the initial effects of opioids generally are calming or dulling, psychomotor agitation and aggressiveness can occur.

Signs of *overmedication*, which may progress to overdose, include [1,15]:

- Unusual sleepiness or drowsiness;
- Mental confusion, slurred speech, or intoxicated behavior;
- Slow or shallow breathing;
- Pinpoint pupils;
- Slow heartbeat and/or low blood pressure; and
- Difficulty waking the individual from sleep.

The most common signs of *opioid overdose* include [1,15]:

- Pale and clammy face;
- Limp body;
- Fingernails or lips turning blue or purple;
- Vomiting or gurgling noises;
- Inability to wake the individual from sleep or, when awakened, the person is unable to speak;
- Very little or no breathing; and
- Very slow or no heartbeat.

Immediate Response

Opioid overdose requires rapid action. Because opioids depress respiratory function and breathing, one telltale sign of an individual in a critical medical state is the "death rattle." Often mistaken for snoring, this sound results from an exhaled breath combined with a very distinct, labored sound coming from the throat. It indicates that emergency resuscitation is required immediately [1,16].

Supporting the patient's respiration is the single most important intervention for opioid overdose and may be life-saving on its own. Ideally, individuals who are experiencing opioid overdose should be ventilated with 100% oxygen before naloxone is administered to reduce the risk of acute lung injury [1,15,16].

If 100% oxygen is not available, *rescue breathing* can be very effective in supporting respiration [16]. Rescue breathing involves the following steps:

- Verify that the airway is clear.
- With one hand on the patient's chin, tilt the head back and pinch the nose closed.
- Place your mouth over the patient's mouth to make a seal and give two slow breaths (the patient's chest should rise, but not the stomach).
- Follow up with one breath every five seconds [1].

Use of Naloxone

In an effort to address the rising number of opioid overdose cases, emergency medical personnel, health care professionals, and patients are being trained in the use of naloxone, a short-acting, parenterally administered, full opioid antagonist with an extremely high affinity for mu-opioid receptors [1,16]. The FDA approved naloxone for this indication in 1971, and the drug is incorporated in the World Health Organization (WHO) List of Essential Medicines [17]. It is widely used by emergency medical services personnel and in emergency rooms across the United States and throughout the world [1,14].

Mechanism of Naloxone's Actions

Naloxone is metabolized in the liver, primarily through glucuronide conjugation, with naloxone-3-glucoronide the major metabolite. For this reason, dose adjustment is required in patients with liver disease, as assessed by the Child-Pugh Score [14–16].

Naloxone's rapid displacement of opioid agonists and blockade of mu-opioid receptors produces an immediate and rapid onset of withdrawal symptoms. It is rapidly distributed throughout the body and readily crosses the placenta. Plasma protein binding occurs but is relatively weak. Plasma albumin is the major binding constituent, but significant binding of naloxone also occurs to plasma constituents other than albumin. It is not known whether naloxone is excreted in human milk [16].

Naloxone Formulations

The following naloxone formulations are available on the U.S. market:

Naloxone hydrochloride (injectable) is available as a sterile solution for intravenous, intramuscular, and subcutaneous administration in 1 mg/mL concentration. It is commercially available as 2 mL single-dose disposable prefilled syringes, in the Min-I-Jet® system or Luer-Jet® Luer-Lock prefilled syringe [16–18].

Naloxone also can be administered *intranasally*, using an atomizer device that delivers a mist of naloxone to nasal mucus membranes [19]. *Narcan*® (naloxone HCl) nasal spray 4 mg is the first and (to date) only FDA-approved nasal formulation of naloxone for use in treating a known or suspected opioid overdose. Nasal injection requires a higher concentration of the drug, at one milligram per milliliter. Its ease of use provides a viable option for at-home opioid overdose rescue by family members and non–emergency services (EMS) personnel [19–21].

The Evzio® epi-pen, which provides an injection of 0.4 mg naloxone, was the first commercially available handheld auto-injector that could be carried in a pocket or stored in a medicine cabinet. Evzio is injected into the muscle (intramuscular) or under the skin (subcutaneous) [21]. Once turned on, the device provides oral instructions, guiding the user in how to deliver the medication, in a manner similar to automated defibrillators. Family members or caregivers should become familiar with all instructions for use before administering to an individual known or suspected to have had an opioid overdose [1].

Naloxone Dosing

An initial dose of 0.4–0.8 mg of naloxone effectively and quickly reverses cardiorespiratory and neurological depression caused by most opioids. When administered intravenously, naloxone takes effect within one to two minutes; when injected into a muscle, it takes effect within five minutes. Naloxone's effects lasts 30–90 minutes, and multiple doses may be required to completely reverse the opioid effect [1,15,16].

Overdoses that involve highly potent opioids (such as fentanyl) or long-acting opioids (such as methadone) may require higher or more frequent doses of naloxone. Patients who fail to respond to multiple doses of naloxone require reassessment as to the cause of their respiratory depression.

Naloxone's Side Effects

Side effects of treatment with naloxone are the symptoms of naloxone-induced opioid withdrawal, including body ache, diarrhea, rapid heartbeat, fever, runny nose, sneezing, sweating, yawning, nausea, vomiting, nervousness, restlessness, irritability, shivering or trembling, stomach cramps, and weakness. In rare cases, ventricular fibrillation, cardiac arrest, and seizures have occurred [16,20,21].

Monitoring the Patient's Response

Patients should be monitored for reemergence of signs and symptoms of opioid toxicity for at least four hours following the last dose of naloxone [1,16].

Most patients respond to naloxone by returning to spontaneous breathing, with mild withdrawal symptoms [16]. The response generally occurs within three to five minutes of naloxone administration. (Rescue breathing should continue while waiting for the naloxone to take effect.)

The duration of effect of naloxone is 30–90 minutes [1]. Patients should be observed after that time for re-emergence of overdose symptoms. The goal of naloxone therapy should be to restore adequate spontaneous breathing, but not necessarily complete arousal [16].

More than one dose of naloxone may be required to revive the patient. Those who have taken longer-acting opioids such as methadone may require further intravenous bolus doses or an infusion of naloxone [16]. Therefore, it is essential to get the person to an emergency department or other source of acute care as quickly as possible, even if he or she responds to the initial dose of naloxone and seems to feel better [1].

Supportive Measures

Whenever possible, general supportive measures—including cardiorespiratory maintenance and stabilization—should be initiated at the same time naloxone is administered [1]. Careful and frequent monitoring of the patient's cardiorespiratory and neurological status is essential until the patient is stabilized and other contributing factors can be excluded or controlled [16].

Other Considerations

Since 2014, the purchase price for Narcan®—the most widely used injectable and intranasal formulations of naloxone—has increased by more than 50% [22]. For this reason, health care professionals face an obvious challenge in finding ways to make naloxone more widely available to individuals who can help save lives (overdose victims cannot administer naloxone to themselves).

To avoid legal challenges, prescribers should employ two different prescription options for overdose prevention and management. These are standing orders (also referred to as non–patient-specific orders) and third-party prescriptions [23,24].

Standing orders generally allow the prescriber to write an order covering administration of a medication by a person other than the patient, who may be unknown to the prescriber at the time of the order. Whenever a patient meets certain criteria, a qualified health care professional, acting under the order, can administer the medication without the physician personally examining the patient. (Examples include influenza vaccinations administered by school nurses.)

A *third-party prescription* is an order written for a medication dispensed to one person with the intention that it will be administered to another person [23,24]. In the context of naloxone, a third-party prescription could be given to a family member of an individual at risk for opioid overdose. The recipient would have the prescription filled in his or her own name so that it is immediately available in the event the at-risk patient actually overdoses.

In the past, state medical practice acts often were ambiguous regarding the reach of standing orders and generally discouraged or prohibited third-party prescriptions. However, concern over the recent escalation in the number of overdose deaths has led a large number of states to pass laws that explicitly permit third-party prescriptions and standing orders for naloxone (see Figure 13.2) [23,24].

Other suggestions for increasing access to naloxone include an application by the manufacturer to make it available as an over-the-counter drug and

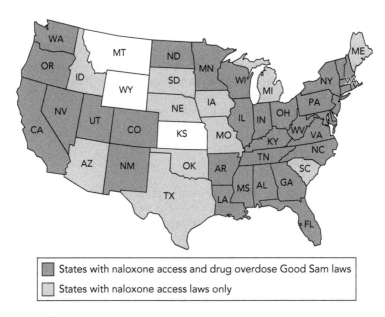

Legend:
- States with naloxone access and drug overdose Good Sam laws
- States with naloxone access laws only

Figure 13.2 *States That Have Adopted Laws to Improve Access to Naloxone, 2016*

Source: Davis C, Chang S, Carr D. Legal interventions to reduce overdose mortality: Naloxone access and overdose Good Samaritan laws. The Network for Public Health Law. 2016. (Accessed at: https://www.networkforphl.org/_asset/qz5pvn/network-naloxone-10-4.pdf.). Reprinted by permission of The Network for Public Health Law.

expanded pharmacy distribution models to provide this lifesaving medication to those who need it most [24].

Conclusion

An opioid overdose is a life-changing and traumatic event. Those who survive an overdose are forced to cope with emotional, personal, and physical consequences. Survivors need medical assistance with immediate (and often prolonged) opioid withdrawal and craving [1].

Most important, they need the support of family and friends to enter and sustain long-term recovery and overdose prevention. Many suffer from untreated chronic pain and substance use disorder and require medication-assisted treatment and nonpharmacological therapies, as well as participation in a mutual support group. Thus it is crucial to involve family members in the recovery and support process [1].

Overdose survivors should be referred to an addiction specialist who offers office-based opioid treatment (OBOT) or to a Federally certified opioid treatment program (OTP) for inpatient or outpatient care [1,13].

The opioid overdose epidemic forces us to create and expand medical treatments for this life-threatening condition, as well as to encourage public–private partnerships that engage medical professionals, families and concerned community members. As citizens, we need to challenge local, state, and Federal agencies to provide access to effective, affordable overdose treatments and to develop and expand education and prevention resources for patients, as well as training resources for health care professionals, first responders, and caregivers in how to employ these life-saving measures.

Note: Federally funded CME courses on opioid overdose are available at no charge at www.OpioidPrescribing.com *(five courses funded by the Substance Abuse and Mental Health Services Administration) and on MedScape (two courses funded by the National Institute on Drug Abuse).*

For More Information on the Topics Discussed:

American Society of Addiction Medicine (ASAM):

Clark AK, Wilder CM, Winstanley EL. A systematic review of community opioid overdose prevention and naloxone distribution programs (Chapter 30—Sidebar). In RK Ries, DA Fiellin, SC Miller, R Saitz, eds. *The ASAM Principles of Addiction Medicine, Fifth Edition.* Philadelphia, PA: Wolters Kluwer; 2014.

Finch JW, Parran TV Jr., Wilford BB, et al. Clinical, ethical, and legal considerations in prescribing drugs with abuse potential (Chapter 111). In RK

Ries, DA Fiellin, SC Miller, R Saitz, eds. *The ASAM Principles of Addiction Medicine, Fifth Edition.* Philadelphia, PA: Wolters Kluwer; 2014.

Substance Abuse and Mental Health Services Administration (SAMHSA):

Opioid Overdose Prevention Toolkit. SMA16-4742. Rockville, MD: SAMHSA, U.S. Department of Health and Human Services; 2016. (Access at or download from: http://store.samhsa.gov/product/Opioid-Overdose-Prevention-Toolkit-Updated-2016/SMA16-4742.)

References

1. Substance Abuse and Mental Health Services Administration (SAMHSA). *Opioid Overdose Toolkit.* Rockville, MD: SAMHSA, U.S. Department of Health and Human Services; 2014. (Accessed at: https://store.samhsa.gov/shin/content/SMA134742/Overdose_Toolkit_2014_Jan.pdf.)
2. Rudd RA, Aleshire N, Zibbell JE, et al. Increases in drug and opioid overdose deaths—United States, 2000–2014. *MMWR.* 2016 Jan 1;64(50):1378–1382. (Accessed at: https://www.cdc.gov/mmwr/preview/mmwrhtml/mm6450a3.htm.)
3. Levy B, Paulozzi L, Mack KA, et al. Trends in opioid analgesic prescribing rates by specialty, U.S., 2007–2012. *Am J Prev Med.* 2015;49(3):409–413.
4. Daubresse M, Chang H, Yu Y, et al. Ambulatory diagnosis and treatment of nonmalignant pain in the United States, 2000–2010. *Med Care.* 2013;51(10):870–878.
5. Rudd RA, Seth P, David F, et al. Increases in drug and opioid-involved overdose deaths—United States, 2010–2015. *MMWR.* 2016 Dec 30;65(5051):1445–1452.
6. Substance Abuse and Mental Health Services Administration (SAMHSA). *Results from the 2015 National Survey on Drug Use and Health: Summary of National Findings.* Rockville, MD: SAMHSA, U.S. Department of Health and Human Services; Dec. 2, 2016.
7. Centers for Disease Control and Prevention (CDC). Vital Signs: Overdoses of prescription opioid pain relievers and other drugs among women—United States, 1999–2010. *MMWR.* 2013;62(26);537–542.
8. Chen LH, Hedegaard H, Warner M. Drug-poisoning deaths involving opioid analgesics: United States, 1999–2011. *NCHS Data Brief No. 166.* Washington, DC: National Center for Health Statistics, U.S. Department of Health and Human Services; 2014.
9. Centers for Disease Control and Prevention (CDC). Vital Signs: Demographic and substance use trends among heroin users, United States, 2002–2013. *MMWR.* 2015 July 10;64(26);719–725.
10. Centers for Disease Control and Prevention (CDC). Increases in fentanyl drug confiscations and fentanyl-related overdose fatalities. *CDC Health Advisory.*

Atlanta, GA: CDC, U.S. Department of Health and Human Services; October 26, 2015. (Accessed at: http://emergency.cdc.gov/han/han00384.asp.)

11. Birnbaum HG, White AG, Schiller M, et al. Societal costs of prescription opioid abuse, dependence, and misuse in the United States. *Pain Med.* 2011;12:657–667.

12. Center for Substance Abuse Treatment (CSAT). *Clinical Guidelines for the Use of Buprenorphine in the Treatment of Opioid Addiction.* Rockville, MD: CSAT, Substance Abuse and Mental Health Services Administration; 2004. (Accessed at: http://www.ncbi.nlm.nih.gov/books/NBK64237/.)

13. Finch JW, Parran TV, Wilford BB, et al. Clinical, legal and ethical considerations in prescribing drugs with abuse potential (Chapter 109). In Ries RK, Alford DP, Saitz R, Miller S, eds. *Principles of Addiction Medicine, Fifth Edition.* Philadelphia, PA: Lippincott, Williams & Wilkins; 2013.

14. LaRochelle MR, Liebschutz JM, Zhang F, et al. Opioid prescribing after non-fatal overdose and association with repeated overdose: A cohort study. *Ann Intern Med.* 2016;164(1):1–9.

15. Beletsky L, Rich JD, Walley AY. Prevention of fatal opioid overdose. *JAMA.* 2012 Nov 14;308(18):1863–1864.

16. Walley AY, Xuan Z, Hackman HH, et al. Opioid overdose rates and implementation of overdose education and nasal naloxone distribution in Massachusetts: interrupted time series analysis. *BMJ* 2013;346:f174. http://www.bmj.com/content/346/bmj.f174

17. World Health Organizations (WHO). *Model List of Essential Medicines.* Geneva, Switzerland: WHO; 2013. (Accessed at: http://www.who.int/selection_medicines/committees/expert/20/EML_2015_FINAL_amended_AUG2015.pdf?ua=1.)

18. Food and Drug Administration (FDA). FDA News Release: FDA approves new hand-held auto-injector to reverse opioid overdose. Rockville, MD: FDA, U.S. Department of Health and Human Services; 2014 April 3. (Accessed at: http://www.fda.gov/NewsEvents/Newsroom/PressAnnouncements/ucm391465.htm.)

19. Robertson TM, Henley GW, Stroh G, et al. Intranasal naloxone is a viable alternative to intravenous naloxone for prehospital narcotic overdose. *Prehosp Emerg Care.* 2009 Oct–Dec;13(4):512–516.

20. Sporer KA. Acute heroin overdose. *Ann Intern Med.* 1999 Apr 6;130(7):584–590.

21. Anonymous. Narcan nasal spray. Radnor, PA: Adapt Pharma; 2016. (Accessed at: http://intranasal.net/OpiateOverdose.)

22. Anonymous. Naloxone. Drugs.com. 2016. (Accessed at: http://www.drugs.com/pro/naloxone.html.)

23. Davis C, Chang S, Carr D. Legal interventions to reduce overdose mortality: Naloxone access and overdose Good Samaritan laws. *The Network for Public Health Law,* 2016. (Accessed at: https://www.networkforphl.org/_asset/qz5pvn/network-naloxone-10-4.pdf.)

24. Fehn J. Issue Brief: Using law to support pharmacy naloxone distribution. *The Network for Public Health Law,* 2014. (Accessed at: https://www.networkforphl.org_asset/qdkn97/Pharmacy-Naloxone-Distributions.pdf.)

SECTION III

TREATING PAIN IN PATIENTS DIAGNOSED WITH, OR AT RISK FOR, CO-OCCURRING ADDICTION

The chapters in **Section III** address the challenges involved in treating pain in patients who either have been diagnosed with a co-occurring substance use disorder—especially one involving opioids—or who appear to be at risk for such a disorder.

- In **Chapter 14**, the authors review opioid pharmacotherapies approved by the U.S. Food and Drug Administration for the management of chronic pain, as well as some agents that are used off-label, such as buprenorphine. The review includes the relative advantages and disadvantages of each agent, as well as any strong indications or clear contraindications.
- The author of **Chapter 15** discusses non-opioid pharmacotherapies for chronic pain, which are appropriate for many pain patients, particularly those at risk for opioid use disorder.
- Non-pharmacological therapies that usually are administered under the supervision of a health care professional are described in **Chapter 16**.
- Approaches to pain treatment that can be self-administered by patients are the subject of **Chapter 17**.
- The authors of **Chapter 18** discuss situations in which the pain treatment plan may need to be revised, or pain treatment ended and the patient referred for other types of care.

Chapter 14

Opioid Pharmacotherapies for Chronic Pain

THIEN C. PHAM, PHARM.D., COURTNEY KOMINEK, PHARM.D., BCPS, CPE, ABIGAIL BROOKS, PHARM.D., BCPS, AND JEFFREY FUDIN, PHARM.D., DAIPM, FCCP, FASHP

Given the need to balance risks and benefits, how do physicians decide who should receive an opioid analgesic for pain? Are opioids more likely to be prescribed for some patients than for others? How can physicians organize their practices to afford protection to themselves and their patients as they pursue the optimal management of pain? This chapter provides a succinct overview of the best available information, while online Appendix B of this Handbook suggests sources of additional information (Box 14.1).

Balancing the Risks and Benefits of Opioid Analgesics

It is a fundamental principle of medicine that the use of any treatment makes sense only when the benefits to the patient outweigh the risks and negative side effects. *Benefit* is suggested when the patient experiences a significant increase in his or her level of functioning, a reduction in or elimination of pain, a more positive and hopeful attitude, and when side effects are minimal or controllable.

BOX 14.1 Related Figures and Tables in Online Appendix B of This Handbook

Online Appendix Figure B-1. Opioid Receptor Affinity and Activity
Online Appendix Figure B-2. Relationship of Opioid Dose to Respiratory Depression
Online Appendix Table B-1. Opioid Metabolism and Detection Times
Online Appendix Table B-2. Opioid Pharmacogenetics in Pain Management
Online Appendix Table B-3. Opioid-Related Adverse Effects
Online Appendix Table B-4. Comparison of Oral Drug Formulations That Deter or Prevent Misuse and Abuse

Risks of opioids include tolerance, hyperalgesia (abnormal sensitivity to pain), hormonal effects (reduced testosterone levels or libido, irregular menses), depression, and suppression of the immune system.

Without careful attention to the balance between risks and benefits, a physician may prescribe opioids to reduce a patient's pain and improve function, but the effect on the patient may be quite the opposite [1].

Actions of Selected Opioids

In order to use opioids effectively and safely when they are indicated, physicians must understand the pharmacological and clinical issues related to opioids and carefully structure a treatment plan that reflects the particular benefits and risks of opioid use for each individual patient. Understanding the mechanisms of action of the various opioid analgesics is key to developing such a plan.

Opioids interact with mu, delta, and kappa receptors in the brain, which are responsible for opioids' analgesic effects as well as associated adverse events (see online Appendix B, Table B-3). Mu-opioid receptors, which are prototypical receptors, are involved with analgesia, respiratory depression, and euphoria. In contrast, dysphoria or analgesia may occur with kappa-opioid receptors, depending on the receptor subtype involved [2].

Opioids act on different types of receptors and can affect those receptors in different ways; for example, as an agonist, partial agonist, antagonist, or agonist/antagonist (see online Appendix B, Figure B-1).

Pure opioid agonists wrap around the receptor tightly. With increasing doses of an opioid agonist, there is increasing analgesia and respiratory depression. Partial agonists result in receptor activation, but to a lesser extent than full opioid agonists. As the dose of a partial agonist increases, its activity eventually plateaus.

Buprenorphine and other partial agonists are safer options for patients who have respiratory conditions because there is a limit to the amount of carbon dioxide that can accumulate and thus a ceiling to respiratory depression.

Agonists/antagonists include pentazocine, which is an agonist at some opioid receptors and an antagonist at others. Naloxone falls into the category of opioid antagonists, which occupy the receptor but do not lead to receptor activity [2].

Buprenorphine and—to a lesser extent—methadone also have high affinity for the opioid receptor. This is clinically useful because other (higher potency, lower affinity) opioids cannot out-compete buprenorphine and methadone for the opioid receptor. Clinically, what this means is that individuals who are on medication-assisted therapy (MAT) with methadone and buprenorphine find high-potency opioids much less euphoric and reinforcing, because the high affinity of methadone and buprenorphine make it relatively difficult for other opioids to bind to the receptor.

The effect of any given opioid can vary markedly, depending on whether or not it is injected (which yields a very fast onset and short duration of action) or given orally (producing a slower onset and longer duration of action), or the drug formulation is altered by embedding the active ingredient in a matrix of insoluble substances so that intestinal absorption is further delayed (leading to even slower onset and longer duration of action); see Table 14.1.

Use of Opioids for Neuropathic Pain

Opioids such as methadone, levorphanol, tapentadol, and tramadol possess analgesic properties that make them suitable treatments for various neuropathic pain syndromes.

Methadone

Methadone is a racemic mixture of R- and S-enantiomers, which are extensively metabolized by the cytochrome (CYP) 450 system. This occurs primarily through CYP3A4 and CYP2B6, with CYP2D6 and CYP2C19 having minimal roles in hepatic metabolism [3]. R-methadone exhibits the preferential mu-opioid agonist analgesic properties and is metabolized predominantly by CYP3A4, while S-methadone is associated with adverse effects such as QTc prolongation and is metabolized by CYP2B6 [3].

Methadone has several characteristics that make it an attractive analgesic for the management of chronic pain. It has good oral bioavailability, high potency, no active metabolite, slow onset to withdrawal syndrome, multiple routes of administration, and an array of analgesic activities consisting of mu-opioid receptor agonism, N-methyl-D-aspartate (NMDA) receptor antagonism,

TABLE 14.1 Classification of Commonly Used Opioid Analgesics

Classification	Opioid Analgesic	Duration of Action (in hours)
Short-acting opioids (SAOs)	Morphine	3–6
	Hydromorphone	3–6
	Oxycodone	4–6
Longer-acting opioids (LAOs)	Controlled-Release (CR) Morphine	8–12
	Controlled-Release (CR) Hydromorphone	8–12
	Controlled-Release (CR) Oxycodone	8–12
Very long-acting opioids (VLAOs)	Methadone	24–36
	Buprenorphine	48–72

Source: Presumably Pham TC; Dr. Pham co-authored an article which features a longer version of this table, http://opioidremsresource.com/articles/exploring-use-chronic-opioid-therapy-chronic-pain-when-how-and-whom#Treatmentinitiationtitrationandmaintenance.

and norepinephrine (NE) reuptake inhibition, making it ideal for neuropathic pain [3].

However, methadone also has limitations, which include variable pharmacokinetics and analgesic response, the need to titer doses very slowly (e.g., no more often than once every seven days), as well as phase I drug interactions, risk of QTc prolongation, and variable opioid dose conversions. Therefore, it is recommended that methadone be prescribed for pain only by clinicians who are very experienced with its use [4].

Levorphanol

Levorphanol is a potent NMDA antagonist. It possesses a higher affinity than methadone for the delta and kappa opioid receptors, and also has a shorter, more predictable plasma half-life (11–16 hours) and longer duration of action than methadone. Moreover, it has no CYP450 or P-gp interactions or associated risk of QTc prolongation [3].

Levorphanol does not require CYP 450 metabolism; instead, it undergoes phase II metabolism to a 3-glucuronide product that is eliminated through the kidneys, which is similar to the phase II metabolic step of other dehydroxylated phenanthrene opioids such as hydrocodone, hydromorphone, oxycodone, and oxymorphone [3].

Tramadol

Tramadol is a racemic mixture of active R-, R- and S-, and S-tramadol metabolites with mu-opioid agonist and weak NE and serotonin (5-HT) reuptake inhibition activity [5].

Unfortunately, tramadol requires CYP2D6 metabolism to its active form (o-desmethyl-tramadol [M1]) in order to achieve clinically relevant binding affinity to the mu-opioid receptor (MOR) [5]. Consequently, tramadol's analgesic efficacy may be hindered, which may increase the risk of adverse effects (such as seizures), rendering it a less than desirable analgesic option.

Tapentadol

Tapentadol possesses mu-opioid agonist and NE reuptake inhibition activity in the parent form, but with a 5-HT activity that is five times less potent than that of tramadol [5]. Unlike tramadol, tapentadol does not require CYP 450 metabolism, as it undergoes phase II metabolism to a non-active metabolite (tapentadol-O-glucuronide) [5]. As a result, variability in genetics, metabolism, and efficacy seldom occur in diverse patient populations.

Opioid Endocrinopathy

Chronic use of opioids and their effects on the hypothalamic-pituitary-gonadal axis (HPGA) and endocrine function have been well established in clinical studies, particularly with ER/LA opioids such as methadone [6,7]. The HPGA is a sophisticated biochemical system that regulates the release of sex hormones through an endogenous negative feedback mechanism that originates in the hypothalamus. Opioids affect the HPGA, where they inhibit the release of gonadotropin-hormone releasing hormone (GnRH), luteinizing hormone (LH), and follicle stimulating hormones (FSH), including testosterone and estrogen.

Specific symptoms arising from these hormonal effects include reduced libido and activity, erectile dysfunction, small or shrinking testes, lowered sperm count (possibly causing infertility), amenorrhea, and hot flashes [8]. Other symptoms include reduced energy, motivation, initiative, and self-confidence; depressed mood; poor concentration and memory; and diminished physical performance [8]. As a result of these hormonal side effects from long-term opioid therapy, quality of life may be diminished for a patient living with a chronic pain syndrome. In such cases, hormone replacement therapy may be considered [9].

Androgen deficiency also can be a problem with opioid analgesics. Given their partial opioid agonist activity, tramadol, tapentadol, and buprenorphine may exert fewer hormonal effects than the pure opioid agonists.

The Morphine-Equivalent Daily Dose

Opioid-related adverse effects, including overdose, have been widely reported over the years, as has the correlation between adverse effects and the morphine-equivalent daily dose, or MEDD. As a result, the Centers for Disease Control and Prevention (CDC) [1] and other health care organizations have published clinical guidelines and recommendations (see online Appendix D) that focus on minimizing opioid-related risks. In addition, multiple states and health care institutions have implemented opioid safety initiatives or stewardship programs to minimize and prevent risks associated with high-dose opioids. Most base their recommendations on the MEDD.

However, the MEDD is not without its own limitations, given that there are no current consensus guidelines for safe, accurate, and consistent opioid conversions when calculating doses [10]. Further, given genetic polymorphisms and assessments for individualized therapy, an individual's clinical response to opioids may be variable and should not be based on the MEDD alone [11].

Extended-Release/Long-Acting (ER/LA) Opioids

When used appropriately, ER/LA agents may provide more consistent analgesia over a 24-hour period and may be safer options compared to immediate-release (IR) formulations, with their blunted peak serum concentration (Cmax). However, according to the CDC's 2016 guideline [1], if an ER/LA opioid is under consideration, agents with predictable pharmacokinetics and pharmacodynamics are preferred in order to minimize unintentional overdose risk. Furthermore, only clinicians who are familiar with methadone's complex pharmacokinetics, as well as the absorption properties of transdermal fentanyl, should consider prescribing them [1].

Abuse-Deterrent Technology (ADT)

Abuse-deterrent opioid formulations are novel options that employ mechanistic barriers to misuse and abuse, in addition to limiting the user's ability to achieve a rapid euphoric effect [12]. ADT strategies include the following:

- Physical barriers used to "shelter" or "entrap" the active drug and control or avert enhancement of delivery;
- Viscosity management with excipients such as water-soluble/swellable cellulose derivatives, polyethylene oxide, gums, clays, and polyacid carbomers that gel or increase in viscosity when the product is crushed and mixed in water or other solvents;
- Aversive agents, which incorporate elements that produce "unpleasant and very noxious effects" in those who intentionally tamper with the product;
- Opioid antagonists that incorporate a sequestered antagonist or un-sequestered naloxone; aversive agents such as laxatives, cutaneous vasodilators, emetics and nauseants, bittering agents; and
- Mucous membrane irritants, which are designed to discourage nonmedical use and reduce the desirability of a tampered product [12].

In online Appendix B, Table B-4 illustrates various mechanisms that have been developed to deter abuse and manipulation of drug delivery.

Ideal candidates for opioids featuring ADT include, but are not limited to, high-risk patients such as those who have a history of SUD (especially abuse of heroin or prescription opioids), elderly patients, or patients whose living conditions may make them targets for theft [13].

At present, there is no clinical evidence to support the effectiveness of ADTs as a lone risk-mitigation agent for deterring or preventing opioid misuse or abuse. Nor do ADTs alone prevent unintentional overdose via the oral administration route. Nevertheless, ADTs can contribute to a comprehensive safety plan that also involves careful patient screening and development of a clear treatment plan, with appropriate monitoring and timely follow-up.

Challenges in Prescribing Opioids for Pain

Challenges that arise when exploring the use of opioids to treat patients include the following [2]:

- *Inaccurate or incomplete marketing to and education of health care professionals and the public about opioids.* Very few drugs have been more heavily marketed to health care professionals and the public than brand-name opioids. This has led to widespread misunderstanding of the pharmacology, safety, and long-term effectiveness of these agents.

- *Opioid effects differ substantially from one individual to another.* Patients who have post-traumatic stress disorder (PTSD), anxiety, depression, and the like have been shown to experience significant changes in the amygdala, hippocampus, and other areas of the limbic system. This is precisely the region of the brain where opioids exert their effects—both analgesic and addictive [14]. This may explain why a disproportionate number of persons with these medical conditions are vulnerable to the addictive potential of opioids.

- *Opioid effects differ substantially, depending on the duration of use.* Most of our understanding of the risks and benefits of opioids is derived from short-term studies whose duration averaged 4–8 weeks [15]. Yet chronic pain patients often are treated with opioids for many months or even years [1]. There is good clinical and research evidence that opioid effects differ dramatically when used for a short versus a long term. Clinically, this means that the short-term desirable effects of opioids (such as improvements in pain, euphoria, etc.) often are very different from—and occasionally the exact opposite of—the harmful effects that occur with long-term use (including hyperalgesia, dysphoria, withdrawal, etc.).

- *Physical dependence on opioids typically develops after a relatively short period of use.* Physical dependence on an opioid reflects a physiological state in which abrupt cessation of the drug, administration of an opioid antagonist, or precipitous lowering of the drug dose will result in a withdrawal syndrome. Such dependence is an expected occurrence in all patients (both those with and without an SUD) after 2–10 days of continuous administration of an opioid [16]. In a patient with acute pain, such dependence generally is not clinically significant, because individuals tend to taper opioids naturally in parallel with gradual reduction in pain as the acute problem (such as post-surgical pain, post-traumatic pain, or medical illness) resolves. However, if pain medications are precipitously reduced or abruptly stopped, a withdrawal syndrome may emerge. The character and intensity of such withdrawal varies, depending on the dose and duration of opioid administration and a variety of host factors.

- *Polymorphisms of the genes that code for the mu-receptor proteins can significantly alter pain tolerance and the risk of addiction.* Murine strains that are bred to have mu receptors with increased opioid binding activity exhibit higher pain tolerance and are more resistant to the reinforcing effects of opioids.

- *The pathophysiology of pain and addiction overlap.* Understanding the concepts of "analgesic tone" and "hedonic tone" can help us appreciate why there is such a significant overlap in the pathophysiology of pain and addiction. The pain literature uses the term *analgesic tone* to describe the ways in which the central nervous system (particularly the limbic system) can enhance or inhibit the experience of pain. This explains why individuals can and do experience different levels of pain from exactly the same pain-inducing experience. Before the brain consciously experiences pain, it is processed by the CNS in ways that can alter both the amount of pain experienced and the level of distress that a given amount of pain will cause. Similarly, an individual's level of *hedonic tone* may affect the severity of the emotional distress and suffering associated with a given event.

The limbic system of the brain plays a key role in mediating *both* hedonic and analgesic tone and also is the principal region of the brain where opioids exert their action. Because of their powerful effect at the receptors in the limbic system, opioids have a remarkable capacity to alter both hedonic and analgesic tone. In fact, the use of opioids in an individual who is addicted to them can be described as an attempt to alter hedonic tone, while the use of opioids to treat pain can be defined as an attempt to alter analgesic tone. The reality is that hedonic tone and analgesic tone are to some extent inseparable, and opioids inevitably affect both.

Conclusion

Opioids have an important role in relieving human suffering. They also have the potential to cause harm. This duality has provoked confusion and concern on the part of policymakers and the public. In addition, it has presented physicians and other caregivers with the dilemma of how to balance the comfort of their patients against the risk that a prescribed opioid will be misused by a patient or given or sold to others. The resulting problems of under- and over-prescribing—which often are described as an "imbalance" in opioid prescribing—pose a major quality assurance and risk-management issue for all physicians.

For More Information on the Topics Discussed:

American Society of Addiction Medicine (ASAM):

Prickett W, Copenhaver DJ, Fishman SM. Legal and regulatory considerations in opioid prescribing (Chapter 99). In RK Ries, DA Fiellin, SC Miller, R Saitz, eds. *The ASAM Principles of Addiction Medicine, Fifth Edition*. Philadelphia, PA: Wolters Kluwer; 2014.

Savage SR. Opioid therapy of pain (Chapter 97). In RK Ries, DA Fiellin, SC Miller, R Saitz, eds. *The ASAM Principles of Addiction Medicine, Fifth Edition*. Philadelphia, PA: Wolters Kluwer; 2014.

Centers for Disease Control and Prevention (CDC):

CDC Guideline for Prescribing Opioids for Chronic Pain. Atlanta, GA: Centers for Disease Control and Prevention; 2016. CDC developed and published this guideline to provide recommendations for the prescribing of opioid pain medication for patients 18 and older in primary care settings. Recommendations focus on the use of opioids in treating chronic pain (pain lasting longer than three months or past the time of normal tissue healing) outside of active cancer treatment, palliative care, and end-of-life care. (Access at: https://www.cdc.gov/drugoverdose/prescribing/guideline.html.)

Acknowledgment and Disclosures

The authors acknowledge with gratitude the valuable contributions to this chapter by Christopher Cavacuiti, M.D., CCFP, M.H.Sc., DFASAM, FCFP, FABAM.

Disclosures: This commentary is the sole opinion of the authors and does not reflect the opinion of employers, employee affiliates, and/or pharmaceutical companies mentioned or specific drugs discussed. It was not prepared as part of official government duties for Drs. Brooks, Kominek, or Pham. Dr. Fudin discloses the following industry relationships: Astra Zeneca (speaker's bureau, advisory board); DepoMed (advisory board); Endo (speaker's bureau, consultant); Kaléo (speaker's bureau, advisory board); Kashiv Pharm (consultant); KemPharm (consultant); Millennium Health LLC (speaker's bureau); Pernix; Remitigate LLC (founder, owner); and Scilex Pharmaceuticals (consultant). Participation by any of the authors does not reflect the opinion of employers, employee affiliates, and/or pharmaceutical companies listed.

References

1. Dowell D, Haegerich TM, Chou R. CDC Guideline for Prescribing Opioids for Chronic Pain—United States, 2016. *JAMA.* 2016 Apr 19;315(15):1624–1645.
2. Cavacuiti C. Personal communication, May 25, 2017.
3. Pham TC, Fudin J, Raffa RB. Is levorphanol a better option than methadone? *Pain Med.* 2015 Sep;16(9):1673–1677.
4. Janicki PK. *Pharmacogenomics of Pain Management. Comprehensive Treatment of Chronic Pain by Medical, Interventional, and Integrative Approach.* Chicago, IL: American Academy of Pain Medicine; 2013.
5. Raffa RB, Buschmann H, Christoph T, et al. Mechanistic and functional differentiation of tapentadol and tramadol. *Expert Opin Pharmacother.* 2012 Jul;13(10):1437–1449.

6. Daniell HW. Hypogonadism in men consuming sustained-action oral opioids. *J Pain*. 2002 Oct;3(5):377–384.

7. Daniell HW. Opioid endocrinopathy in women consuming prescribed sustained-action opioids for control of nonmalignant pain. *J Pain*. 2008 Jan;9(1):28–36.

8. Smith HS. Opioid metabolism. *Mayo Clin Proc*. 2009 Jul;84(7):613–624.

9. Bhasin S, Cunningham GR, Hayes FJ, et al. Testosterone therapy in men with androgen deficiency syndromes: An Endocrine Society clinical practice guideline. *J Clin Endocrinol Metab*. 2010 Jun;95(6):2536–2559.

10. Rennick A, Atkinson T, Cimino NM, et al. Variability in opioid equivalence calculations. *Pain Med*. 2016 May 1;17(5):892–898.

11. Fudin J, Pratt Cleary J, Schatman ME. The MEDD myth: The impact of pseudoscience on pain research and prescribing-guideline development. *J Pain Res*. 2016;9:153–156.

12. Mastropietro DJ, Omidian H. Abuse-deterrent formulations: Part 1— Development of a formulation-based classification system. *Expert Opin Drug Metab Toxicol*. 2015 Feb;11(2):193–204.

13. Stanos SP, Bruckenthal P, Barkin RL. Strategies to reduce the tampering and subsequent abuse of long-acting opioids: Potential risks and benefits of formulations with physical or pharmacologic deterrents to tampering. *Mayo Clin Proc*. 2012 Jul;87(7):683–694.

14. Juurlink DN, Dhalla IA. Dependence and addiction during chronic opioid therapy. *J Med Toxicol*. 2012;8(4):393–399.

15. Earnshaw V, Smith L, Copenhaver M. Drug addiction stigma in the context of methadone maintenance therapy: An investigation into understudied sources of stigma. *Int J Ment Health Addict*. 2013;11(1):110–122.

16. Portenoy RK, Hagen NA. Breakthrough pain: Definition, prevalence and characteristics. *Pain*. 1990 Jun;41(3):273–281.

Chapter 15

Non-Opioid Pharmacotherapies for Chronic Pain

JAMES A. D. OTIS, M.D., FAAN, DABPM

Medications can provide effective pain management in most patients. Choosing the appropriate medication requires that the pain state be correctly diagnosed and classified as somatic, visceral, or neuropathic.

Non-steroidal anti-inflammatory drugs (NSAIDs) and opioids are the principal medications for somatic pain, while adjuvant medications such as antidepressants, anticonvulsant/antiepileptic drugs (AEDs), anesthetics, and adrenergic agents are useful for neuropathic pain. Severe pain, whether somatic or neuropathic, usually requires opioid therapy.

Once the appropriate class of medication has been selected, the choice of a specific drug is determined by its side effects, route of administration, and individual patient characteristics. Balancing the benefits of a drug with the patient's ability to take it is the art of drug therapy. Other treatment modalities include interventional techniques and physical modalities. In the management of chronic pain, these are adjuncts to primary therapy and are not substitutes for pharmacotherapy.

This chapter provides an overview of these methods and their indications. (Psychosocial approaches, which are integral to a multidisciplinary approach to pain management, are reviewed in Chapter 3 of this Handbook. Use of opioid medications to treat pain is discussed in Chapter 14.)

Non-Opioid Pharmacotherapies

Many of the medications used to treat pain are not primarily analgesics, but have analgesic efficacy under certain conditions. Such medications are classified as *adjuvant analgesics*. They include AEDs, antidepressants, adrenergic agonists, local anesthetics, and muscle relaxants. Other medications are *primary analgesics*, but are not in the opioid class. Appropriate use of both types of medications can greatly improve analgesia as well as overall pain management.

Non-Steroidal Anti-Inflammatory Drugs (NSAIDs)

NSAIDS are the most widely used analgesics and are indicated to treat somatic pain of mild intensity. They are most useful in bone and joint pain, but also can be used in conjunction with opioids for all forms of pain. The first NSAID, aspirin, remains the model for all others. Newer compounds have the same presumed mechanism of action but offer advantages in their side effect profiles and ease of use.

Although the exact mechanism of NSAID analgesia is unclear, it is thought to be related to the inhibition of cyclo-oxygenase activity, which in turn inhibits prostaglandin production [1]. *Prostaglandins* sensitize peripheral nerve endings to noxious stimuli and are the key to the inflammatory cascade. There also is evidence that NSAIDs play a role in modulating pain in the central nervous system, particularly at the spinal cord level [2], independent of their anti-inflammatory action [3]. It is not clear which mechanism is more important clinically.

All NSAIDs are well absorbed in the gastrointestinal (GI) tract. Most undergo some hepatic conjugation and are excreted in urine. For this reason, hepatic and renal impairment can lead to drug accumulation, and doses need to be adjusted accordingly.

There is a ceiling level to the analgesic effect of NSAIDs, beyond which increasing doses do not improve analgesia. Unfortunately, this ceiling level varies from patient to patient, requiring individualized titration of dose. Patients also have variable responses to the different classes of NSAIDs: some patients do not respond at all to one class, but have excellent results with a different class.

The toxicity of NSAIDs is well recognized. In older adults and patients with renal, hepatic, and hematological disease, several of the side effects are enhanced. For this reason, the usual guidelines regarding dose need to be adjusted and sometimes disregarded.

Nausea and diarrhea are common GI side effects of NSAIDs. Several studies suggest that the rate of significant GI problems is about 10% [4]. Gastric and duodenal ulceration, although less common, are clinically more important. The effects of NSAIDs on the GI tract are thought to be due to *prostaglandin inhibition*, because prostaglandins have a protective effect on the gastric mucosa. It does not appear that NSAIDs produce ulceration by a local effect alone, since the decline in prostaglandins is seen throughout the entire GI tract.

It is difficult to predict which patients will develop GI ulceration. Nausea and abdominal pain are poor warning symptoms of toxicity. Prophylaxis with misoprostol can be useful, but it is expensive, and its long-term effects are unknown. Consequently, it should be reserved for patients who have a known sensitivity to NSAIDs.

Renal damage is another major toxic side effect of NSAIDs, particularly for patients with compromised renal function [5,6]. NSAIDs should be used very cautiously in these patients. A useful "rule of thumb" is to avoid the use of NSAIDs in any patient with proteinuria and reduced glomerular filtration rate.

Hematological toxicity due to NSAIDs can be particularly problematic. The major toxicity of this type is platelet dysfunction. Most NSAIDs produce inhibition of platelet aggregation and prolonged bleeding time; these effects usually last about one week. Choline trisalicylate has minimal anti-platelet effect and can be used in patients with platelet dysfunction who would benefit from an NSAID. However, it is expensive, and compliance with it is poor.

Other side effects associated with NSAIDs are not well characterized. For example, headache is a common complaint in patients maintained on NSAIDs, as is dizziness, but the mechanism behind these is not well understood and appears to be dose-related. Skin reactions also can occur, usually as an allergic response. Treatment should be discontinued and the patient re-challenged with a different class of NSAID if clinically necessary.

Significant interactions between NSAIDs and other medications are common. The most important of these involve the potentiation of renal and hepatic toxicity of co-administered drugs and the changes NSAIDs can produce in anticonvulsant levels. There is no known interaction between NSAIDs and anti-retroviral medications.

While the major indication for NSAIDs is the treatment of mild to moderate somatic pain (<3 on the visual analog scale), these drugs often are used in conjunction with low-potency opioids for more severe pain. Bone and joint pain is very responsive to the use of NSAIDs, but neuropathic pain usually is not. In the author's experience, diffuse myalgias also are resistant to these medications, except in the setting of fever. Patients with advanced disease and pain sufficiently severe to interfere with activities of daily living will require additional medications.

Cox-2 Selective NSAIDs

Cox-2 selective inhibitors have been developed as part of an effort to reduce the toxicity of traditional NSAIDs. Whereas older NSAIDs inhibit both Cox-1 (which is protective to the gut) and Cox-2 (which is involved in inflammation and pain), Cox-2 selective NSAIDs affect only the inflammatory pathway.

Two Cox-2 selective agents, *celecoxib* and *rofecoxib*, currently are indicated for the management of acute pain associated with rheumatoid arthritis and osteoarthritis, as well as painful dysmenorrhea. Initial reports suggested that both agents were extremely safe, but as their use has increased, it has become clear that they may have significant adverse effects on renal and cardiovascular function (although they have fewer GI side effects than traditional NSAIDs). Until more data are available, their use should be restricted to the lowest possible dose, and then only in otherwise healthy patients. In the elderly, care should be taken to monitor for fluid retention and accelerated hypertension [7].

Adjuvant Analgesics

Medications that have a primary indication other than analgesia, but have analgesic properties under certain conditions, are termed *adjuvant analgesics*. Most of these medications enhance the body's own pain-modulating mechanisms or the effectiveness of other analgesics. Several different classes of medications are used as adjuvants, including antidepressants, antiepileptic drugs, oral local anesthetics, and adrenergic agonists.

Antidepressants

The *tricyclic antidepressants* (TCAs) have been used for many years for the management of neuropathic pain. Their analgesic effect appears to be independent of their antidepressant actions. There is evidence to suggest that their mode of action is to enhance the body's own pain modulating pathways and to enhance opioid effect at the opioid receptors [8,9]. Their onset of action is slow, requiring several weeks for the full drug effect to be achieved. They are most effective for continuous, burning, or dysesthetic pain [10].

Although tricyclic antidepressants are a first-line therapy for many forms of neuropathy, there is some question about their efficacy in HIV neuropathy [11]. This may be due to the rapid degeneration of fibers in HIV.

The greatest analgesic effect is seen with the older, tertiary amine antidepressants, such as amitriptyline, imipramine, and doxepin. Secondary amine tricyclics, such as desipramine and nortriptyline, also are effective and have less sedating and anticholinergic side effects [12].

The newer antidepressants of the selective serotonin reuptake inhibitor (SSRI) class do not seem to be as effective for neuropathic pain [13]. Nevertheless, they can be helpful in managing associated depression and insomnia.

Tricyclics are well-absorbed from the GI tract and have few interactions with antiretroviral agents. However, they do have a significant number of side effects, the most common of which is sedation. In many cases, this can be avoided by starting at a low dose and instructing the patient to take the medication 10–12 hours before arising, rather than at bedtime. The usual starting dose for amitriptyline is between 10 mg and 25 mg, and most patients find benefit at ranges between 50 mg and 150 mg (some patients do well with doses above and below this range).

Many of the other side effects seen with tricyclic antidepressants are related to their anticholinergic properties. These include dry mouth, visual blurring, urinary retention, hypotension, and cardiac arrhythmias. Many patients become tolerant to these after some time. Starting at a low dose of 10 mg and escalating at weekly intervals reduces the likelihood of significant discomfort.

TCAs are contraindicated in patients with glaucoma and cardiac arrhythmias and should be used with caution in patients with urinary outlet obstruction. Some patients are not able to tolerate TCAs and may benefit from some of the newer antidepressants. *Paroxetine*, in particular, has been found useful in certain forms of painful peripheral neuropathy [14]. Similar evidence does not exist for other SSRIs.

Anticonvulsants

Carbamazepine, phenytoin, and several other AEDs have efficacy in paroxysmal neuropathic pain, although their exact mechanism of action is unclear. It is suspected that AEDs may help to reduce pain by reducing neuronal excitability and local neuronal discharges. These drugs appear to be helpful in pain syndromes that are characterized by paroxysmal or lancinating pain [15].

Phenytoin has been used for the management of a variety of neuropathic pain syndromes, including trigeminal neuralgia and post-herpetic neuralgia [16]. The average dose is 300 mg per day. A loading dose of one gram can be used for acute pain management. Phenytoin has significant drug interactions with a variety of protein-bound medications, including rifampin, methadone, and several antifungal agents.

Dizziness and somnolence are common with phenytoin and usually are dose-related. Serious skin reactions such as Stevens-Johnson syndrome can occur, necessitating discontinuation of the drug. Leukopenia and thrombocytopenia can occur as idiosyncratic reactions. Elevation of liver enzymes is common.

Carbamazepine has been well studied and used successfully in a variety of neuropathic pain states [15,17]. It appears to be more effective than phenytoin but has several significant side effects, including dizziness, somnolence, and significant leukopenia. Hyponatremia also can occur as an idiosyncratic reaction.

Starting at a dose of 100 mg and gradually escalating in 100 mg increments every three to seven days can minimize the dizziness. Close monitoring of the blood count is necessary and limits the utility of this drug in HIV patients.

Valproic acid has been used for the management of lancinating pain, with mixed results. There are no large studies suggesting its long-term effectiveness. The numerous drug interactions and significant hepatic dysfunction that can occur with this drug make it a second-line choice.

Several AEDs have been found to be useful in treating neuropathic pain. *Gabapentin,* in particular, has been found to be effective in both lancinating and continuous dysesthetic pain [18–21]. It is a remarkably well-tolerated drug, with few interactions and a good side effect profile. Treatment usually is started at 100 mg three times per day and then escalated in increments of 100 to 300 mg every three to five days. Most patients have a response at 300 mg thrice daily (TID). There is some evidence that doses above 3600 mg to 4800 mg are not well absorbed, so doses above this range are of questionable utility [22]. The most common reported side effect is somnolence, which resolves after the first two weeks of therapy.

Clonazepam is a benzodiazepine with anticonvulsant properties that has been used for lancinating pain. It has utility in the treatment of muscle spasms as well as myoclonus [23,24]. Because it produces significant sedation, it is best used in patients who have anxiety or difficulty sleeping. It can produce significant dysphoria and should be used cautiously when depression is present. The usual starting dose is 0.5 mg in the evening, escalating to 2 mg TID.

Oral Anesthetics and Alpha-Agonists

Neuropathic pain has been found to respond to high doses of intravenous local anesthetics, such as lidocaine [25,26]. The mechanism of action is different from that of the peripheral effect of local anesthetics. It seems that systemic administration suppresses the activity of dorsal horn cells, which respond to noxious stimulation. Spontaneous firing of damaged cells and axons also is suppressed [27].

Tocainide and *mexiletine* are oral local anesthetics used for cardiac arrhythmias that have been useful for neuropathic pain. Mexiletine has fewer side effects and has been studied more thoroughly. It is useful for continuous dysesthetic pain [28]. The starting dose is 150 mg per day, increasing in 150 mg increments every three to five days, up to a dose of 300 mg TID or until side effects occur.

The most common side effects are dose-related and include nausea, dizziness, and tremors. Hematological reactions are idiosyncratic and rare. In this regard, oral local anesthetics may be a good alternative in patients with blood dyscrasias.

Adrenergic agonists are another type of adjuvant analgesic. Alpha$_2$-adrenergic agonists in particular have proved useful in a variety of pain syndromes. The mechanism of action is presumed to be an enhancement of endogenous pain-modulating systems.

The best studied adrenergic agonist is *clonidine*, which has been found to be effective in neuropathic pain. It can be administered epidurally, intrathecally, orally, or transdermally. For chronic pain, the starting dose is 0.1 mg per day. Gradually escalating the dose to 0.3 mg per day can produce enhanced analgesia.

The major limiting factor in the use of clonidine is its hypotensive effects. Although these are not pronounced in otherwise healthy patients, in the presence of neuropathy, blood pressure fluctuations can be increased. There are few if any other side effects. For patients who have dysesthetic pain, clonidine can be a useful adjunct to other analgesics.

Topical Agents

Topical agents are useful for several types of continuous dysesthetic pain. In general, they are most effective in pain states that have a predominantly peripheral cause. These include painful neuropathies, herpetic and post-herpetic neuralgia, and—occasionally—painful arthropathies. Topical agents alone usually are insufficient to produce total pain relief, but they can be helpful in patients who experience adverse effects from other adjuvant drugs.

Capsaicin, a naturally occurring pepper extract, has proved useful in reducing neuropathic pain in diabetics [29]. The capsaicin preparation is applied to the area of greatest discomfort several times a day. Pain relief does not occur for several days. On initial application, many patients complain of markedly worsened pain and burning. This resolves after several applications and may be due to the local release of Substance P. Unfortunately, the burning can be severe and patients often are not able to tolerate it.

EMLA (eutectic mixture of local anesthetics) is a 1:1 mixture of prilocaine and lidocaine, which can penetrate the skin and produce local anesthesia. It has been helpful in patients with peripheral nerve lesions and in reducing pain associated with blood drawing. EMLA has been particularly helpful in post-herpetic neuralgia [30]. In the author's experience, the combination of EMLA applied first, followed by capsaicin, has been better tolerated than capsaicin alone and may be more effective.

Compounded ointments of salicylates and NSAIDs also have been used for neuropathic pain, but the data regarding their efficacy are unclear [31]. Large trials currently are under way for treatment of a variety of neuropathic pain states.

Muscle Relaxants

Several different classes of medications have muscle relaxant properties. Spasmolytic agents such as baclofen, tizanidine, and benzodiazepines are useful for conditions that produce flexor and extensor spasms because of neural injury, as well as chronic muscle spasm.

A group of diverse agents also are classified as muscle relaxants, although their exact mode of action is poorly understood. These include cyclobenzaprine, carisoprodol, methocarbamol, and chlorzoxazone. The latter group has no clear spasmolytic action, but they may exert their action through central nervous system (CNS) depression.

Baclofen is a gabaminergic drug with affinity for the presynaptic GABA-B receptors. It suppresses excitatory transmitter release and action at the spinal cord level. There is some evidence that it also blocks transmitter release at cutaneous nociceptive nerve endings [32]. It is indicated for pain secondary to spasms of CNS origin. Patients with spasticity related to multiple sclerosis or upper motor neuron lesion from trauma, cerebrovascular disease, or degenerative disease might benefit from baclofen. There is some anecdotal literature suggesting that it also may be useful for facial pain.

The major side effects of baclofen are sedation and liver dysfunction. Abrupt discontinuation can result in seizures.

Intrathecal administration of baclofen can be useful in patients who develop systemic side effects to the oral form [33]. It also is indicated in cerebral palsy, multiple sclerosis, and spastic hemiplegia from trauma or cerebrovascular accident (CVA). However, patients may require additional antispasmodic medications.

Tizanidine, a newer spasmolytic agent, is a centrally acting alpha$_2$ adrenergic agonist. Clinical experience suggests that it has antinociceptive properties, particularly in muscle and soft tissue pain [34]. It is as effective as baclofen in decreasing spasticity, but produces less muscle weakness. However, it can be sedating and should not be administered with other adrenergic agonists.

Cyclobenzaprine is a tricyclic agent that has been marketed as a muscle relaxant. Its major site of action appears to be in the brainstem, although the exact mechanism of action is unclear. It is indicated for short-term use only. It is quite sedating and should be used carefully with other CNS depressants.

Methocarbamol, carisoprodol, and *chlorzoxazone* are older agents whose exact mode of action remains unclear. All have significant CNS depressant effects. There are no controlled studies demonstrating clear efficacy for these medications as analgesic agents. Because of their potential for abuse, they should be avoided.

Interventional Procedures

Anesthetic procedures have become a mainstay of pain management. Although there are many effective procedures for acute pain, chronic pain procedures are somewhat more limited. They include infusions and local blocks with anesthetic agents, administration of epidural steroids, implantable drug delivery systems, and implantable neural stimulators.

Anesthetic Infusions

Intravenous (IV) or oral administration of local anesthetics can produce systemic analgesic effects. It is postulated that the mechanism of action for this phenomenon is the interruption of local reflex arcs, vasodilatation, and low-level anesthesia of susceptible nerve endings [35]. This technique has been particularly helpful in the diagnosis and treatment of neuropathic pain syndromes.

The usual method is to infuse lidocaine at a rate of 5mg/kg of body weight over 30 minutes in a monitored setting. The patient usually experiences relief of paresthesias and lancinating pain within one hour of the infusion; this relief can persist for several days [36,37]. Repeat infusions can be used, although their efficacy may decline. Oral anesthetic agents such as mexiletine also can be used after a loading dose of IV lidocaine. IV lidocaine also has been found helpful in certain forms of vascular headache [38].

Trigger Point Injections

Local injection of anesthetic into tender areas in muscle, referred to as "trigger points," can provide temporary relief in acute and chronic soft tissue pain. The main indication for these injections is myofascial pain. Considerable controversy exists as to which agents should be injected and how often. In general, a dilute solution of a short-acting local anesthetic (with or without steroid) is injected into the trigger point. Dry needling, or mechanical disruption of the tender area, also can be employed, although it usually is poorly tolerated.

The techniques of trigger point injection are described in several texts [39,40]. The injections usually are given in conjunction with physical therapy; this maximizes the efficacy of muscle stretching techniques and reduces pain during the recovery phase from an acute injury.

Local Neural Blockade

Local neural blockade is used principally for the relief of acute pain and for diagnostic purposes. Sequential blocks of individual nerves or spinal levels can help to pinpoint sites of pain generation, but they do not identify the specific disease state that may be producing the pain [41].

Neurolytic blocks are reserved for the most intractable cases and for patients with a limited life expectancy [42]. The risk of developing a deafferentation pain syndrome is high and increases over time. The local vascular effects and soft tissue damage require that these procedures be performed only by clinicians who have ample clinical expertise in their use.

Phenol and absolute alcohol are the most commonly used agents. Both work by destroying peripheral myelin and producing irreversible conduction block. Prolonged administration also is toxic to poorly myelinated axons. Because collateral sprouting can occur, and the peripheral myelin rarely is repaired, ectopic generators can develop lysed nerves, which may produce a return of the pain locally. This phenomenon, coupled with the frequency of recurrent central pain, limits the utility of these agents.

Spinal Steroid Injections and Facet Injections

Local steroid injections into either the epidural space or the facet joints have been used in the treatment of mechanical neck and back pain. Although the indications remain controversial, epidural steroids are used in the management of acute or recurrent pain resulting from root irritation with clinical evidence of radicular dysfunction and in non-operative spinal stenosis [43–45]. Facet blocks are useful in patients with neck or back pain with a mechanical component but without radicular signs, presumably arising in the spinal column [46–49].

The technique of epidural steroid injections is well described in several standard texts [50]. Usually, triamcinolone (at a dose of 50 mg) or methylprednisolone (at a dose of 40 mg to 80 mg) is injected into the epidural space after dilution with either normal saline or a short-acting local anesthetic agent. The injection is performed at the disc level adjacent to the affected nerve roots, and sufficient fluid is given to bathe the adjacent nerve roots.

Complications are uncommon and usually result from either local irritation or a persistent dural leak. Rare complications include radicular irritation and infection [51]. Improvement usually is noted within a week and may persist for several months. A course of three injections generally is given, until pain relief or treatment failure is reached.

Efficacy is variable, with most series indicating short-term improvement of acute back pain. Patients who are most likely to benefit have pain of less than six months' duration or radicular signs [52–54]. Benefits are less convincing in pain related to spinal stenosis [55].

Facet blocks are performed with fluoroscopic guidance. Local anesthetic, either 0.5% bupivicaine or 2% lidocaine, is injected at the base of the superior articular process. Relief of pain suggests that the pain generator is within the facet joint [47]. Efficacy is quite variable, with prolonged relief usually obtained only after radiofrequency ablation.

Sympathetic Blockade

Sympathetic blockade is indicated for pain involving the sympathetic nervous system and the viscera. Nociceptive input from the upper extremities, head, and neck can be blocked by infiltrating the stellate ganglion. Thoracic sympathetic paravertebral ganglia receive input from the cardiac and thoracic viscera; their blockade can be helpful in pain originating at those sites. The abdominal viscera are innervated by the celiac ganglion, while the urogenital viscera are supplied by the superior hypogastric plexus and the ganglion impar. Deep visceral pain can be relieved by blocking the appropriate location.

Finally, the lumbar sympathetic ganglia are involved in mediating pain in the lower extremities. Lumbar sympathetic blockade can be very useful in managing ischemic limb pain and neuropathic pain from failed back surgery, as well as chronic regional pain syndromes.

The exact mechanisms of involvement of the sympathetic nervous system in peripheral pain are not fully understood. In addition, there is poor correlation between the degree of sympathetic dysfunction and response to pain blockade. Therefore, for practical purposes, response to sympathetic blocks is based on the patient's report of pain relief and on changes in skin temperature [56]. The indications for stellate ganglion blocks are painful conditions affecting the head, neck, and upper extremities. Both blind and radiographically guided approaches can be used [57], as can repeated blocks. Neurolysis or spinal cord stimulation can be used if significant relief is obtained from temporary blocks.

Lumbar sympathetic blockade is used in the diagnosis and therapy of painful and other conditions, presumably associated with a dysfunction of the sympathetic nervous system. These include complex regional pain syndrome types I and II, herpes zoster, amputation stump pain, and inoperable peripheral vascular and vasospastic diseases of the lower extremities. Other indications include selected cases of pelvic pain in which superior hypogastric nerve block cannot be performed [58].

Celiac and superior hypogastric blocks, as well as ganglion impar blocks, are used for chronic painful visceral conditions. There are no long-term effectiveness studies of any of these procedures. Radiographic imaging and guidance are mandatory to ensure appropriate anesthetic placement. The major indication for these blocks is chronic cancer-related pain [59,60].

Spinal Cord Stimulation

Spinal cord stimulation (SCS) for the management of pain was introduced in 1967. The actual mechanism of action of SCS is not known, but there are several theories for the analgesic efficacy of this treatment. For example, it is postulated that the electrical stimulation produces antidromic blocking of painful information at the spinal cord level, spinothalamic tract conductance blocking, and activation of supraspinal pain processing nuclei [61,62]. There also is good evidence from cerebrospinal fluid (CSF) markers of chemical neuromodulatory mechanisms. Studies have shown an increase in serotonin, Substance P, and gamma-aminobutyric acid (GABA) release, as well as a reduction in the presence of excitatory amino acids in response to SCS [63].

There are multiple reports of the efficacy of SCS for widely differing chronic pain syndromes [64,65]. Generally, it is agreed that SCS is effective in treating pain of neuropathic origin, particularly sympathetically mediated pain and pain emanating from ischemic origin. It appears that SCS has no efficacy in acute pain or pain of nociceptive origin. Because it is known that SCS causes vasodilatation in animal studies, clinicians have used this modality for the treatment of pain resulting from peripheral vascular disease and visceral pain. Peripheral vascular disease remains the leading indication for SCS in Europe today. There are promising results in the use of SCS in pancreatic and pelvic pain, but no large-scale studies of SCS for these indications [66].

SCS implantation is expensive and labor-intensive. Because it usually requires surgical intervention, it should be reserved for patients who have failed more conservative therapies.

Conclusion

Patients who have co-occurring opioid use disorder and chronic pain may, from time to time, require more intensive treatment and monitoring. This could involve additional counseling or mental health services, referral to a specialized opioid treatment program (OTP), or consultation with an addiction medicine specialist (preferably one who is knowledgeable about and experienced in managing patients with comorbid pain conditions).

While every clinician has his or her own criteria in deciding when a change is needed, evidence that a patient is engaged in aberrant medication-taking behaviors or that the medications being used to treat the patient's chronic pain are not effective both are strong indications of the need for consultation or referral.

Consultation with pain management experts also may be indicated for the otherwise stable patient who begins to experience intense pain [67].

For More Information on the Topics Discussed:

American Society of Addiction Medicine (ASAM):

Otis JAD, Perloff M, Deck GM. Non-opioid pharmacotherapy of pain (Chapter 96). In RK Ries, DA Fiellin, SC Miller, R Saitz, eds. *The ASAM Principles of Addiction Medicine, Fifth Edition.* Philadelphia, PA: Wolters Kluwer; 2014.

Interventional Pain Management:

Jain S, Gupta R. Neurolytic agents in clinical practice. In SD Waldman, AP Winnie, eds. *Interventional Pain Management.* Philadelphia, PA: W.B. Saunders; 2001.

Myofascial Pain and Dysfunction:

Travell JG, Simon DG. *Myofascial Pain and Dysfunction: The Trigger Point Manual.* Baltimore, MD: Williams & Wilkins; 1983.

References

1. Vane JR. Inhibition of prostaglandin synthesis as a mechanism of action for aspirin-like drugs. *Nature.* 1971;234:231–238.
2. McCormack K, Brune K. Dissociation between the antinociceptive and anti-inflammatory effects of the non-steroidal anti-inflammatory drugs. *Drugs.* 1991;41:533–547.
3. Willer JC, DeBroucker T, Bussel B, et al. Central analgesic effect of ketoprofen in humans. *Pain.* 1989;38:1–7.
4. Loeb DS, Ahlquist DA, Talley NJ. Management of gastroduodenopathy associated with the use of nonsteroidal anti-inflammatory drugs. *Mayo Clin Proc.* 1992;67:354–364.
5. Kincaid-Smith P. Effects of non-narcotic analgesics on the kidney. *Drugs.* 1986; 32(Suppl 4):109–128.
6. Porile JL, Bakris L, Garella S. Acute interstitial nephritis with glomerulopathy due to non-steroidal anti-inflammatory agents: A review of its clinical spectrum and effects of steroid therapy. *J Clin Pharmacol.* 1990;30:468–475.
7. Bell GM. Cox-2 inhibitors and other nonsteroidal anti-inflammatory drugs in the treatment of pain in the elderly. *Clin Geriatr Med.* 2001;17(3):489–502.
8. Feinmann C. Pain relief by antidepressants: Possible modes of action. *Pain.* 1985;23(1):1–8.
9. Fields H. Pain modulation and the action of analgesic medications. *Ann Neurol.* 1994; 35(Suppl):S42–S45.
10. Galer BS. Painful polyneuropathy: Diagnosis, pathophysiology, and management. *Semin Neurol.* 1994;14(3):237–246.

11. Kieburtz K, Simpson D, Yiannoutsos C, et al. A randomized trial of amitriptyline and mexiletine for painful neuropathy in HIV infection. AIDS Clinical Trial Group 242 Protocol Team. *Neurology*. 1998;51:1682–1688.
12. Godfrey RG. A guide to the understanding and use of tricyclic antidepressants in the overall management of fibromyalgia and other chronic pain syndromes. *Arch Intern Med*. 1996;156(10):1047–1052.
13. Max MB, Lynch SA, Muir J, et al. Effects of desipramine, amitriptyline, and fluoxetine on pain in diabetic neuropathy. *NEJM*. 1992;326(19):1250–1256.
14. Sindrup SH, Gram LF, Brosen K, et al. The selective serotonin reuptake inhibitor paroxetine is effective in the treatment of diabetic neuropathy symptoms. *Pain*. 1990;42:135–144.
15. Galer BS. Neuropathic pain of peripheral origin: Advances in pharmacologic treatment. *Neurology*. 1995;45(12 Suppl 9):S17–S25.
16. McQuay H, Carroll D, Jadad AR, et al. Anticonvulsant drugs for management of pain: A systematic review. *BMJ*. 1995;311(7012):1047–1052.
17. Moosa RS, McFadyen ML, Miller R, et al. Carbamazepine and its metabolites in neuralgias: Concentration-effect relations. *Eur J Clin Pharmacol*. 1993;45(4):297–301.
18. Chapman R, Suzuki HL, Chamarette LJ, et al. Effects of systemic carbamazepine and gabapentin on spinal neuronal responses in spinal nerve ligated rats. *Pain*. 1998;75(2–3):261–272.
19. Houtchens MK, Richert JR, Sami A, et al. Open label gabapentin treatment for pain in multiple sclerosis. *Mult Scler*. 1997;3(4):250–253.
20. Segal AZ, Rordorf G. Gabapentin as a novel treatment for postherpetic neuralgia. *Neurology*. 1996;46(4):1175–1176.
21. Rowbotham M, Harden N, Stacey B, et al. Gabapentin for the treatment of postherpetic neuralgia: A randomized controlled trial. *JAMA*. 1998;280:1837–1842.
22. Elwes RD, Binnie CD. Clinical pharmacokinetics of newer antiepileptic drugs. Lamotrigine, vigabatrin, gabapentin and oxcarbazepine. *Clin Pharmacokinet*. 1998;30(6):403–415.
23. Bartusch SL, Sanders BJ, D'Alessio JG, et al. Clonazepam for the treatment of lancinating phantom limb pain. *Clin J Pain*. 1996;12(1):59–62.
24. Eisele Jr. JH, Grigsby EJ, Dea J. Clonazepam treatment of myoclonic contractions associated with high-dose opioids: Case report. *Pain*. 1992;49(2):231–232.
25. Glazer S, Portenoy RK. Systemic local analgesics in pain control. *J Pain Symptom Manag*. 1991;6:30–39.
26. Rowbotham MC, Reisner L, Fields HL. Both IV lidocaine and morphine reduce the pain of post-herpetic neuralgia. *Neurology*. 1991;41:1024–1028.
27. Woolf CJ, Wiesenfeld-Hallin Z. The systemic administration of local anesthetic produces a selective depression of C-afferent evoked activity in the spinal cord. *Pain*. 1985;23:361–374.
28. Chabel C, Jacobson L, Mariano A, , et al. The use of oral mexiletine for the treatment of pain after peripheral nerve injury. *Anesthesiology*. 1992;76:513–517.
29. Capsaicin Study Group. Treatment of painful diabetic neuropathy with topical capsaicin. *Arch Intern Med*. 1991;151(11):2225–2229.

30. Stow PJ, Glynn CJ, Minor B. EMLA cream in the treatment of post herpetic neuralgia: Efficacy and pharmacokinetic profile. *Pain*. 1989;39:301–305.
31. Rowbotham MC. Topical analgesic agents. In HL Fields, JC Liebskind, eds. *Pharmacological Approaches to the Treatment of Chronic Pain*. New York: IASP Press; 1994:211–229.
32. Hwang AS, Wilcox GL. Baclofen, gamma aminobutyric acid B receptors and substance P in the mouse spinal cord. *J Pharmacol Exper Ther*. 1989;248:1026–1033.
33. Pirotte B, Heilporn A, Joffrey A, et al. Chronic intrathecal baclofen in severely disabling spasticity: Selection, clinical assessment and long-term benefit. *Acta Anesthesiol Belg*. 1995;95(4):216–225.
34. Coward DM. Tinazidine: Neuropharmacology and mechanism of action. *Neurology*. 1994;44(Suppl 9):6–11.
35. Bigelow N, Harrison I. General analgesic effects of procaine. *J Pharmacol Exper Ther*. 1944;81:368.
36. Boas RA, Covino BG, Shahnarian A. Analgesic responses to IV lignocaine. *Br J Anaesth*. 1982;54:501.
37. Kastrup J, Petersen P, Dejgard A, et al. Intravenous lidocaine infusion: A new treatment of painful diabetic neuropathy. *Pain*. 1987;28:69.
38. Edwards WT, Habib F, Burney RG, et al. Intravenous lidocaine in the management of various chronic pain states. *Reg Anesth*. 1985;10:1.
39. Maciewicz R, Chung RY, Strassman A, et al. Relief of vascular headache with intravenous lidocaine. *Cincinnati J Pain*. 1988;4:11.
40. Rachlin ES, ed. *Myofascial Pain and Fibromyalgia*. St. Louis, MO: Mosby-Year Book; 1994:143–382.
41. Travell JG, Simon DG. *Myofascial Pain and Dysfunction: The Trigger Point Manual*. Baltimore, MD: Williams & Wilkins; 1983.
42. Winnie AP. Differential neural blockade for the diagnosis of pain mechanisms. In SD Waldman, AP Winnie, eds. *Interventional Pain Management*. Philadelphia, PA: W.B. Saunders; 2001.
43. Jain S, Gupta R. Neurolytic agents in clinical practice. In SD Waldman, AP Winnie, eds. *Interventional Pain Management*. Philadelphia, PA: W.B. Saunders; 2001:19–67.
44. Abram SE. Risk versus benefit of epidural steroids: Let's remain objective. *Am Pain Soc Bull*. 1994;3:28–29.
45. Weinstein SM, Herring SA. Contemporary concepts in spine care: Epidural steroid injections. *Spine*. 1995;20:1842–1846.
46. Rowlingson JC. Epidural steroids: Do they have a place in pain management? *Am Pain Soc Bull*. 1994;3:20–27.
47. Bogduk N. International Spinal Injection Society guidelines for the performance of spinal injection procedures, part I: Zygapophyseal joint blocks. *Clin J Pain*. 1997;13:285–302.
48. Dwyer A, Aprill C, Bogduk N. Cervical zygapophyseal joint pain patterns: A study in normal volunteers. *Spine*. 1990;15:453–457.
49. Mooney V, Robertson J. The facet syndrome. *Clin Orthoped*. 1976;115:149–156.

50. Cousins MJ, Veering BT. Epidural neural blockade. In MJ Cousins, PO Bridenbaugh, eds. *Neural Blockade, 4th Edition*. Philadelphia, PA: Lippincott-Raven; 1998;11:241–295.
51. Nelson DA. Intraspinal therapy using methylprednisolone acetate: Twenty-three years of clinical controversy. *Spine*. 1993;18:278.
52. Bowman SJ, Wedderburn L. Outcome assessment after epidural corticosteroid injection for low back pain and sciatica. *Spine*. 1993;18:1345.
53. Watts RW, Silagy CA. A meta-analysis on the efficacy of epidural corticosteroids in the treatment of sciatica. *Anaesth Intens Care*. 1995;23:564–569.
54. Koes BW, Scholten RJPM, Mens JM, et al. Efficacy of epidural steroid injections for low-back pain and sciatica: A systematic review of randomized clinical trials. *Pain*. 1995 Dec;63:279–288.
55. Fukusaki M, Kobayashi I. Symptoms of spinal stenosis do not improve after epidural steroid injection. *Clin J Pain*. 1998;14:148–151.
56. Tahmoush AJ, Malley J, Jennings JR. Skin conductance, temperature and blood flow in causalgia. *Neurology*. 1983;33:1483–1486.
57. Aesbach A, Nagy M. Common nerve blocks in chronic pain management. *Anesthesiol Clin North Am*. 2000;18(2):429–459.
58. Cousins MJ, Reeve TS, Glynn CJ, et al. Neurolytic lumbar sympathetic blockade: Duration of denervation and relief of rest pain. *Anaesth Intens Care*. 1979;7:121.
59. Plancarte R, Amescua C, Patt RB, et al. Superior hypogastric plexus block for pelvic cancer pain. *Anesthesiology*. 1999;73:236–239.
60. Plancarte R, DeLeon-Cassola OA, El-Helaly M, et al. Neurolytic superior hypogastric plexus block for chronic pelvic pain associated with cancer. *Reg Anesth*. 1997;22:562–568.
61. Broggi G, Franzini A, Parati E, et al. Neurochemical and structural modifications related to pain control induced by spinal cord stimulation. In *Neurostimulation: An Overview*. New York: Futura Publishing; 1985:87–95.
62. Saade NE, Tabet MS, Souiedan SA, et al. Supraspinal modulation of nociception in awake rats by stimulation of the dorsal column nuclei. *Brain Res*. 1986;369:307–310.
63. Meyerson BA, Brodin E, Linderoth B. Possible neurohumoral mechanisms in CNS stimulation for pain suppression. *Appl Neurophysiol*. 1985;48:175–180.
64. Spiegelmann R, Friedman WA. Spinal cord stimulation: A contemporary series. *Neurosurgery*. 1991;28:65–70.
65. Kumar K, Nath RK, Toth C. Spinal cord stimulation is effective in the management of reflex sympathetic dystrophy. *Neurosurgery*. 1997;40:503–509.
66. Kemler MA, Barendse GA, van Kleef M, et al. Spinal cord stimulation in patients with chronic reflex sympathetic dystrophy. *NEJM*. 2000;343(9):618–624.
67. Olsen Y. Personal communication, June 1, 2017.

Chapter 16

Professionally Directed Non-Pharmacological Management of Chronic Pain

PETER PRZEKOP, D.O., PH.D.

Healing is a matter of time, but it is sometimes also a matter of opportunity.
                                                    —HIPPOCRATES

Over the past two decades, new research has made it clear that chronic pain is fundamentally different from acute pain. Chronic pain is a disease process in which the brain has changed, reorganized, and is capable of generating pain spontaneously [1]. Chronic pain also is recognized as very complex; therefore, effective treatments must consider the brain, mind, body, and spirit [2]. The current lack of such treatments has left many physicians in a difficult position, especially those who treat patients with chronic pain and co-occurring substance use disorder (SUD) [3].

Non-pharmacological treatments range from mind-body therapies, to psychosocial treatments, to technology-based therapies, all of which can offer the possibility of healing to complex patients [2]. These treatments are effective and popular because they support 12-Step recovery, add balance and well-being, and are devoid of adverse effects. An estimated 62% of Americans use them at some point in their lives [4].

The Nature of Chronic Pain

The incidence of chronic pain is increasing rapidly. For example, experts estimate that half of all patients with SUDs also have chronic pain [5]. Patients who have co-occurring chronic pain and SUDs are very difficult to treat with conventional medical methods because they need help for more than their physical pain. Many also seek relief from anxiety, depression, chronic stress, and the culmination of adversity they experienced in the past and continue to suffer. These complex patients often are placed on chronic opioid therapy in an attempt to relieve their physical pain but for many, this is not the appropriate treatment [3].

Historically, such patients have been excluded from opioid clinical trials. Thus, there is virtually no evidence to guide opioids as a treatment choice. Pain must be adequately treated in these patients because studies have found that 60% report that pain has significantly contributed to the development of their SUD [5]. Without adequate treatment, such individuals are likely to experience repeated episodes of relapse. However, effective treatment can normalize the changes that occur in the brain as a result of chronic pain [6].

Patients with Co-Occurring Chronic Pain and Substance Use Disorder

In approaching a patient with chronic pain and SUD, it is important for the clinician to realize that the patient's brain, mind, body, and spirit have been transformed and reorganized. The structural, functional, and connectivity changes in the brain that arise because of chronic pain and SUDs have been well documented [2]. Research studies show that they contribute to reorganization of neural networks involved in goal-directed behavior, attention, internal surveillance, emotional regulation, and the ability to enjoy natural rewards, all of which produce significant changes in the patient's thinking, regulation of emotion, behavior, and overall outlook [7].

Patients with chronic pain and SUD live with biased acquisition and processing of information, which distort their thinking, thus continuing to activate and sustain both disease states. These patients have lost attentional control, in that their attention has been captured by the pain signal, making it difficult for them to disengage from drug-related cues. This results in a bias toward pain-related and drug-related thinking. Moreover, their self-referential thoughts focus on their poor health and lack of well-being. This contributes to a loss of emotional regulation so that emotions are negative and thinking is skewed toward prolonged suffering, poor self-efficacy, pain catastrophizing, and fear of future pain [7].

Patients with both pain and SUDs report high levels of current suffering that is driven by self-reported unresolved adversity. This results in a dysregulated stress response that becomes chronic. Patients display poor coping skills and report a lack of optimism. All of these factors should be considered when evaluating and treating such patients [8].

Approach to the Patient

The recommended approach involves multiple steps.

History of Present Illness (HPI)

In evaluating the patient, it is important to consider how the patient has changed as a result of chronic pain and SUD. The best approach is to consider the whole person and inquire about all factors that may be contributing to the patient's suffering. In addition to a comprehensive history of the present illness (HPI), patients should be asked about their:

1. Coping style (internalization and avoidance);
2. Ability to access and process emotions;
3. Hope and motivation for change and healing;
4. Fear of attempting new treatments;
5. Perception of the effectiveness of their current and past treatments;
6. The last time they felt well;
7. How long they have been under stress;
8. Present level of stress;
9. Quality of sleep, exercise routines, and mindfulness activities;
10. Barriers to change;
11. Sense of self-worth and self-esteem;
12. What they think may be contributing to their suffering; and
13. Their ability to achieve a quiet mind [9].

Note: It is appropriate to use a scale ranging from 0 (not at all) to 10 (extreme) to answer the foregoing questions.

Patients also should be asked when they began to: (1) feel anxious, (2) experience a lack of well-being, and (3) experience bad feelings inside of their body.

In addition to a comprehensive HPI, the health care team should obtain a past medical history, social history, family history, and medication list from the patient. In assessing medications currently being used, consideration should be given to drug interactions, adverse effects, and the potential for dependence or addiction [10].

Physical Examination

A complete physical examination is important and should include special attention to any asymmetrical findings in terms of muscle bulk, muscle strength, deep tendon reflexes, and sensations.

Muscle groups should be palpated for signs of spasms, reduced range of motion, allodynia, and hyperalgesia. Allodynia can be assessed by having the patient sit in a chair. Using an index and middle fingers to apply gentle pressure bilaterally to the middle of the trapezius muscles helps to determine whether the patient perceives minimal pressure as excessively painful [11].

Non-Pharmacological Treatment Options

On completion of the patient assessment just described, the treating physician will have the information needed to select one or more non-pharmacological therapies, as follows.

Movement Therapies

Movement therapies are available and effective. Among the oldest and most extensively studied are qi gong, tai chi, and yoga. All involve movement, breathing, mindfulness, and the ability to focus energy to achieve healing. Each has the ability to help the patient to regain a sense of self-efficacy and optimism, as well as to improve physical and psychological strength [12].

Internal qi gong is an ancient method of healing that uses *qi* ("life energy"), movement, and a meditative state to promote healing. Individuals who practice qi gong are able to increase *qi* and promote healing by allowing the body, mind, and spirit to employ their innate healing mechanisms. Qi gong has been tested in a multi-modal program and found to help patients with chronic pain and SUD [13].

Tai chi ("Ultimate Supreme") is a form of exercise that promotes psychological and physiological health. Like qi gong, it uses movement, breathing, and qi energy. It is a form of martial arts that has been used to help patients with chronic pain [14].

Yoga is based on a series of spiritual and physical beliefs and practices that are used to promote awareness and healing. Yoga employs breathing, exercise, and physical stances to promote health. Numerous studies have shown the benefits of yoga in helping patients with chronic pain [15].

Martial arts are a viable option for patients who are interested in achieving healing through mindfulness, meditative states, *qi* energy, and a disciplined lifestyle. Martial arts classes are relatively easy to access, but physicians should proceed with caution to be certain that the instructors are promoting the art and not the fighting techniques [16].

Other forms of exercise, movement, and stretching have been explored to help individuals with chronic pain, and positive results have been reported. However, it is best to explore each type of movement before recommending it to patients.

Energy Therapies

Therapeutic touch/healing touch is related to the ancient technique of laying on of hands. The goal of this technique is to balance the vital energy fields that exist in the body. The idea is that the practitioner's healing touch can positively influence health. A limited number of studies have shown positive results for use of this technique to treat chronic pain [17].

Reiki is a Japanese term that translates to "universal life energy." Reiki practitioners are trained to channel spiritual energy. Through this process, patients gain spiritual healing. Reiki has been shown to reduce pain [18].

External qi gong practitioners can move energy and use it to help patients heal. Practitioners are able to channel their own energy, the patient's energy, and universal healing energy. *Qi* activates the natural ability of the mind, body, brain, and spirit to heal. External qi gong has been successfully used to treat patients with chronic pain and SUD [19].

Acupuncture and acupressure are techniques that increase the flow of *qi* in the body. With acupuncture, needles are inserted at specific acupuncture points, while acupressure uses pressure applied at specific points. Both have been used extensively to help patients with chronic pain [20].

Psychosocial Treatments

Psychosocial treatments are designed to motivate the patient to change while increasing his or her insight into the contribution of cognition, emotions, and behaviors to illness.

Motivational interviewing is a patient-centered approach that offers encouragement to the patient to undergo behavior change through choice and empowerment [21]. The idea is to help the patient realize that targeted behavioral change is of benefit and can help eliminate maladaptive thoughts and behaviors that lead to poor choices and reduced self-efficacy.

Cognitive restructuring is based on the idea that positive adaptive thoughts lead to increased optimism, mood, adaptive behaviors, and a healthy lifestyle. The treatment involves increasing the patient's awareness of cognition and how to recognize it to control positive or negative effects on behavior and health.

Patients are encouraged to replace any maladaptive thoughts with adaptive ones [22].

Cognitive-behavioral therapy (CBT) is a broad category of well-studied treatment regimens that include cognitive therapy as a primary component. CBT emphasizes changes in thoughts and behaviors. It includes coping skills, relaxation skills, pacing/activity/rest cycling, exercise, and enjoyment [23].

Acceptance-based cognitive therapy (ACT) is a modification of CBT that incorporates acceptance techniques to emphasize a separation of self from thoughts and feelings in relation to the pain experience. The treatment emphasizes cognitive flexibility and moment-to-moment non-judgmental attentiveness to the pain experience. Acceptance-based therapies include acceptance and commitment therapy, contextual cognitive behavioral therapy, and mindfulness-based cognitive therapy [24].

Operant training is based on the belief that behaviors are repeated because they are reinforced. Behaviors that are followed by negative reinforcers should decrease in frequency. The idea is that if pain persists and becomes chronic, there are behavioral reinforcers that are keeping it present [25].

Hypnosis helps the patient focus attention on a single sensory experience. Suggestions are offered to encourage changes in thoughts, emotions, attention, sensory experience, and behaviors, and then a number of post-hypnotic suggestions are offered. Hypnosis can reduce the patient's pain experience [26].

Relaxation training teaches the patient to experience relaxation. Relaxation techniques such as progressive muscle relaxation, biofeedback, and autogenic training have been shown to reduce chronic pain [27].

Mindfulness/meditation is discussed in Chapter 21 of this Handbook. A number of meditation and mindfulness techniques are able to quiet the mind and reduce suffering [28].

Other Treatments

Chiropractic treatments use high-velocity and low-velocity forces to realign structural abnormalities in the body. Chiropractic treatments are comparable in their effectiveness to conventional treatments for chronic pain [29].

Osteopathic manipulation and craniosacral therapy engage the body's natural ability to heal while restoring blood flow and structural integrity. Craniosacral therapy attempts to restore the body's natural rhythm and enhance healing. Both techniques have been used to help patients with chronic pain and SUD [30].

Massage therapy involves a trained masseuse using the hands in a therapeutic way to promote healing. There are many different styles of massage, ranging from very gentle to deep tissue techniques. Massage is used to promote muscle relaxation, as well as to achieve stress reduction and a silent mind. Several studies have shown that massage improves chronic pain [31].

Pulsed electromagnetic fields use generator units to produce pulsed electromagnetic charges. These units are thought to promote healing by increasing blood flow to affected tissues. They have been shown to significantly reduce headaches [32].

Cranial electrotherapy stimulation involves the steady delivery of low-output electrical current to painful areas of the body. It is hypotheized that the electrical current engages neurophysiological and neurochemical systems to relieve pain. Favorable outcomes have been reported using this technique [33].

Trans-epidermal nerve stimulation (TENS) is a self-contained unit that can be applied to the skin. It is thought to work by reducing nociceptive input and activating central inhibition pain pathways. Multiple studies have shown its effectiveness [34].

Transcranial magnetic stimulation (TMS) uses an electromagnet to generate a magnetic field. The unit is placed over the scalp and can result in small sustained reductions in electrical activity in the area of the brain that is stimulated. It has been used successfully for the treatment of chronic pain [35].

Conclusion

Physicians should become familiar with the services available in their area of practice and consider studying and becoming proficient in some of the recommended therapies. This can add to a physician's personal program of self-care, while allowing him or her to provide first-hand expertise to his or her patients [9].

Once a physician becomes knowledgeable about non-pharmacological options and recognizes their value, he or she will be able to integrate a full range of therapies into the patients' treatment plan. This will lead to improved care and additional options for care, which can help reduce patients' suffering and improve their lives [26,36].

No patient is too old or too ill to engage in any of these treatment modalities [6]. It is necessary to inform the patient that he or she should enter at a level that feels comfortable. Many modalities can be initiated from a chair or even a bed.

More information about non-pharmacological treatments can be obtained on the Internet, at a bookstore, and through continuing medical education (CME) courses. Information about mindfulness, movement therapy, pain blogs, and Internet groups is available online.

For More Information on the Topics Discussed:

American Society of Addiction Medicine (ASAM):

Gallagher RM, Koob G, Popescu A. The pathophysiology of chronic pain and clinical interfaces with addiction (Chapter 93). In RK Ries, DA Fiellin,

SC Miller, R Saitz, eds. *The ASAM Principles of Addiction Medicine, 5th Edition.* Philadelphia, PA: Wolters Kluwer; 2014.

Chapters 55 to 68 (Behavioral Interventions) in RK Ries, DA Fiellin, SC Miller, R Saitz, eds. *The ASAM Principles of Addiction Medicine, 5th Edition.* Philadelphia, PA: Wolters Kluwer; 2014.

References

1. Apkarian AV, Baliki MN, Geha PY. Towards a theory of chronic pain. *Prog Neurobiol.* 2009 Feb;87(2):81–97.
2. Gatchel RJ, Peng YB, Peters ML, et al. The biopsychosocial approach to chronic pain: Scientific advances and future directions. *Psychol Bull.* 2007;4:581–624.
3. Pohl M, Smith L. Chronic pain and addiction: Challenging co-occurring disorders. *J Psychoact Drug.* 2012;44:119–124.
4. Nahin RL, Barnes PM, Stussman BJ, et al. *Costs of complementary and alternative medicine (CAM) and frequency of visits to CAM practitioners: United States, 2007.* Hyattsville, MD: National Center for Health Statistics Report; 2009 Jul 30;(18):1–14.
5. Morasco BJ, Gritzner S, Lewis L, et al. Systematic review of prevalence, correlates, and treatment outcomes for chronic non-cancer pain in patients with comorbid substance use disorder. *Pain.* 2011;152:488–497.
6. Przekop P, Haviland MG, Oda K, et al. Prevalence and correlates of pain interference in older adults: Why treating the whole body and mind is necessary. *J Body Mov Ther.* 2015;19:217–225.
7. Melzack R. From the gate to the neuromatrix. *Pain.* 1999;82:S121–S126.
8. Gold PW. The organization of the stress system and its dysfunction in depressive illness. *Mol Psychiatry.* 2015;20:32–47.
9. Miller WR, Rollnick S. *Motivational interviewing: Preparing people for change.* New York: Guilford Press; 2002.
10. Federation of State Medical Boards (FSMB). *Model Policy on the Use of Opioid Analgesics in the Treatment of Chronic Pain.* Euless, TX: The Federation; July 2013.
11. Parran TV, McCormick RA, Delos Reyes C. Assessment (Chapter 20). In RK Ries, DA Fiellin, SC Miller, R Saitz, eds. *The ASAM Principles of Addiction Medicine, 5th Edition.* Philadelphia, PA: Wolters Kluwer; 2014.
12. Seminowicz DA, Wideman, TH, Naso L, et al. Effective treatment of chronic low back pain in humans reverses abnormal brain anatomy and function. *J Neurosci.* 2011;31:7540–550.
13. Bai Z, Guan Z, Fan Y, et al. The effects of Qigong for adults with chronic pain: Systematic review and meta-analysis. *Am J Chin Med.* 2015;43(8):1525–1539.

14. Kong LJ, Lauche R, Klose P, et al. Tai Chi for chronic pain conditions: A systematic review and meta-analysis of randomized controlled trials. *Sci Rep.* 2016 Apr 29;6:25325.
15. Holtzman S, Beggs RT. Yoga for chronic low back pain: A meta-analysis of randomized controlled trials. *Pain Res Manag.* 2013 Sep–Oct;18(5):267–272.
16. Lee C, Crawford C, Schoomaker E, for the Active Self-Care Therapies for Pain (PACT) Working Group. Movement therapies for the self-management of chronic pain symptoms. *Pain Med.* 2014 Apr;15(Suppl 1):S40–S53.
17. Marletta G, Canfora A, Roscani F, et al. The complementary medicine (CAM) for the treatment of chronic pain: Scientific evidence regarding the effects of healing touch massage. *Acta Biomed.* 2015 Sep 9;86(Suppl 2):127–133.
18. Furrer S. Reiki to relieve chronic pain. *Krankenpfl Soins Infirm.* 2015;108(12):74–76.
19. Lee MS, Pittler MH, Ernst E. External qigong for pain conditions: A systematic review of randomized clinical trials. *J Pain.* 2007 Nov;8(11):827–831.
20. Eshkevari L. Acupuncture and chronic pain management. *Annu Rev Nurs Res.* 2017 Jan;35(1):117–134.
21. Alperstein D, Sharpe L. The efficacy of motivational interviewing in adults with chronic pain: A meta-analysis and systematic review. *J Pain.* 2016 Apr;17(4):393–403.
22. Elman I, Borsook D, Volkow ND. Pain and suicidality: Insights from reward and addiction. *Prog Neurobiol.* 2013;109:1–27.
23. Ehde DM, Dillworth TM, Turner JA. Cognitive-behavioral therapy for individuals with chronic pain: Efficacy, innovations, and directions for research. *Am Psychol.* 2014 Feb-Mar;69(2):153–166.
24. Baranoff J, Hanrahan SJ, Kapur D, et al. Acceptance as a process variable in relation to catastrophizing in multidisciplinary pain treatment. *Eur J Pain.* 2013 Jan;17(1):101–110.
25. Gatzounis R, Schrooten MG, Crombez G, et al. Operant learning theory in pain and chronic pain rehabilitation. *Curr Pain Headache Rep.* 2012 Apr;16(2):117–126.
26. Adachi T, Fujino H, Nakae A, et al. A meta-analysis of hypnosis for chronic pain problems: A comparison between hypnosis, standard care, and other psychological interventions. *Int J Clin Exp Hypn.* 2014;62(1):1–28.
27. Blödt S, Pach D, Roll S, et al. Effectiveness of app-based relaxation for patients with chronic low back pain (Relaxback) and chronic neck pain (Relaxneck): Study protocol for two randomized pragmatic trials. *Trials.* 2014 Dec 15;15:490.
28. La Cour P, Petersen M. Effects of mindfulness meditation on chronic pain: A randomized controlled trial. *Pain Med.* 2015 Apr;16(4):641–652.
29. Peterson CK, Bolton J, Humphreys BK. Predictors of improvement in patients with acute and chronic low back pain undergoing chiropractic treatment. *J Manipulat Physiol Ther.* 2012 Sep;35(7):525–533.
30. Franke H, Franke JD, Fryer G. Osteopathic manipulative treatment for nonspecific low back pain: A systematic review and meta-analysis. *BMC Musculoskelet Disord.* 2014 Aug 30;15:286.

31. Kamali F, Panahi F, Ebrahimi S, et al. Comparison between massage and routine physical therapy in women with subacute and chronic nonspecific low back pain. *J Back Musculoskelet Rehabil.* 2014;27(4):475–480.
32. Stocchero M, Gobbato L, De Biagi M, et al. Pulsed electromagnetic fields for postoperative pain: A randomized controlled clinical trial in patients undergoing mandibular third molar extraction. *Oral Surg Oral Med Oral Pathol Oral Radiol.* 2015 Mar;119(3):293–300.
33. Thomas AW, Graham K, Prato FS, et al. A randomized, double-blind, placebo-controlled clinical trial using a low-frequency magnetic field in the treatment of musculoskeletal chronic pain. *Pain Res Manag.* 2007 Winter;12(4):249–258.
34. Vance CG, Dailey DL, Rakel BA, et al. Using TENS for pain control: The state of the evidence. *Pain Manag.* 2014 May;4(3):197–209.
35. Young NA, Sharma M, Deogaonkar M. Transcranial magnetic stimulation for chronic pain. *Neurosurg Clin N Am.* 2014 Oct;25(4):819–832.
36. Breivik H. *World Health Organization supports global effort to relieve chronic pain.* Geneva, Switzerland: WHO Media Centre; Oct. 11, 2004.

Chapter 17

Self-Directed Non-Pharmacological Management of Chronic Pain

STEPHEN COLAMECO, M.D., M.ED.,
DFASAM, AND STEPHEN F. GRINSTEAD,
A.D., LMFT, ACRPS, CADC-II

Successful treatment of chronic pain requires a comprehensive approach that combines medical interventions and occupational and physical therapies that are focused on improving function, as well as self-care and psychological, psychosocial, and alternative/complementary approaches. Unfortunately, many patients with chronic pain do not have access to integrated multidisciplinary care. Under these circumstances, self-management of pain often is essential to recovery, through its ability to facilitate improvement in physical and social functioning [1].

Self-management approaches include psychological self-help, behavioral approaches, online support, group support, nutrition, graded exercise, the use of devices such as Trans-Epidermal Nerve Stimulation (TENS), self-guided movement therapies, and many other alternative and complementary approaches.

Because clinical outcomes from any intervention are influenced by the patient's beliefs, physicians should discuss with their patients the potential benefit of incorporating self-management strategies, including alternative and complementary or spiritual practices, in the comprehensive treatment plan. Such a discussion should be sensitive to and respectful of the patient's belief system, religion, and culture.

Self-Management of Pain Flare-ups

In the context of pain self-management, a pain flare-up is characterized by a temporary increase in pain intensity [2]. This should be distinguished from significant disease progression or a new condition that would prompt medical interventions. Some patients experience flare-ups when they are anxious. Such episodes can be viewed as a possibly new, serious condition; anxiety itself can increase pain intensity. It is important for clinicians to explain that most patients experience flare-ups and to describe the factors that contribute to pain flare-ups, as well as how to use self-management interventions when they occur. Factors that contribute to flare-ups include excessive exercise/overuse, poor posture, insomnia, and anxiety [2].

Some patients will want to manage flare-ups through increased medication use or will seek reassurance through diagnostic testing. Helping patients sort through the difference between a pain flare-up and a new or worsening condition is necessary in order to engage patients in pain self-management. Self-care techniques that can be used to manage flare-ups include heat, ice, distraction, relaxation, and rest, followed by appropriate levels of activity.

Spirituality

Chronic pain is a multifaceted mind-body-spirit problem. On one hand, spirituality can be adversely affected by chronic pain; on the other, spirituality may play a critical role in recovery from such pain [3].

Spiritual healing should be an integral component of a comprehensive approach to pain treatment. Many individuals have found that spiritual interventions such as prayer and meditation help ease their suffering.

Experts emphasize the importance of treating chronic pain patients holistically, rather than focusing primarily on the biomedical aspects of pain care and management. They maintain that chronic pain requires patients to find a path to living as full a life as possible despite their pain. For some patients, improved quality of life is achieved through spiritual practice. Therefore, incorporating spiritual discussions into interactions with patients may create an opportunity for increased clinical effectiveness in managing the patient's pain [4].

Sleep Hygiene

Sleep disorders are among the most common conditions among persons living with chronic pain [5]. Unfortunately, in many cases, sleep medication is the initial medical intervention. While medication-assisted treatment is the ideal response in some instances, in many cases improving the patients' sleep hygiene is a more effective and self-directed intervention.

One very helpful resource in this regard is found in the Mayo Clinic's online patient care and information section. An article posted there, "Sleep Tips: 7 Steps to Better Sleep," outlines the following steps: (a) stick to a sleep schedule; (b) pay attention to what you eat and drink; (c) create a bedtime ritual; (d) get comfortable; (e) limit daytime naps; (f) include physical activity in your daily routine; and (g) manage stress [6].

Another helpful resource is an online article titled "Twelve Simple Steps to Improve Your Sleep," published by the Division of Sleep Medicine at Harvard Medical School and WGBH Educational Foundation [7].

Nutrition

Nutrition is both a "mainstream" and a complementary/integrative intervention for the treatment of chronic pain, depending on the foods, vitamins, or supplements consumed. At a basic level, good nutrition involves eating a balanced, healthy diet. Many individuals with chronic pain have unhealthy lifestyles that include overeating, consuming "junk food" or excessive caffeinated drinks, and heavy use of alcohol and/or nicotine. (See Chapter 26 of this Handbook for a discussion of the link between obesity and chronic pain, and Chapter 27 for a description of the relationship between cigarette smoking and chronic pain.) For these reasons, dietary counseling and smoking cessation are part of comprehensive pain management.

Obesity increases the risk of many medical disorders, including degenerative disc disease, back strain, and arthritis of the lower back, hips, and knees [8]. Based on pre-clinical research and theoretical assumptions, some researchers recommend a high-protein, low glycemic index diet to avoid weight gain and to promote strength, movement, energy, and mental function [9], but there is insufficient evidence to recommend a specific diet.

According to the National Center for Complementary and Integrative Health (NCCIH; an agency of the National Institutes of Health), there is insufficient evidence to recommend dietary supplements for painful conditions, including glucosamine or chondroitin for the treatment of arthritis [10]. Dietary supplements may be recommended to prevent osteopenia and osteoporosis. There is not sufficient evidence to support higher than the recommended daily amounts of vitamin D for the purpose of pain management; however, vitamin D deficiency has been linked to muscle weakness and pain [11].

In addition, excessive caffeine consumption can cause muscle tension and insomnia—symptoms that often accompany chronic pain [12].

Research studies have shown that smokers and ex-smokers have higher rates of chronic pain than those who never smoked; also, smokers are more likely than non-smokers to report that their pain is intense and is associated with greater occupational and social impairment [13].

Exercise

Physical exercise is an essential component of a comprehensive pain program. Exercise may be part of physical therapy treatment or aftercare within the context of "movement therapies," or may involve less structured physical activities [14]. Individualized exercise therapy has been associated with clinically significant functional improvement in patients with many disorders [15]. However, patients should be dissuaded from the "no pain/no gain" approach they may have followed in the past, as this can lead to exacerbation of pain or "crash and burn" cycles.

In general, exercise should follow a gradual approach, starting out slowly and increasing incrementally in very small steps. If pain is severe, the patient may need to start out with just a few minutes of gentle movement or stretching. Aqua therapy (such as walking in a warm pool or gentle swimming) often is a good first step [16]. Graded exercise therapy helps correct the negative cycle of inactivity and deconditioning to which many patients have succumbed; in contrast, structured exercise programs are a significant component of pain management therapy [17].

Acupressure

Acupressure is based on the same meridian theory as acupuncture, which proposes that pressure stimulates a network of energy pathways throughout the body to increase the flow of bioenergy (*qi*). Acupressure involves applying pressure to specific points of the body through the use of finger, hand, elbow, rods, or proprietary acupressure bands that have protruding plastic pressure knobs [18].

Studies of the efficacy of acupressure for symptom management have been a focus of research in recent years, but there are few well-controlled studies involving the application of acupressure in the management of chronic pain, so there is little evidence of benefit. As a result, acupressure treatment is not included in current evidence-based chronic pain treatment guidelines.

In 2014, Chen and Wang [19] published a systematic review of the use of acupressure in the treatment of various pain disorders, including dysmenorrhea, labor pain, low back pain, chronic headache, and traumatic pain. The authors found results that begin to establish a credible evidence base for the use of acupressure in relieving pain; however, they acknowledge the need for higher quality research to determine whether acupressure can be shown to be an evidence-based practice.

12-Step Groups for Chronic Pain

While very few 12-Step groups for chronic pain sufferers are available, there is telephone access to meetings through a dial-in conference call service [20]. Other patients may find support in Pills Anonymous meetings [21].

Also, 12-Step pain recovery books are available in print and e-book versions; these address the problem of pain complicated by a substance use disorder (SUD) [22]. Individuals already working an Alcoholics Anonymous or Narcotics Anonymous program may find the application of the 12 Steps to chronic pain, as described in these books, an important adjunct to their overall recovery.

In addition, support groups are available online and in person for various disease states that are accompanied by significant pain, such as lupus, fibromyalgia, irritable bowel syndrome, and many others [23].

Conclusion

It is important for patients to understand the nature of chronic pain, as opposed to acute pain, and to accept the fact that chronic pain cannot be "cured," but rather must be managed through a combination of medical and nonmedical interventions [24]. In fact, over-reliance on medical interventions, particularly pharmacotherapies with opioid analgesics, places patients at risk for poor outcomes, including addiction.

(Note that psychological approaches, movement therapies, and acupressure are discussed in Chapter 16 of this Handbook.)

For More Information on the Topics Discussed:

American Society of Addiction Medicine (ASAM):

Auerbach S. Sleep disorders related to alcohol and other drug use (Chapter 80). In RK Ries, DA Fiellin, SC Miller, R Saitz, eds. *The ASAM Principles of Addiction Medicine, Fifth Edition*. Philadelphia, PA: Wolters Kluwer; 2014.

Gallanter M. Spirituality in the recovery process (Chapter 71). In RK Ries, DA Fiellin, SC Miller, R Saitz, eds. *The ASAM Principles of Addiction Medicine, Fifth Edition*. Philadelphia, PA: Wolters Kluwer; 2014.

Nace EP. Twelve-Step programs in addiction recovery (Chapter 69). In RK Ries, DA Fiellin, SC Miller, R Saitz, eds. *The ASAM Principles of Addiction Medicine, Fifth Edition.* Philadelphia, PA: Wolters Kluwer; 2014.

National Center for Complementary and Integrative Health (NCCIH): Complementary health approaches for chronic pain. NCCIH Clinical Digest for Health Professionals. Bethesda, MD: NCCIH, National Institutes of Health; 2016. (Access at: https://nccih.nih.gov/health/providers/digest/chronic-pain.)

References

1. Griffin ML, McDermott KA, McHugh RK, et al. Longitudinal association between pain severity and subsequent opioid use in prescription opioid dependent patients with chronic pain. *Drug Alcohol Depend.* 2016 Jun 1;163:216–221.
2. Suri P, Saunders KW, Von Korff M. Prevalence and characteristics of flare-ups of chronic non-specific back pain in primary care: A telephone survey. *Clin J Pain.* 2012 Sep;28(7):573–580.
3. Siddall PJ, Lovell M, MacLeod R. Spirituality: What is its role in pain medicine? *Pain Med.* 2015 Jan;16(1):51–60. Review.
4. Kress HG, Aldington D, Alon E, et al. A holistic approach to chronic pain management that involves all stakeholders: Change is needed. *Curr Med Res Opin.* 2015;31(9):1743–1754. Review.
5. Davin S, Wilt J, Covington E, et al. Variability in the relationship between sleep and pain in patients undergoing interdisciplinary rehabilitation for chronic pain. *Pain Med.* 2014 Jun;15(6):1043–1051.
6. Mayo Clinic. *Sleep Tips: 7 Steps to Better Sleep.* (Accessed at: http://www.mayoclinic.org/healthy-lifestyle/adult-health/in-depth/sleep/art-20048379.)
7. Harvard Medical School Division of Sleep Medicine. *Twelve Simple Steps to Improve Your Sleep.* Boston, MA: Harvard Medical School and WGBH Educational Foundation. (Accessed at: http://healthysleep.med.harvard.edu/healthy/getting/overcoming/tips.)
8. Narouze S, Souzdalnitski D. Obesity and chronic pain: Systematic review of prevalence and implications for pain practice. *Reg Anesth Pain Med.* 2015 Mar–Apr;40(2):91–111. Review.
9. Narouze S, Souzdalnitski D. Obesity and chronic pain: Opportunities for better patient care. *Pain Manag.* 2015;5(4):217–219. Review.
10. National Center for Complementary and Integrative Health (NCCIH). Complementary health approaches for chronic pain. *NCCIH Clinical Digest for Health Professionals.* Bethesda, MD: NCCIH, National Institutes of Health; 2016. (Accessed at: https://nccih.nih.gov/health/providers/digest/chronic-pain.)
11. Huang W, Shah S, Long Q, et al. Improvement of pain, sleep, and quality of life in chronic pain patients with vitamin D supplementation. *Clin J Pain.* 2013 Apr;29(4):341–347.

12. Derry CJ, Derry S, Moore RA. Caffeine as an analgesic adjuvant for acute pain in adults. *Cochrane Database Syst Rev.* 2014 Dec 11;(12):CD009281. Review.
13. Petre B, Torbey S, Griffith JW, et al. Smoking increases risk of pain chronification through shared corticostriatal circuitry. *Hum Brain Map.* 2015 Feb;36(2):683–694.
14. Lee C, Crawford C, Schoomaker E. Active Self-Care Therapies for Pain (PACT) Working Group: Movement therapies for the self-management of chronic pain symptoms. *Pain Med.* 2014 Apr;15(Suppl 1):S40–S53.
15. Naugle KM, Fillingim RB, Riley JL 3rd. A meta-analytic review of the hypoalgesic effects of exercise. *J Pain.* 2012 Dec;13(12):1139–1150.
16. Fisken A, Keogh JW, Waters DL, et al. Perceived benefits, motives, and barriers to aqua-based exercise among older adults with and without osteoarthritis. *J Appl Gerontol.* 2015 Apr;34(3):377–396.
17. National Center for Complementary and Integrative Health (NCCIH). *Yoga: In Depth.* Bethesda, MD: NCCIH, National Institutes of Health, June 2013. (Accessed at: https://nccih.nih.gov/health/yoga/introduction.htm.)
18. Chen CL, Wang CW, Ho RT, et al. Qigong exercise for the treatment of fibromyalgia: A systematic review of randomized controlled trials. *J Altern Complement Med.* 2012;18(7):641–646.
19. Chen YW, Wang HH. The effectiveness of acupressure on relieving pain: A systematic review. *Pain Manag Nurs.* 2014;15(2):539–550.
20. Chronic Pain Anonymous. (Accessed at: https://www.chronicpainanonymous.org/.)
21. Pills Anonymous. (Accessed at: www.pillsanonymous.org/.)
22. Cleveland M. *Chronic Illness and the Twelve Steps: A Practical Approach to Spiritual Resilience.* Center City, MN: Hazelden Publishing; 2013.
23. Ruehlm LS, Karoly P, Enders C. A randomized controlled evaluation of an online chronic pain self management program. *Pain.* 2012;(153):319–330.
24. Lee C, Crawford C, Hickey A, for the Active Self-Care Therapies for Pain (PACT) Working Group. Mind-body therapies for the self-management of chronic pain symptoms. *Pain Med.* 2014 Apr;15(Suppl 1):S21–S39. Review.

Chapter 18

Revising the Treatment Plan and/or Ending Pain Treatment

MARK A. WEINER, M.D., DFASAM AND
HERBERT L. MALINOFF, M.D., FACP, DFASAM

Many patients who suffer from chronic non-malignant pain (CNMP) are placed on short- and long-acting opioids as part of a pain management program. However, only a small minority of patients (and their physicians) find this form of medication management satisfactory. Lack of functional improvement, intolerable adverse effects, inadvertent or intentional opioid overdose, opioid misuse, drug diversion, worsening pain, and psychological symptoms are common in the chronic pain patient who is managed exclusively with opioid therapy.

The term "opioid treatment failure" should be applied to this population of patients with CNMP. Recent reviews estimate that more than 75% of patients placed on an opioid for CNMP will be classified as treatment failures at five years [1].

Identifying opioid treatment failure often is difficult, and it may require significant time and many clinical encounters. Lack of progress in functional improvement—accompanied by higher doses of opioids, drug seeking or misuse, and the perception of worsening pain—is a familiar clinical scenario [2].

Usefulness of an Opioid Taper

Whenever a pain patient has failed treatment with high doses of opioids (i.e., more than 60 mg morphine equivalents per day), ending opioid therapy should be considered. However, abruptly discontinuing opioids almost always precipitates an uncomfortable abstinence syndrome, which may persist for many weeks [3]. In such cases, it is reasonable to consider a tapering strategy. Such strategies are based on the theory that opioid tolerance can be reversed and withdrawal avoided if the opioid dose is reduced gradually, thereby avoiding the dysphoria and exacerbation of pain associated with opioid withdrawal [4,5].

Although there is no universal consensus to guide a tapering schedule, it is not unreasonable to attempt an opioid taper if it is done with proper forethought and in close collaboration with the patient. Following a successful taper, the patient could be returned to a much more stable treatment regimen without the risk involved in adding more medications [6].

Challenges in Tapering Opioids

Opioid tapers are most likely to be successful in patients who are on relatively low doses of opioids or who have been treated with opioids for relatively short periods of time. The presence of psychological or psychiatric disorders, or a history or signs of SUD, suggest a greater likelihood that tapering strategies will fail. Even in patients without those conditions, tapering strategies can fail if the patient develops intolerable symptoms of pain or withdrawal, a significant loss of function, and/or a reduction in quality of life.

Emerging evidence suggests a neurobiochemical basis for the failure of tapering approaches [7]. In animal models, long-term exposure to opioids sometimes leads to permanent downregulation in dopaminergic fibers that serve the nucleus accumbens. In such cases, some experts hypothesize that patients experience significant dysphoria that does not readily return to baseline [8]. Such patients need long-term opioid replacement therapy or some other pharmacological or nonpharmacological therapy to address this syndrome.

At present, one practical approach is the use of buprenorphine in these patients [4,5]. Therefore, the remainder of this chapter addresses the use of buprenorphine as an exit strategy.

Stratification of Risk

When it becomes clear that a patient is not benefiting from pain treatment with opioids, it is essential to formulate an appropriate plan of action. However, development of evidence-based protocols for managing patients who are trapped on high doses of opioids is in its infancy. Some research suggests that traditional tapering methods result in poor outcomes when used in these patients [9].

On the other hand, there is notable success in weaning patients from opioids and sedatives with minimal use of pharmacotherapy. This strategy appears to be most effective when carried out in a structured setting, using an interdisciplinary approach [10]. In highly specialized residential rehabilitation centers, patients undergo intensive daily counseling for several weeks, in combination with techniques such as psychological counseling (see Chapter 15 of this Handbook) and mindfulness therapy (see Chapter 21 of this Handbook).

The exit strategy discussed in this chapter is designed for the clinician who is managing patients in a standard outpatient practice (occasionally involving brief hospitalization). As emphasized earlier, many patients require interdisciplinary care [11].

The first step in identifying a specific exit strategy is determining the patient's level of pain and the medical resources required to address it. Whenever central nervous system (CNS) depressants such as opioids or sedatives are stopped, psychiatric instability may emerge. As a result, extreme care should be taken in treating patients who have undergone multiple psychiatric hospitalizations, especially if any of those are recent (e.g., within the past few months). In the best possible circumstance, such a patient already will be in the care of a psychiatrist who can provide insight into the patent's stability.

This scenario illustrates the point that, before beginning a taper, the clinician must determine whether clearance by other specialists is required. For example, in patients who are receiving medications from a psychiatrist, it is imperative to involve that psychiatrist in the process and, ideally, obtain a letter of clearance. As in any medical interaction, the highest priority is the patent's safety [12]. One potential risk inherent in not involving the patent's psychiatrist is that unmasking the patent's depression or mania could lead to harm or death to the patient or another.

In many circumstances, the services of a psychologist or psychiatrist with special knowledge of pain can be helpful in determining "next steps" for patients with psychiatric comorbidities. Similarly, in patients with a significant medical comorbidity (such as a recent coronary event, stroke, etc.), it may be best to obtain clearance from a cardiologist and wait a specified period of time (e.g., six months) before beginning a medical transition. The same is true of patients who have had recent surgery, severe or worsening chronic obstructive pulmonary disease (COPD) (on chronic oxygen therapy), or any recent active medical problem. The rule here is not to proceed with transition until the patient is relatively stable, *unless* failing to proceed with the transition would lead to further harm [7].

In complex patients, a brief hospitalization often is advisable. Since patients may present with active addiction in the setting of chronic pain and opioid toxicity, attention must be paid to both disorders [13]. A general rule regarding active substance use disorder (SUD) is that it must be relatively quiescent or in remission before treatment of pain can begin. Patients who are actively alcoholic and unable to stop drinking, or patients who are actively involved in cocaine or heroin use, are best treated for pain after they have completed an intensive outpatient or residential treatment program. Once they have completed such treatment, they are much better candidates for pharmacotherapy to address their chronic pain.

At the other end of the risk spectrum, if a patient is taking a relatively low dose of benzodiazepines, all that may be needed is to work with the patient's primary care practitioner and to clarify expectations with the patient [14].

Managing Opioid Withdrawal in the Medical Office

When a patient is diagnosed with an SUD involving opioids and/or benzodiazepines, it is essential to decide whether withdrawal from those medications can be safely conducted in an office-based setting or whether a brief hospitalization is advisable.

Office-based treatment is intended to be carried out on an outpatient basis in a general medical office setting. With proper risk stratification, it is rare for a patient undergoing office-based withdrawal to have a poor outcome or to be medically compromised. Nevertheless, it is recommended that the entire office staff know how to obtain medical help in the event of an emergency.

For patients who are dependent on both opioids and benzodiazepines, it is recommended that the benzodiazepine be discontinued before the opioid use is addressed, because concurrent use of benzodiazepines and opioids (including buprenorphine) can lead to unpredictable central nervous system and respiratory depression. In fact, in the relatively few cases of buprenorphine-associated deaths, co-ingestion of benzodiazepines often has been implicated [15].

In patients who are on low doses of benzodiazepines and benzodiazepine-like substances (e.g., zolpidem [Ambien®]) 10 mg at nighttime or alprazolam 0.5 mg three times a day), the standard approach is to discontinue the benzodiazepine and replace it with phenobarbital. In many cases, phenobarbital 30–60 mg once or twice a day will suffice [16]. Other useful medications include gabapentin and oxcarbazepine.

It is further recommended that patients be withdrawn from benzodiazepines and then be medically stable for two weeks before addressing their opioid use. However, this needs to be determined on a case-by-case basis, depending primarily on how well a particular patient is handling discontinuation of the sedative. Once such patients are stabilized, it is appropriate to address the opioid.

At present, research into specific pharmacotherapies for use in this process is limited. For patients with chronic pain, with or without the presence of addiction, the use of buprenorphine has received much attention [17]. Recently the use of low-dose naltrexone also has been suggested as a pharmacotherapy for these patients [18]. However, there is not yet sufficient research-based evidence for naltrexone to be a standard recommendation.

Treatment with Buprenorphine

The following discussion focuses on the use of buprenorphine for patients who are experiencing opioid tolerance, dependence, and hyperalgesia. It is important to inform such patients of the rationale for selecting buprenorphine, the risks and benefits involved, and the off-label use of sublingual buprenorphine in the treatment of chronic pain. This information should be carefully documented in the patient's chart [19].

Patients for whom outpatient transition from another opioid to buprenorphine is appropriate generally use only short-acting opioids (such as hydrocodone, morphine, and oxycodone), with morphine equivalents of less than 80 mg per day. Such patients typically are instructed to discontinue their short-acting opioid 12 hours before induction onto buprenorphine [20].

The induction process is similar to buprenorphine induction with patients who have an SUD without pain. Patients should be monitored for three to four hours after the first dose of buprenorphine and their vital signs taken three or four times during that period. Regardless of the patient's customary opioid dose, very small amounts of buprenorphine are given initially, with starting doses generally 0.5 mg of buprenorphine (one-quarter of a 2 mg buprenorphine tablet), taken sublingually [21]. It is better to under-treat patients during their first exposure to buprenorphine, because there is an opportunity to increase the dose, whereas induction with too large a dose often leads to nausea, headache, and vomiting. Because many patients have experienced chronic pain for a very long time, a slow, thoughtful approach is the best way to ensure success.

Some clinicians have reported good results with transdermal buprenorphine, which has a very slow onset of action. The major drawback of transdermal buprenorphine is that it takes about three days to achieve a steady state, and there is no possibility of demand dosing under which patients can take less buprenorphine on days when they feel better and more on days when they feel more pain. This and other examples underscore the point that matching the right pharmacotherapy to the needs of a given patient requires considerable experience and careful consideration of multiple factors [22].

Once a patient has completed induction onto buprenorphine, he or she can adopt a very low-dose stable regimen (such as one-half to 1 mg of buprenorphine sublingually three to four times a day). Unlike patients with opioid use disorders, patients who have chronic pain often derive significant benefit from small doses of buprenorphine ingested more frequently. The duration of buprenorphine's analgesic effect is in the range of four to eight hours and varies sharply from one patient to another [23].

An alternative approach is to begin the patient on a gentle upward escalation of dose, such as 0.5 mg twice a day for two days, followed by 0.5 mg three times a day for two days, followed by 0.5 mg four times a day for two days, followed by 1 mg sublingually four times a day. In some patients, such a slow escalation of dose can reduce the side effects of nausea and headache [24].

Regardless of the induction strategy used, close follow-up is important; for example, having the patient return every two to three weeks until he or she is relatively stable on the buprenorphine regimen. Although the buprenorphine dose is fairly easily adjusted, it is strongly suggested that patients be kept on a low dose for a period of a few weeks, until the risk of opioid-induced hyperalgesia has passed. This is because many patients ultimately require only very small doses of buprenorphine to manage their pain. However, if the buprenorphine dose escalates rapidly, based solely on the patient's reports of pain within the first few weeks, it is possible that the patient eventually will need higher doses of buprenorphine than he or she otherwise would. In this context, a slow hand often reaps benefits.

Managing Opioid Withdrawal in a Hospital Setting

As noted earlier, a fair number of pain patients present with ongoing or recent medical, surgical, or psychiatric instability that requires hospital-based care. Moreover, for patients on very high-dose opioids and possibly also high-dose sedatives, hospital-based transition to buprenorphine is recommended to maintain the patient's safety [5]. Depending on the severity of the patient's instability or the medical questions left unanswered, referral to inpatient care on a unit specializing in psychiatry, neurology, neurosurgery, orthopedic surgery, gastroenterology, cardiology, oncology, or pulmonary medicine may be very helpful.

When preparing the patient and his or her family for hospitalization, it is extremely important to clearly explain the process and give the patient and family members sufficient time to ask questions and voice their anxieties. The process of explaining the need for hospital-based care may begin at the very first visit, and usually continues through a subsequent visit or two so that the patient and family have time to process the information and thus enter the process with ease and comfort. In this regard, providing the patient and family with patient education materials in addition to the verbal description can be extremely helpful [25]. It also is appropriate (when possible) to refer the patient for educational programs delivered by nursing staff and hospitalists.

Many patients who have been treated for long periods of time with high-dose opioids and sedatives fear that they will be abandoned if they are hospitalized. Although they may have some understanding that the medications they have been taking have been harming them, such patients often have a deeply conditioned fear of changing to new medications. Thus, taking the time to address patient expectations with careful, easy-to-understand explanations and having the entire transition team work in concert can help this process move along more smoothly.

Once a date for buprenorphine induction has been set, the patient should be advised to remain on the medications he or she currently is taking, under the care of the physician who prescribed them, up to the point of entering the hospital. Some patients may express enthusiasm about discontinuing their medications, but if they begin the process in florid withdrawal, or fatigued by lack of sleep, or medically compromised by abrupt discontinuation of their medication, the process of withdrawal can become much more difficult.

Discontinuing Current Medications

At the time of admission, the first step is for the patient to discontinue use of current opioids and all other medications, followed by stabilization. This can be accomplished by having the patient discontinue use of current drugs while in the hospital and replacing them with a patient-controlled hydromorphone anesthesia pump.

If the patient is on relatively low-dose opioids and sedatives, a patient-controlled analgesia (PCA) pump may not be needed. However, for patients who are taking more than 80 mg of morphine equivalent per day, the suggested starting dose is 0.2 mg hydromorphone infused every hour, with 0.2 mg infused on demand (with a six-minute lockout) [26]. For most patients taking sustained-release opioids, including morphine and oxycodone, an appropriate "wash-out time" (i.e., time for the opioid to clear the patient's system) is approximately 36–48 hours. In patients who are using transdermal fentanyl, the wash-out time may be three to four days, because fentanyl is deposited in subcutaneous and subdermal fat [27]. For methadone, the wash-out time can be even longer because of individual variability in methadone metabolism [28]. For such patients, evaluating methadone levels daily and waiting for results to drop below 25 ng/ml often is appropriate.

Induction onto Buprenorphine

When initiating induction onto buprenorphine, the hydromorphone PCA pump usually is discontinued in the morning and the patient instructed to alert a nurse when he or she begins to experience opioid withdrawal.

Buprenorphine can be started either sublingually or intramuscularly, but only after the patient begins to experience some objective signs of withdrawal. After the initial dose of buprenorphine, the patient should be monitored in a hospital setting for approximately 24 hours to determine whether he or she is medically stable and free from any side effects of the buprenorphine. If the patient also is dependent on a benzodiazepine or benzodiazepine-like substance, those drugs should be continued until the patient is hospitalized under the care of a specialist. Upon hospitalization, the medication(s) should be discontinued and phenobarbital or similar agents substituted.

In a hospital setting, higher doses of phenobarbital, gabapentin, or other substances can be administered under close nursing supervision, with the patient monitored carefully for signs of excess sedation [24].

Once stabilized, patients usually are discharged after a hospital stay of three to five days (again, somewhat longer for fentanyl and much longer for methadone). Patients should be followed in an outpatient setting for one to two weeks after release from the hospital to allow ongoing assessment and reassurance [29].

The Importance of Aftercare

An intensive aftercare program is essential to obtaining optimal outcomes. For the practitioner, this involves meeting with the patient every one to two weeks until the patient is appropriately stabilized. Patients who have been on high-dose opiates and sedatives also may need intensive psychological or psychiatric counseling [7,8].

With many patients, it appears that once high-dose opioids and sedatives have been discontinued, emotions and memories that have been repressed for long periods of time—even decades—reemerge. These may present as psychiatric comorbidities or be transformed into perceptions of physical pain. In such cases, careful discussion with the patient, accompanied by steady reassurance and a hesitation to accelerate pharmacotherapy, typically enhances the success rate.

In some cases, family counseling is necessary. For patients who have co-occurring pain and SUDs, it is extremely important to engage the patient in creating a recovery plan. Many such patients benefit from individual or group counseling or referral to a 12-Step or other self-help program during this period; ideally, such patients will develop a long-term relationship with their support program.

Conclusion

The approach to the pain patient who has failed treatment with high doses of opioids (i.e., more than 60 mg morphine equivalents per day) has been problematic because "weaning" or tapering patients from opioids can lead to worsening pain and dysfunction [2].

Moreover, abruptly discontinuing opioids almost always precipitates an uncomfortable abstinence syndrome, which may persist for weeks [3]. The partial opioid agonist buprenorphine is a valuable clinical tool in treating such patients. As a partial mu agonist with modest intrinsic mu-agonist activity and high mu-receptor affinity, buprenorphine represents a means of discontinuing opioids safely, quickly, and tolerably [4,5].

An intensive aftercare program is essential to obtaining optimal outcomes.

For More Information on the Topics Discussed:

American Society of Addiction Medicine (ASAM):

Covington EC, Kotz MM. Psychological issues in the management of pain (Chapter 94). In RK Ries, DA Fiellin, SC Miller, R Saitz, eds. *The ASAM Principles of Addiction Medicine, Fifth Edition*. Philadelphia, PA: Wolters Kluwer; 2014.

Savage SR. Opioid therapy of pain (Chapter 97). In RK Ries, DA Fiellin, SC Miller, R Saitz, eds. *The ASAM Principles of Addiction Medicine, Fifth Edition*. Philadelphia, PA: Wolters Kluwer; 2014.

Substance Abuse and Mental Health Services Administration (SAMHSA):

The Facts About Buprenorphine (patient education brochure) SMA09-4442. Rockville, MD: SAMHSA, Department of Health and Human Services, rev. 2011. (Access at: http://store.samhsa.gov/shin/content/SMA09-4442/SMA09-4442.pdf.)

Veterans Administration (VA):

VA Buprenorphine Helpline Resource Guide, Version 9. Washington, DC. VA, Department of Defense, June 2009. (Access at: http://www.mental-health.va.gov/providers/sud/docs/VA_Bup_Resource_Guidev9-1.pdf.)

References

1. Saper JR, Lake AE, Bain PA, et al. A practice guide for continuous opioid therapy for refractory daily headache: Patient selection, physician requirements, and treatment monitoring. *Headache*. 2010;50:1175–1193.
2. Holliday S, Hayes C, Dunlop A. Opioid use in chronic non-cancer pain— Part 1: Known knowns and known unknowns. *Aust Fam Physician*. 2013 Mar;42(3):98–102. (Review article)
3. Tetrault JM, O'Connor PG. Management of opioid intoxication and withdrawal (Chapter 45). In RK Ries, DA Fiellin, SC Miller, R Saitz, eds. *The ASAM Principles of Addiction Medicine, Fifth Edition*. Philadelphia, PA: Wolters Kluwer; 2014.

4. Malinoff HL, Barkin RL, Wilson G. Sublingual buprenorphine is effective in the treatment of chronic pain syndrome. *Am J Ther*. 2005 Sep–Oct;12(5):379–384.

5. Berland DW, Malinoff HL, Weiner MA, et al. When opioids fail in chronic pain management: The role for buprenorphine and hospitalization. *Am J Ther*. 2013 Jul–Aug;20(4):316–321.

6. Wang H, Akbar M, Weinsheimer N, et al. Longitudinal observation of changes in pain sensitivity during opioid tapering in patients with chronic low-back pain. *Pain Med*. 2011 Dec;12(12):1720–1726.

7. Berna C, Kulich RJ, Rathmell JP. Tapering long-term opioid therapy in chronic noncancer pain: Evidence and recommendations for everyday practice. *Mayo Clin Proc*. 2015 Jun; 90(6):828–842. (Review)

8. Turk DC, Swanson KS, Tunks ER. Psychological approaches in the treatment of chronic pain patients—When pills, scalpels, and needles are not enough. *Can J Psychiatry*. 2008 Apr; 53(4):213–223. (Review)

9. Stanos S, Calisoff RL. Rehabilitation approaches to pain management (Chapter 95). In RK Ries, DA Fiellin, SC Miller, R Saitz, eds. *The ASAM Principles of Addiction Medicine, Fifth Edition*. Philadelphia, PA: Wolters Kluwer; 2014.

10. Huffman KL, Sweis GW, Gase A, et al. Opioid use 12 months following interdisciplinary pain rehabilitation with weaning. *Pain Med*. 2013 Dec;14(12):1908–1917.

11. Gallagher RM, Koob G, Popescu A. The pathophysiology of chronic pain and clinical interfaces with addiction (Chapter 93). In RK Ries, DA Fiellin, SC Miller, R Saitz, eds. *The ASAM Principles of Addiction Medicine, Fifth Edition*. Philadelphia, PA: Wolters Kluwer; 2014.

12. Hamza M, Doleys D, Wells M, et al. Prospective study of 3-year follow-up of low-dose intrathecal opioids in the management of chronic nonmalignant pain. *Pain Med*. 2012 Oct;13(10):1304–1313.

13. Gowing L, Ali R, White J. Buprenorphine for the management of opioid withdrawal. *Cochrane Database Syst Rev*. 2000;(3):CD002025 (Review). Update in: *Cochrane Database Syst Rev*. 2002;(2):CD002025.

14. Lader M, Tylee A, Donoghue J. Withdrawing benzodiazepines in primary care. *CNS Drugs*. 2009;23(1):19–34.

15. Cunningham JL, Evans MM, King SM, et al. Opioid tapering in fibromyalgia patients: Experience from an interdisciplinary pain rehabilitation program. *Pain Med*. 2016 Sep;17(9):1676–1685.

16. Younger J, Parkitny L, McLain D. The use of low-dose naltrexone (LDN) as a novel anti-inflammatory treatment for chronic pain. *Clin Rheumatol*. 2014 Apr;33(4):451–459.

17. Saleh MI. Predictors of long term opioid withdrawal outcome after short-term stabilization with buprenorphine. *Eur Rev Med Pharmacol Sci*. 2014;18(24):3935–3942.

18. Mannelli P, Patkar AA, Peindl K, et al. Very low dose naltrexone addition in opioid detoxification: A randomized, controlled trial. *Addict Biol*. 2009 Apr;14(2):204–213.

19. Huang A, Azam A, Segal S, et al. Chronic postsurgical pain and persistent opioid use following surgery: The need for a transitional pain service. *Pain Manag*. 2016 Oct;6(5):435–443.

20. Lee M, Silverman SM, Hansen H, et al. A comprehensive review of opioid-induced hyperalgesia. *Pain Physician*. 2011 Mar–Apr;14(2):145–161. (Review article)

21. Rosenblum A, Cruciani RA, Strain EC, et al. Sublingual buprenorphine/naloxone for chronic pain in at-risk patients: Development and pilot test of a clinical protocol. *J Opioid Manag*. 2012 Nov–Dec;8(6):369–382.

22. Chou R, Ballantyne JC, Fanciullo GJ, et al. Research gaps on use of opioids for chronic noncancer pain: Findings from a review of the evidence for an American Pain Society and American Academy of Pain Medicine clinical practice guideline. *J Pain*. 2009;10(2):147–159.

23. James IG, O'Brien CM, McDonald CJ. A randomized, double-blind, double-dummy comparison of the efficacy and tolerability of low-dose transdermal buprenorphine (BuTrans seven-day patches) with buprenorphine sublingual tablets (Temgesic) in patients with osteoarthritis pain. *J Pain Symptom Manag*. 2010 Aug;40(2):266–278.

24. Raffa RB, Haidery M, Huang HM, et al. The clinical analgesic efficacy of buprenorphine. *J Clin Pharm Ther*. 2014 Dec;39(6):577–583.

25. Rose P, Sakai J, Argue R, et al. Opioid information pamphlet increases postoperative opioid disposal rates: A before versus after quality improvement study. *Can J Anaesth*. 2016 Jan;63(1):31–37.

26. Rapp SE, Egan KJ, Ross BK, et al. A multidimensional comparison of morphine and hydromorphone patient-controlled analgesia. *Anesth Analg*. 1996 May;82(5):1043–1048.

27. Mercadante S, Villari P, Ferrera P, et al. Opioid plasma concentrations during a switch from transdermal fentanyl to methadone. *J Palliat Med*. 2007 Apr;10(2):338–344.

28. Breivik H. Tapering and discontinuation of methadone for chronic pain. *J Pain Palliat Care Pharmacother*. 2015 Jun;29(2):185–186.

29. Mellbye A, Karlstad Ø, Skurtveit S, et al. The duration and course of opioid therapy in patients with chronic non-malignant pain. *Acta Anaesthesiol Scand*. 2016 Jan;60(1):128–137.

TREATING OPIOID USE DISORDER IN PATIENTS DIAGNOSED WITH CHRONIC PAIN

In **Section IV**, the chapters address the management of patients who have a documented chronic pain condition and who also are diagnosed with an opioid use disorder.

- In **Chapter 19**, the authors describe pain medications approved by the U.S. Food and Drug Administration, along with their potential for interaction with medications approved for the treatment of opioid use disorder.
- The author of **Chapter 20** reviews non-pharmacological therapies for opioid use disorder, which often are indicated in the management of patients with preexisting chronic pain.
- The author of **Chapter 21** describes mindfulness and related therapies as potential components of treatment for chronic pain or addiction.
- Preventing avoidable work disability related to chronic pain and/or addiction is the focus of **Chapter 22**.
- The authors of **Chapter 23** describe situations in which the treatment plan for an opioid use disorder may need to be revised or treatment ended and the patient referred for another—usually more structured—type of care.

Chapter 19

Opioid Pharmacotherapies
for Substance Use Disorders
and Addiction

JASON BAKER FIELDS, M.D., DABAM,
WILLIAM F. HANING, III, M.D., DFASAM, DFAPA,
YNGVILD OLSEN, M.D., M.P.H., DFASAM, AND
BONNIE B. WILFORD, M.S.

Treatment with opioid agonists is an effective, accepted medical treatment for opioid use disorder, especially if chronic pain also is present. In fact, there is considerable consensus among addiction experts that treatment with opioid agonists or partial agonists (broadly, "pharmacological therapies" or "medication-assisted treatment" [MAT]) should be considered for every patient whose substance use disorder (SUD) involves opioids [1,2].

However, no single treatment approach is appropriate for every patient at all times. For this reason, in formulating a treatment plan for each patient, the treating physician should consider the risks and benefits of medication-assisted treatment in general, as well as with each potential treatment agent, and compare the risks associated with each medication to the risks of no treatment or treatment without medication [2,3].

As described later, two medications have gained U.S. Food and Drug Administration (FDA) approval for use in office-based treatment of opioid use disorders: the partial agonist *buprenorphine* (which is available as buprenorphine alone and as buprenorphine in combination with naloxone) and the antagonist *naltrexone*, which is available in both oral form and as an extended-release injectable formulation. These medications differ in terms of their route and frequency of administration, as well as in the regulatory restrictions on their use.

In addition, the opioid agonist *methadone* has a long history in the treatment of opioid addiction, but it is not available for use in office-based treatment; federal law limits its use for that indication to federally certified opioid treatment programs (OTPs).

Treatment with Buprenorphine

Buprenorphine's unique combination of pharmacological properties (as described in Chapter 8 of this Handbook) appears to offer significant advantages for office-based treatment of opioid use disorder [2,4,5]. Through its tight binding to opioid receptors, buprenorphine relieves patients' opioid craving, prevents opioid withdrawal, and partially blocks the effects of euphoria-inducing opioids [6–10]. This allows patients to focus on recovery-oriented activities. Although more than a pharmacological therapy is needed to help patients achieve the lasting changes required for recovery from opioid dependence, medications such as buprenorphine make it possible for such patients to participate in counseling, peer and family support, and community alliances [11,12].

Requirements for the Use of Buprenorphine in Office-Based Treatment

Physicians who wish to use buprenorphine in office-based treatment of opioid use disorder must apply to the Center for Substance Abuse Treatment (CSAT), a component of the Substance Abuse and Mental Health Services Administration (SAMHSA), for a waiver of the Controlled Substance Act that will enable them to treat patients for the disorder in their medical offices [13,14]. Physicians typically are eligible for a waiver if they meet at least one of the following criteria [15,71]:

- Certification in Addiction Medicine or Addiction Psychiatry through training approved by the American Board of Medical Specialties (ABMS) and the Accreditation Council on Graduate Medical Education (ACGME); or
- Completion of at least eight hours of approved training in the treatment or management of patients who are physically dependent on or addicted to opioids; or
- Other training or experience that demonstrates their ability to treat and manage opioid-dependent patients.

Physicians who wish to obtain a waiver also must certify that they can provide (or refer patients for) ancillary services such as behavioral counseling, mental health care, and case management [16].

BOX 19.1 New Federal Regulations Increase Buprenorphine Limit to 275 Patients

Under recently adopted federal regulations, physicians who have prescribed buprenorphine to at least 100 patients for one year or more are allowed to submit an application to increase their patient limit to 275 patients. For more information, send an email to infobuprenorphine@samhsa.hhs.gov or phone 1-866-287-2728.

To be considered for the higher limit, physicians must complete a form titled "Online Request for Patient Limit Increase."

To learn more about the new rule, see the following publications, which are available on SAMHSA's website at: https://www.samhsa.gov/medication-assisted-treatment/treatment/buprenorphine.

- *SAMHSA's Letter on the Expansion of Access to Medication-Assisted Treatment for Opioid Use Disorder—2016.*
- *Understanding the Final Rule for a Patient Limit of 275–2016*, a guidance document to help determine your eligibility for the new, higher patient limit based on your credentials or features of your practice setting.
- *Medication-Assisted Treatment for Opioid Use Disorders*, the final rule, as announced in the Federal Register.

Source: Substance Abuse and Mental Health Services Administration (SAMHSA), U.S. Department of Health and Human Services; 2017.

In addition, federal regulations limit the number of patients who can be treated at one time, and stipulate specific prescribing, dispensing, record-keeping, drug storage, and inspection requirements (Box 19.1).

Indications for Treatment with Buprenorphine

An ideal candidate for office-based treatment with buprenorphine is an individual who has been carefully assessed and diagnosed with opioid use disorder, who has the capacity to consent freely, who is willing to follow safety precautions for treatment, who can be expected to adhere to the treatment plan, who has no contraindications to buprenorphine therapy, and who agrees to treatment with buprenorphine after his or her physician reviews all appropriate treatment options [17].

Given the long-term nature of medication-assisted treatment and the potential for toxicity, a high degree of certainty regarding the diagnosis is

required before recommending maintenance treatment with any opioid agonist or partial agonist, including buprenorphine [18]. If the diagnosis cannot
be confirmed through observation of opioid withdrawal, injection sites, or confirmation of previous treatment, then treatment should be initiated cautiously
and with very close monitoring. In such a situation, lack of intoxication from
opioid agonists will provide direct evidence of opioid tolerance [19].

Contraindications to Treatment with Buprenorphine

The only *absolute* contraindication to the use of buprenorphine is hypersensitivity to buprenorphine or naloxone [20,21].

An important *relative* contraindication is the concurrent use of monoamine oxidase inhibitors (MAOIs) and selective serotonin reuptake inhibitors
(SSRIs), because the use of these agents in combination with buprenorphine
poses the risk of life-threatening serotonin syndrome [22]. Other relative contraindications include liver failure or the use of benzodiazepines or other central nervous system (CNS) depressants. Somnolence that may preclude driving
or operating equipment is another warning cited by the manufacturer [21].

Cautions in the Use of Buprenorphine

Special caution should be exercised when buprenorphine treatment is considered for patients with any of the following clinical conditions [21].

High-Risk Poly-Substance Use

Patients with SUDs complicated by concomitant use of other substances should
be evaluated carefully for the substances' identities and dosages. A particular
concern is that those who use substances in addition to opioids may need more
structure than can be provided in outpatient care [23].

Severe Hepatic Impairment

Physicians should use their clinical judgment when prescribing buprenorphine to patients with significant hepatic impairment because buprenorphine
is metabolized in the liver. If buprenorphine is prescribed, the patient's liver
function should be monitored closely (with tests at initiation of treatment and
every three to six months thereafter). Note that simply being positive for hepatitis B or C does *not* indicate severe hepatic impairment.

Pregnancy

The FDA classifies buprenorphine (like methadone) as a Pregnancy Category C medication [21]. Until recently, the recommended treatment for opioid-dependent pregnant women was methadone maintenance. While methadone continues to be used for this purpose, recent data from the MOTHER Study indicate that buprenorphine is safe and effective for use in pregnancy [24].

Experts recommend that any pregnant woman seeking treatment should receive a comprehensive assessment for appropriateness of buprenorphine versus methadone. Note that, as of this writing, only the *buprenorphine monoproduct* is advised for use with pregnant women [21].

Breastfeeding Women

The literature on safety of buprenorphine use by lactating women is limited. Generally speaking, buprenorphine's poor oral bioavailability in infants, the low levels found in breast milk, and the low levels found in the serum and urine of breastfed infants lead to the conclusion that its use is acceptable in nursing mothers [21].

Other Medical Conditions

Because buprenorphine is an opioid, it should be used only with extreme caution in patients who have a recent head injury (which raises the possibility of increased intracranial pressure) and those with severely compromised respiratory function [25].

Non-Tolerant Patients

Patients who are not fully tolerant to opioids, but who are at high risk of relapse and wish to begin treatment, should be started on the lowest possible dose of buprenorphine.

Patients Being Transferred from Methadone Maintenance

Buprenorphine may precipitate withdrawal in patients transferring from methadone. This is most likely to occur in patients on higher doses of methadone. With such patients, protocols that slowly reduce methadone and gradually introduce the buprenorphine should be followed [25,26].

Other Considerations When Using Buprenorphine

Several additional factors require caution in the use of buprenorphine.

Significant Current Pain

The sublingual formulations of buprenorphine are not FDA-approved for the treatment of pain. Therefore, buprenorphine is not recommended as a first-line choice for the treatment of pain, but it often is used off-label for this diagnosis. Patients who have co-occurring significant pain and opioid use disorder must be evaluated on an individual basis. Some of these patients can achieve adequate pain control with buprenorphine (often dosed two to four times per day) in combination with non-opioid medications such as nonsteroidal anti-inflammatory drugs (NSAIDs). Those previously maintained with buprenorphine should be returned to buprenorphine (or buprenorphine/naloxone) as soon as feasible [26].

Seizures

Buprenorphine does not control seizures caused by withdrawal from alcohol or other sedative-hypnotics. When buprenorphine is used concurrently with anti-seizure medications (such as phenytoin, carbamazepine, or valproic acid), the metabolism of either or both medications may be altered [15]. In addition, the relative risk of interactions between buprenorphine and sedative-hypnotics (such as phenobarbital and clonazepam) should be kept in mind. For this reason, plasma levels of anti-seizure medications should be carefully monitored [16].

High Tolerance to Opioids

Patients who have a very high level of tolerance to opioids ultimately may need a full agonist (such as methadone) to stabilize. There is no reliable comparative measure of tolerance, however, so a therapeutic trial with buprenorphine is appropriate until lack of efficacy has been demonstrated [27].

Concurrent Use of Alcohol

Individuals with active, current, severe alcohol use disorder rarely are appropriate candidates for office-based treatment with buprenorphine. However, it may be possible to treat such patients through initial, intensive services that effectively detoxify the patient from alcohol while sequentially initiating buprenorphine in a more structured (inpatient or residential) treatment setting [11,28,29].

Concurrent Use of Sedative-Hypnotics

Use of sedative-hypnotic medications (benzodiazepines, barbiturates, etc.) is a relative contraindication to treatment with buprenorphine because the combination—especially in overdose—has been associated with deaths. Taken in combination, sedative-hypnotics and buprenorphine accelerate depression of the central nervous system and should be avoided [11,28].

Concomitant Acute Psychiatric Conditions

Buprenorphine treatment should not be initiated in anyone with acute psychosis or other psychiatric condition whose severity compromises the patient's ability to give informed consent for treatment [15,16].

Dosing and Administration

In several studies [30,31], most patients remained stable on doses of 8–24 mg of buprenorphine per day. Increasing the buprenorphine dose to 24 mg per day or more has been shown to prolong the duration of drug effects and usually is necessary if patients are to be dosed every second day, an option sometimes required by special circumstances. Such an increase does not appear to increase buprenorphine's agonist effects [32].

Induction and Stabilization

The goal of induction and stabilization is to find the lowest dose of buprenorphine at which the patient discontinues or markedly reduces the use of other opioids without experiencing withdrawal symptoms, significant side effects, or uncontrollable craving for a drug [33,34].

Induction Phase

The induction process requires more attention and monitoring than the later maintenance phase [11]. During induction, patients should be assessed at least once a day for signs of over- or under-medication, and dose adjustments should be made as needed [35].

Induction should not begin until moderate signs and symptoms of opioid withdrawal appear, to avoid inadvertently triggering a significant withdrawal episode. A standard opioid withdrawal scale can be used to evaluate the severity of the patient's withdrawal [36]. Attention should be given to the timing of the initial dose of buprenorphine/naloxone so as to minimize untoward outcomes, including loss of confidence on the part of the patient. Morning often is the most suitable time for dosing.

Induction protocols differ according to whether the patient is dependent on a short- or long-acting opioid and whether the patient is in active withdrawal at the time of induction [15].

Because buprenorphine is a partial agonist with a ceiling effect, a buprenorphine induction regimen can be more aggressive than induction with a full agonist such as methadone. In most cases, the initial induction dose is 2–4 mg, with individual titration up to a total first-day dose of 8 mg. The timing of buprenorphine induction requires care to avoid overdose (for example, in a patient who has been using CNS depressants such as alcohol or benzodiazepines in addition to opioids) or under-dose (which can trigger re-emergence of opioid craving) [11].

Stabilization Phase

With every patient, the major objective of the stabilization phase is to find the right dose. A patient is fully stabilized when the dose of buprenorphine allows him or her to conduct activities of daily living and to be aware of his or her surroundings, without either intoxication or withdrawal symptoms (including drug craving) [36,37].

There is no precise way to predict the optimal dose for a particular patient [32,38]. Most patients stabilize on doses of 8–24 mg of buprenorphine per day [17]. Dose adjustments generally can be made in increments of 2 mg per day. Because buprenorphine has a long plasma half-life and an even longer duration of action at the mu opioid receptor, five to seven days should elapse between dose adjustments [32].

Blood concentrations of buprenorphine stabilize after approximately seven days of consistent dosing [38]. If withdrawal symptoms subsequently emerge during any 24-hour dosing interval, the dose should be increased, after first considering other causes such as diversion; however, it is noteworthy that little reduction in buprenorphine levels is seen with co-administration of other medications [16,28].

Patients should be monitored for symptoms of withdrawal precipitated by the naloxone component of the combination product. Such symptoms include sweating, anxiety, cravings, and gastrointestinal symptoms such as abdominal cramps, diarrhea, and/or nausea. Symptoms may appear within 90 minutes of buprenorphine dosing, peak between 90 minutes and three hours, and diminish thereafter [39]. This syndrome differs from withdrawal caused by under-dosing of buprenorphine, which usually occurs during the latter part of a 24-hour dosing interval [16]. The patient on an inadequate dose of buprenorphine typically describes symptoms that include muscle aches; hot flashes; an "electric," restless or uncomfortable feeling; nausea; yawning; fatigue; and irritability. The onset of symptoms is delayed with each dose increase [40].

Patients should be advised to avoid driving or operating machinery until their dose is stabilized and they are familiar with the effects of a particular dose of buprenorphine [32].

Safety and Adverse Effects

Buprenorphine exhibits a ceiling effect for respiratory depression, but emerging evidence suggests lack of a ceiling effect for analgesia. Coma and respiratory arrest have been reported with combinations of buprenorphine and benzodiazepines.

Adverse Effects

The most commonly reported adverse effects of buprenorphine include headache, constipation, reduced sexual function, nausea, dizziness, and drowsiness [11,32]. Dose reductions may alleviate some of these symptoms, but such reductions should be balanced against the risk of relapse.

Patients are at risk for serious adverse effects—such as overdose or treatment dropout—if they are undertreated with buprenorphine and attempt to manage symptoms of withdrawal on their own through use of methadone, other opioids, alcohol or sedative-hypnotics [41]. Under-medication or over-medication can be avoided through a flexible approach to dosing (which sometimes requires higher doses of treatment medication) and by considering the effects of setting and anxiety on the symptoms reported by the patient [36,42]. Use of the Clinical Opiate Withdrawal Scale (COWS) can guide the medication response [72]. On the second day of induction, if withdrawal symptoms are present, increases of 2–4 mg may be given, up to a total of 12–16 mg.

Treatment with Naltrexone

Developed in the early 1970s, naltrexone is a long-acting competitive antagonist at opioid receptors that blocks the subjective and objective responses produced by an opioid challenge [43]. Naltrexone and its active metabolite 6-β-naltrexol are pure opiate receptor antagonists—that is, they are competitive antagonists at the mu- and kappa-opioid receptors and, to a lesser extent, at the delta-opioid receptors [44–46]. Naltrexone is thought to block glutamate and may reduce craving for alcohol through that mechanism.

Oral Naltrexone

An oral formulation of naltrexone (Revia®) was approved by the FDA in 1984 "for the blockade of the effects of exogenously administered opioids" [46]. (Oral naltrexone also is approved for the treatment of alcohol use disorder.)

Taken orally, naltrexone is rapidly absorbed, with peak blood levels achieved about one hour after oral administration. It has a relatively short plasma half-life of four hours [47]. Naltrexone is metabolized primarily in the liver to a metabolite, 6-β-naltrexol, which has a plasma half-life of about 10 hours and also is an opioid antagonist. For this reason, liver function tests are recommended before and during naltrexone treatment to identify liver impairment [48].

Extended-Release Injectable Naltrexone (XR-NTX)

The extended-release injectable formulation of naltrexone (Vivitrol®) was approved by the FDA in 2006 "for the treatment of alcohol dependence in patients who are able to abstain from alcohol in an outpatient setting prior to the initiation of treatment with Vivitrol" [46]. In 2010, the FDA expanded the indication for extended-release, injectable naltrexone (XR-NTX) to include "prevention of relapse to opioid dependence, following opioid detoxification" [49].

Because XR-NTX is a pure opioid antagonist, patients cannot develop tolerance to or dependence on the medication [49]. The drug appears to be generally well tolerated, and any adverse effects tend to be mild [50]. The most frequently reported adverse events include hepatic enzyme abnormalities, injection site pain, symptoms of the common cold, insomnia, and toothache. Nausea, vomiting, muscle cramps, dizziness, sedation, decreased appetite, and an allergic form of pneumonia also have occurred in patients treated with XR-NTX [49].

XR-NTX is a microsphere-based formulation of naltrexone incorporated into a biodegradable matrix of polylactide-co-glycolide for intramuscular use. This formulation, which contains 380 mg of naltrexone, releases naltrexone at levels above 1 ng/mL for about four to five weeks, with no need to adjust the dose for weight, age, gender, or health status [46]. It is administered intramuscularly in the gluteal region.

Studies suggest that XR-NTX benefits persons with opioid use disorder who are at risk for opioid use immediately after detoxification [51]. Individuals who are experiencing increased stress or other events that place them at elevated risk of relapse (such as visiting sites of previous drug use, loss of a spouse, or loss of employment) may find that they benefit from the reassurance the blockade provides [52,53]. Individuals who have a shorter or less severe history of opioid use disorder and who thus do not require opioid agonist therapy may be good candidates for injectable naltrexone [51]. For patients who must demonstrate to professional boards, supervisors, drug court judges, or other authorities that their risk of using a non-prescribed opioid is low, the extended-release formulation provides an option that reduces the risk of relapse without relying on adherence to an oral medication regimen [43].

Indications for Treatment with XR-NTX

There is no definitive research to identify patients who would benefit most from XR-NTX; however, current research suggests that patients in the following categories may be good candidates:

- *Patients who have a high level of motivation for abstinence:* Individuals who are highly motivated to achieve and maintain abstinence from opioids may be good candidates for XR-NTX [52,54]. This includes persons who are required to demonstrate abstinence with drug screens, such as individuals in programs for impaired health care providers, airline pilots, parolees, and probationers [43]. Preliminary results from an ongoing study of U.S. health care professionals diagnosed with opioid use disorder suggest that this treatment can be successful for up to one year [55,56].
- *Patients who have not had treatment success with methadone or buprenorphine:* Depending on the reasons for treatment failure, individuals diagnosed with opioid use disorder who have not found success with methadone or buprenorphine may benefit from extended-release injectable naltrexone [57].
- *Patients who have been successful on agonists who wish to change their medication, or patients who are not interested in agonist therapy to treat their opioid addiction:* Some patients may be successful on agonist treatment and want continued pharmacological help to prevent relapse, but would prefer a type of treatment other than methadone [57]. Other patients may never be interested in agonist therapy. The latter group could include: (a) Individuals who feel they are discriminated against, or who are embarrassed or ashamed, because they are on methadone maintenance, or those who previously experienced such emotions while undergoing methadone therapy [58]; (b) those who would like to reduce the time devoted to daily or multiple OTP visits per week, which usually is required for treatment with methadone [59]; (c) individuals who prefer to receive office-based treatment in a primary medical care setting, rather than treatment in a specialty clinic or treatment center [60,61]; or (d) those who believe that agonist therapy is at variance with their desired culture of recovery, such as Narcotics Anonymous.
- *Physician preference:* Some physicians are reluctant to prescribe agonists to treat opioid use disorder because of their treatment philosophy,

difficulty in tapering patients off these medications, or the potential for
diversion of agonist medications [62]. Physicians with these concerns
may be more comfortable prescribing an antagonist, such as naltrexone,
rather than an agonist.

Contraindications to Treatment with XR-NTX

Although individual cases vary, the following patients generally are *not* considered good candidates for treatment with XR-NTX [43,46,63]:

- *Patients who are at risk for overdose:* Such individuals are not good
  candidates for oral naltrexone, although they may be very good
  candidates for extended-release injectable naltrexone. This includes
  patients with a history of overdose or those who have stopped
  naltrexone and resumed opioid use, but whose level of tolerance is not
  known. As part of the evaluation of an opioid-dependent patient, the
  physician should ask about any history of overdose, in the same way
  that a clinician assessing a depressed patient would ask about a history
  of suicide attempts. Also, the opportunity should be taken to educate
  the patient about the phenomenon of lost tolerance and the associated
  overdose risk.
- *Patients who do not tolerate extended opioid-free periods:* A patient who is
  not tolerating detoxification is better managed with a partial agonist
  (buprenorphine) or an agonist (methadone).
- *Patients who fail to complete detoxification.*
- *Patients with protracted abstinence symptoms following detoxification.*
- *Patients with worsening psychiatric symptoms.*
- *Patients whose chronic pain is being treated with opioid analgesics:*
  Naltrexone maintenance is not an option for patients whose pain is
  being treated with opioids. For acute pain (such as that associated
  with dental work, surgery, or traumatic injury), the use of non-opioid
  strategies such as regional blocks is recommended. If opioids are
  needed, higher doses can be used to override the naltrexone blockade,
  but this should be done in a controlled setting where staff can monitor
  the patient for respiratory depression.
- *Patients with advanced liver disease, impending liver failure, or acute
  hepatitis:* Extended-release injectable naltrexone generally is safe
  in patients with chronic hepatitis B or C, so long as they are not
  approaching liver failure. Patients with elevated but stable liver enzyme
  levels usually do well on naltrexone [1,43].

Use of either oral naltrexone or XR-NTX is *contraindicated* in patients with
acute hepatitis, decompensated liver disease (jaundice, encephalopathy), or
liver failure [47,49].

Children and adolescents should be referred to an addiction specialist for initial assessment and recommendations before treatment is initiated. Collaboration with a child and adolescent psychiatrist is strongly recommended.

Essential Patient Information

Physicians should discuss the following topics with patients who are candidates for treatment with XR-NTX, and reinforce the information throughout the course of treatment [43]:

1. How XR-NTX is administered, how it works, and its advantages and disadvantages.
2. The duration of treatment with XR-NTX, its cost, and associated routines.
3. Known side effects of XR-NTX.
4. Issues related to pregnancy and contraception (Pregnancy Category C).

Dosing and Administration

The recommended dose of XR-NTX is 380 mg, delivered intramuscularly approximately once a month. The injection should be administered by a health care professional as an intramuscular gluteal injection, using the carton components provided, and alternating buttocks for each subsequent injection.

The needles provided in the carton are customized, and XR-NTX must not be injected using any other needle. The needle lengths (either 1.5 or 2 inches) may not be adequate in every patient because of body habitus, which should be assessed in every patient prior to each injection to assure that needle length is adequate for intramuscular administration.

The injection volume is 4 ml. and often is associated with pain at the injection site. The clinician should verify that the naltrexone injection has been given correctly, and should consider alternate treatment for patients whose body habitus precludes an intramuscular gluteal injection with one of the needles provided. The drug *must not be administered* intravenously or subcutaneously [49].

Missed doses: If a patient misses a dose, he or she should be instructed to receive the next dose as soon as possible. Pretreatment with oral naltrexone is not required before using XR-NTX in such a situation [49].

Adverse Events with Naltrexone

Unintended consequences and adverse events associated with naltrexone include the following:

- *Pain at the injection site*: Such pain generally resolves in two to five days. Persistent induration and erythema are possible but usually resolve. To prevent problems, staff should be trained in proper techniques for intramuscular injections.
- *Testing the blockade*: Patients should be cautioned that testing the blockade can be dangerous. Most patients try a small opioid dose, experience no effect, and stop. Very rarely, a patient may try to override the blockade. However, no fatalities associated with testing the blockade have been documented.
- *Increased use of alcohol or other drugs*: Increased use of alcohol or other drugs calls for more intensive counseling. However, because naltrexone also has efficacy in managing alcohol use disorder, the more common response is a reduction in alcohol intake. Also, disulfiram may be prescribed for alcohol use, along with monitoring of hepatic enzymes.
- *Dysphoria*: Many opioid-dependent patients are depressed or anxious when starting treatment; this usually improves on naltrexone. In a recent review of naltrexone induction and maintenance in newly abstinent opioid-dependent individuals, no worsening of depression was associated with naltrexone treatment [61]. However, studies supported by the National Institute on Drug Abuse (NIDA) [62] demonstrate that it can be difficult to discern whether symptoms of depression are related to drug withdrawal or an underlying, comorbid psychiatric disorder. If dysphoria persists, the patient should be assessed for mood or anxiety disorders and treated appropriately.
- *Opioid overdose*: Overdose is a significant risk in any opioid-dependent patient, regardless of the treatment approach. Both the patient and family need to be educated about this risk.
- *Elevated liver enzymes*: Opioid-dependent patients often have elevated liver enzymes from viral hepatitis or alcohol use that is not related to their treatment medication.

The "black box" warning that naltrexone may be hepatotoxic is based on studies that used very high doses (higher than those used to treat opioid dependence). In doses typically used to treat opioid dependence (e.g., 50 mg oral per day or 380 mg injectable per month), liver toxicity is unusual. Nevertheless, caution should be exercised in treating patients with compromised liver function.

Reversing the Naltrexone Blockade of Opioid Receptors

When surgeries or procedures are planned for patients who use XR-NTX, it may be safest to delay the procedure until naltrexone blood levels are low enough to restore opioid receptor availability. The manufacturer also suggests considering use of regional analgesia or non-opioid analgesics [49].

In emergencies, it is possible to reverse the opioid receptor blockade created by XR-NTX. However, higher-than-usual doses of a rapidly acting opioid medication may be needed to achieve pain relief if the patient still has some level of opioid tolerance. These higher doses increase the risk of respiratory depression. For that reason, patients who are given such doses should be closely monitored by professionals trained in the use of anesthetic drugs, management of respiratory depression, and cardiopulmonary resuscitation [46,49].

Patients who are treated with XR-NTX should be encouraged to wear medical alert bracelets or carry a disclosure card to help emergency personnel provide pain management safely if the patient is unable to communicate.

Reinduction onto Naltrexone

Following a relapse, many patients express a desire to resume naltrexone treatment. However, such patients need to be cautioned that physiological dependence occurs within days of renewed heroin use; therefore, resuming naltrexone can precipitate withdrawal.

Clinical experience to date has been that patients who relapse and then return to naltrexone tend to remain in treatment a relatively short time. After multiple relapses, the clinician should seriously consider whether it is appropriate to continue naltrexone treatment, as it is preferable to actively manage cessation of naltrexone treatment than for individuals to be lost to follow-up. This is the point at which discussion of opioid agonist therapy should be reopened.

Whenever the best clinical course is not clear, consultation with another practitioner may be helpful. The results of the consultation should be discussed with the patient and any written consultation reports added to the patient's record [11].

Patients with more serious or persistent problems may benefit from a consultation with or referral to a specialist in psychiatry or addiction psychiatry [63]. In other instances, aberrant or dysfunctional behaviors may indicate the need for more vigorous engagement in peer support, counseling, or psychotherapies, or possibly enrollment in a more structured treatment setting [29]. With such patients, alternatives such as methadone or buprenorphine maintenance therapy may be better options [49,64,65].

Treatment with Methadone

Methadone is the agent with the longest history of use for medication-assisted treatment (MAT) of opioid use disorder. A synthetic agent, methadone works by occupying the mu opioid brain receptor sites affected by chronic use of other opioids. (See Chapter 8 for a discussion of the pharmacology of methadone.) As noted earlier, federal law does not allow the use of methadone to treat opioid addiction outside of federally certified opioid treatment programs.

In multiple studies, patients undergoing maintenance treatment with methadone have reported a high incidence of pain: 39% reported moderate to severe pain, while 61% reported a current pain condition [66]. Up to 88% of patients enrolled in or seeking entry to methadone maintenance treatment reported having experienced pain in the preceding week. When compared to individuals in the general population, 31% of those surveyed reported having a current chronic pain condition, while 26% reported pain in the preceding month [67].

The presence of pain affects both the health and the quality of life of patients enrolled in treatment with methadone, as evidenced by the following [68]:

- Over-utilization of health care due to physical illnesses leading to surgery; and other mental illnesses (commonly depression, anxiety, and somatization);
- Lower than average social and physical functioning;
- Disruption in relationships, employment, and normal activities of daily living;
- Increase in non-opioid drug use during and after treatment;
- Reduced satisfaction with treatment; and
- Lower likelihood of reporting that an adequate dose of methadone was received.

Finding the appropriate dose of methadone for maintenance treatment of opioid use disorders in patients with pain is complicated by the following factors [69]:

- Increased pain sensitivity (hyperalgesia) caused by chronic opioid use;
- Increased opioid tolerance;
- Increased licit and illicit use of opioids by patients to manage pain;
- Inappropriate attitudes toward pain and addiction on the part of patients and health care professionals.

Pain management is important in methadone patients if therapy is to be successful. Clinicians' misunderstanding of the pharmacology of methadone and other opiates is a common barrier to adequate analgesia in this population. One of the most common misperceptions is that the dose of methadone taken for maintenance is, in and of itself, adequate to provide relief of pain. While methadone can be an effective analgesic, patients who are being treated with methadone for opioid addiction typically have developed tolerance to the drug's analgesic effects, thereby underscoring the need for a different dosing strategy or different analgesic to obtain relief of pain [70].

Conclusion

The goal of office-based opioid treatment (OBOT) is to bring more individuals with opioid use disorders into treatment and to engage more physicians in the care of these patients. While multiple studies have indicated that OBOT is achieving the goal of bringing new patients into treatment, there also is general agreement that efforts to date have not enlisted enough physicians to meet the growing need.

As in the treatment of any chronic medical disorder, physicians who offer addiction treatment in their office practices must understand the natural history of the underlying disorder; the specific actions, cautions, and contraindications for each of the available medications; and the importance of careful treatment matching and monitoring, with the objective of a long-term physician–patient relationship.

For More Information on the Topics Discussed:

American Society of Addiction Medicine (ASAM):

Stine SM, Kosten TM. Pharmacologic interventions for opioid dependence (Chapter 49). In RK Ries, DA Fiellin, SC Miller, R Saitz, eds. *The ASAM Principles of Addiction Medicine, Fifth Edition*. Philadelphia, PA: Wolters Kluwer; 2014.

Martin J, Zweben JE, Payte JT. Opioid maintenance treatment (Chapter 50). In RK Ries, DA Fiellin, SC Miller, R Saitz, eds. *The ASAM Principles of Addiction Medicine, Fifth Edition*. Philadelphia, PA: Wolters Kluwer; 2014.

ASAM National Practice Guideline for the Use of Medications in the Treatment of Addiction Involving Opioid Use. Chevy Chase, MD: ASAM, June 1, 2015. (Access at: https://www.asam.org/docs/default-source/practice-support/guidelines-and-consensus-docs/asam-national-practice-guideline-supplement.pdf?sfvrsn=24.)

Substance Abuse and Mental Health Services Administration (SAMHSA):

Treatment Advisory: An Introduction to Extended-Release Injectable Naltrexone for the Treatment of Persons with Opioid Addiction. (Volume 11, Issue 1 [SMA] 12-4682.) Rockville, MD: SAMHSA; 2012.

Clinical Guidelines for the Use of Buprenorphine in the Treatment of Opioid Addiction. Treatment Improvement Protocol (TIP) 40. Rockville, MD: SAMHSA; 2004. (Access at: https://www.ncbi.nlm.nih.gov/books/NBK64245/pdf/Bookshelf_NBK64245.pdf.)

Buprenorphine Treatment Practitioner Locator. Find physicians who hold federal waivers that authorize them to treat opioid use disorders with buprenorphine, by State. (Access at: https://www.samhsa.gov/medication-assisted-treatment/physician-program-data/treatment-physician-locator.)

Behavioral Health Treatment Services Locator. SAMHSA's Behavioral Health Treatment Services Locator is a confidential source of information for persons seeking information about federally certified programs that treat opioid abuse and addiction, as well as co-occurring mental health problems, anywhere in the United States or U.S. Territories. (Access at: https://www.findtreatment.samhsa.gov/.)

References

1. Federation of State Medical Boards of the United States (FSMB). *Model Policy Guidelines for Opioid Addiction Treatment in the Medical Office.* Dallas, TX: The Federation; 2013.
2. Amato L, Minozzi S, Davoli M, et al. Psychosocial and pharmacological treatments versus pharmacological treatments for opioid detoxification. *Cochrane Database Syst Rev* Sep 7, 2011;(9):CD005031.
3. Gunderson EW, Fiellin DA. Office-based maintenance treatment of opioid dependence: How does it compare with traditional approaches? *CNS Drugs.* 2008;22(2):99–111.
4. Strain EC. Efficacy and safety of buprenorphine. In JA Renner, Jr., P Levounis, eds. *Handbook of Office-Based Buprenorphine Treatment of Opioid Dependence.* Washington, DC: American Psychiatric Publishing; 2011.
5. Fiellin DA. The first three years of buprenorphine in the United States: Experience to date and future directions. *J Addict Med.* 2007 Jun;1(2):62–67.
6. Elkader A, Sproule B. Buprenorphine: Clinical pharmacokinetics in the treatment of opioid dependence. *Clin Pharmacokinet.* 2005;44(7):661–680.
7. Stein MD, Cioe P, Friedmann PD. Buprenorphine retention in primary care. *J Gen Intern Med.* 2005 Nov;20(11):1038–1041.
8. Kreek MJ, Bart G, Lilly C, et al. Pharmacogenetics and human molecular genetics of opiate and cocaine addictions and their treatments. *Pharmacol Rev.* 2005 Mar;57(1):1–26. Review.
9. Heidbreder CA, Hagan JJ. Novel pharmacotherapeutic approaches for the treatment of drug addiction and craving. *Curr Opin Pharmacol.* 2005 Feb;5(1):107–118.
10. Fudala PJ, Woody GW. Recent advances in the treatment of opiate addiction. *Curr Psychiatry Rep.* 2004 Oct;6(5):339–346.
11. McNicholas LF. Clinical guidelines for the use of buprenorphine in the treatment of opioid addiction. *A Tool for Buprenorphine Care.* 2008 May;1(12):12.
12. Loxterkamp D. Helping "Them"—Our role in recovery from opioid dependence. *Ann Fam Med.* 2006;4(2):168–171.

13. Substance Abuse and Mental Health Services Administration (SAMHSA). Opioid drugs in maintenance and detoxification of dispensing restrictions for buprenorphine and buprenorphine combination as used in approved opioid treatment medications. Final rule. *Fed Regist.* 2012 Dec 6;77(235):72752–72761.

14. O'Connor PG, Fiellin DA. Pharmacologic treatment of heroin-dependent patients. *Ann Intern Med.* 2000;133:40–54.

15. Center for Substance Abuse Treatment (CSAT). *Clinical Guidelines for the Use of Buprenorphine in the Treatment of Opioid Addiction.* Treatment Improvement Protocol (TIP) Series 40. DHHS Publication No. (SMA) 04-3939. Rockville, MD: CSAT, Substance Abuse and Mental Health Services Administration; 2004.

16. Jones HE. Practical considerations for the clinical use of buprenorphine. *Sci Pract Perspect.* 2004 Aug;2(2):4–20. Review.

17. Gordon AJ, Krumm M, for the Buprenorphine Initiative in the VA (BIV). *Buprenorphine Resource Guide, Version 8.* Washington, DC: Department of Veterans Affairs, April 2008.

18. World Health Organization (WHO). *Guidelines for the Psychosocially Assisted Pharmacological Treatment of Opioid Dependence.* Geneva, Switzerland: WHO; 2009.

19. National Institute on Drug Abuse (NIDA). *Principles of Drug Addiction Treatment, Third Edition.* NIH Publication No. 12–4180. Rockville, MD: NIDA, National Institutes of Health; 2012.

20. O'Brien CP. Toward a rational selection of treatment for addiction. *Curr Psychiatry Rep.* 2007 Dec;9(6):441–442.

21. Reckitt Benckiser Pharmaceuticals, Inc. *Full prescribing information: Suboxone.* (Package Insert 1-1202-019-U.S.-0812, Revised.) Richmond, VA: Reckitt-Benckiser; August 2010.

22. Saber-Tehrani AS, Bruce RD, Altice RL. Pharmacokinetic drug interactions and adverse consequences between psychotropic medications and pharmacotherapy for the treatment of opioid dependence. *Am J Drug Alcohol Abuse.* 2011 Jan;37(1):1–11.

23. Casadonte PP, for the Physician Clinical Support System for Buprenorphine (PCSS-B). *PCSS-B Guidance on Buprenorphine Induction.* East Providence, RI: American Academy of Addiction Psychiatry; October 27, 2009.

24. Jones HE, Finnegan LP, Kaltenbach K. Methadone and buprenorphine for the management of opioid dependence in pregnancy. *Drugs.* 2012;72(6):747–757.

25. Breen CL, Harris SJ, Lintzeris N, et al. Cessation of methadone maintenance treatment using buprenorphine: Transfer from methadone to buprenorphine and subsequent buprenorphine reductions. *Drug Alcohol Depend.* 2003 Jul 20;71(1):49–55.

26. Fiellin DA, Friedland GH, Gourevitch MN. Opioid dependence: Rationale for and efficacy of existing and new treatments. *Clin Infect Dis.* 2006;43:S173–S177.

27. Umbricht A, Huestis M, Cone EJ, et al. Effects of high-dose intravenous buprenorphine in experienced opioid abusers. *J Clin Psychopharmacol.* 2004 Oct;24(5):479–487.

28. McCance-Katz EF, Sullivan LE, Nallani S. Drug interactions of clinical importance among the opioids, methadone and buprenorphine, and other frequently prescribed medications: A review. *Am J Addict.* 2010 Jan–Feb;19(1):4–16.

29. Fishman MJ, Mee-Lee D, Shulman GD, et al., eds. *Supplement to the ASAM Patient Placement Criteria on Pharmacotherapies for the Management of Alcohol Use Disorders*. Philadelphia, PA: Lippincott, Williams & Wilkins; 2010.

30. Maremmani I, Rolland B, Somaini L, et al. Buprenorphine dosing choices in specific populations: Review of expert opinion. *Expert Opin Pharmacother*. 2016 Sep;17(13):1727–1731.

31. Jacobs P, Ang A, Hillhouse MP, et al. Treatment outcomes in opioid dependent patients with different buprenorphine/naloxone induction dosing patterns and trajectories. *Am J Addict*. 2015 Oct;24(7):667–675.

32. Kraus ML, Alford DP, Kotz MM, et al. Statement of the American Society of Addiction Medicine Consensus Panel on the use of buprenorphine in office-based treatment of opioid addiction. *J Addict Med*. 2011 Dec;5(4):254–263.

33. Strain EC, Harrison JA, Bigelow GE. Induction of opioid-dependent individuals onto buprenorphine and buprenorphine/naloxone soluble films. *Clin Pharmacol Ther*. 2011 Mar;89(3):443–449.

34. Caldiero RM, Parran TV, Adelman CL, et al. Inpatient initiation of buprenorphine maintenance vs. detoxification: Can retention of opioid-dependent patients in outpatient counseling be improved? *Am J Addict*. 2006 Jan–Feb;15(1):1–7.

35. Center for Substance Abuse Treatment (CSAT). *Clinical Guidelines for the Use of Buprenorphine in the Treatment of Opioid Addiction*. Treatment Improvement Protocol (TIP) Series 40. DHHS Publication No. (SMA) 04-3939. Rockville, MD: CSAT, Substance Abuse and Mental Health Services Administration; 2004.

36. Baxter LE, chair, for the ASAM Methadone Action Group. Clinical guidance on methadone induction and stabilization. *J Addict Med*. 2013 Nov-Dec;7(6):377–386.

37. Joseph H, Stancliff S, Lagrod J. Methadone maintenance treatment (MMT): A review of historical and clinical issues. *Mt Sinai J Med*. 2000 Oct–Nov;67(5–6):347–364. Review.

38. Chiang CN, Hawks RL. Pharmacokinetics of the combination tablet of buprenorphine and naloxone. *Drug Alcohol Depend*. 2003 May 21;70(2 Suppl):S39–S47. Review.

39. Lintzeris N, Ritter A, Panjari M, et al. Implementing buprenorphine treatment in community settings in Australia: Experiences from the Buprenorphine Implementation Trial. *Am J Addict*. 2004;13(Suppl 1):S29–S41.

40. Marsch L, Bickel W, Badger G, et al. Buprenorphine treatment for opioid dependence: The relative efficacy of daily, twice and thrice weekly dosing. *Drug Alcohol Depend*. 2005 Feb 14;77(2):195–204.

41. Stephenson DK, for the CSAM Committee on Treatment of Opioid Dependence. *Guidelines for Physicians Working in California Opioid Treatment Programs*. San Francisco, CA: California Society of Addiction Medicine; 2008.

42. Leavitt SB, Shinderman M, Maxwell S, et al. When "enough" is not enough: New perspectives on optimal methadone maintenance dose. *Mt Sinai J Med*. 2000 Oct–Nov; 67(5–6):404–411. Review.

43. O'Brien CP, for the Expert Panel. *Treatment Advisory: An Introduction to Extended-Release Injectable Naltrexone for the Treatment of Persons With Opioid Addiction*. (Volume 11, Issue 1 [SMA] 12-4682.) Rockville, MD: SAMHSA; 2012.

44. Sigmon SC, Bisaga A, Nunes EV, et al. Opioid detoxification and naltrexone induction strategies: Recommendations for clinical practice. *Am J Drug Alcohol Abuse*. 2012;38(3):187–199.

45. Xuyi W, Juelu W, Xiaojun X, et al. Phase I study of injectable, depot naltrexone for the relapse prevention treatment of opioid dependence. *Am J Addict*. 2014 Mar–Apr;23(2):162–169.

46. Food and Drug Administration (FDA). Vivitrol [naltrexone for extended-release injectable suspension: NDA 21-897C]—Briefing document/background package. Pharmacologic Drugs Advisory Committee Meeting. Rockville, MD: FDA; 2010.

47. Bell J, Kimber J, Lintzeris N, et al. *National Drug Strategy: Clinical Guidelines for the Use of Naltrexone in the Management of Opioid Addiction*. Canberra, Australia: Department of Health and Ageing; 2003.

48. National Institute for Health and Clinical Excellence (NICE), National Health Service. Naltrexone for the Management of Opioid Addiction (Technology Appraisal Guidance No. 115). London, UK: NICE; 2010.

49. Alkermes, Inc. Vivitrol prescribing information (Revised). Waltham, MA: Author; 2013.

50. Kranzler HR, Wesson DR, Billot L, et al., for the Drug Abuse Sciences Naltrexone Depot Study Group. Naltrexone depot for treatment of alcohol dependence: A multicenter, randomized, placebo-controlled clinical trial. *Alcohol Clin Exp Res*. 2004;28(7):1051–1059.

51. Syed YY, Keating GM. Extended-release intramuscular naltrexone (Vivitrol®): A review of its use in the prevention of relapse to opioid dependence in detoxi-fied patients. *CNS Drugs*. 2013 Oct;27(10):851–861.

52. Gastfriend DR. Intramuscular extended-release naltrexone: Current evidence. *Ann NY Acad Sci*. 2011;1216:144–156.

53. Sullivan MA, Bisaga A, Mariani JJ, et al. Naltrexone treatment for opioid dependence: Does its effectiveness depend on testing the blockade? *Drug Alcohol Depend*. 2013 Nov 1;133(1):80–85.

54. Krupitsky EM, Nunes EV, Ling W et al. Injectable extended-release naltrexone for opioid dependence: A double-blind, placebo-controlled, multicentre ran-domised trial. *Lancet*. 2011;377:1506–1513.

55. National Institute on Drug Abuse (NIDA). *Topics in Brief: Medication-Assisted Treatment for Opioid Addiction*. Washington, DC: National Institutes of Health; April 2012.

56. Gastfriend DR. Extended-release naltrexone (XR-NTX) for opioid addiction. Presentation at the American Society of Addiction Medicine's 42nd Annual Medical-Scientific Conference, Washington, DC, April 2011.

57. Gryczynski J, Jaffe JH, Schwartz RP, et al. Patient perspectives on choosing buprenorphine over methadone in an urban, equal-access system. *Am J Addict*. 2013 May–Jun;22(3):285–291.

58. Fishman MJ, Winstanley EL, Curran E, et al. Treatment of opioid dependence in adolescents and young adults with extended release naltrexone: Preliminary case-series and feasibility. *Addiction*. 2010 Sep;105(9):1669–1676.

59. National Institute on Drug Abuse (NIDA). *Principles of Drug Addiction Treatment, Second Edition*. NIH Publication No. 09-4180. Rockville, MD: NIDA, National Institutes of Health; 2009.

60. Comer SD, Sullivan MA, Yu E, et al. Injectable, sustained-release naltrexone for the treatment of opioid dependence: A randomized, placebo controlled trial. *Arch Gen Psychiatry*. 2006 Feb;63(2):210–218.

61. Korthuis PT, Gregg J, Rogers WE, et al. Patients' reasons for choosing office-based buprenorphine: Preference for patient-centered care. *J Addict Med*. 2010 Dec;4(4):204–210.

62. O'Brien CP. Toward a rational selection of treatment for addiction. *Curr Psychiatry Rep*. 2007 Dec;9(6):441–442.

63. Institute for Research, Education and Training in Addiction (IRETA). *Best Practices in the Use of Buprenorphine. Final Expert Panel Report*. Pittsburgh, PA: Community Care Behavioral Health Organizations; October 18, 2011.

64. Gibson AE, Degenhart LJ. Mortality related to pharmacotherapies for opioid dependence: A comparative analysis of coronial records. *Drug Alc Rev*. 2007 Jul;26:405–410.

65. Bruce RD. Medical interventions for addictions in the primary care setting. *Topics HIV Med*. 2010 Feb–Mar;18(1):8–12.

66. Alford DP, Compton P, Samet J. Acute pain management for patients receiving maintenance methadone or buprenorphine therapy. *Ann Intern Med*. 2006:144(2):127–134.

67. Stine SM, Kosten TM. Pharmacologic interventions for opioid dependence (Chapter 49). In RK Ries, DA Fiellin, SC Miller, R Saitz, eds. *The ASAM Principles of Addiction Medicine, Fifth Edition*. Philadelphia, PA: Wolters Kluwer; 2014.

68. Hooten WM, Timming R, Belgrade M, et al. *Assessment and Management of Chronic Pain*. Institute for Clinical Systems Improvement. Updated November 2013.

69. Bart G. Maintenance medication for opiate addiction: The foundation of recovery. *J Addict Dis*. 2012;31(3):207–225.

70. Krueger C. Methadone for pain management. *Practical Pain Management*. 2012;12(2):1–3.

71. Current SAMHSA Physician Criteria for buprenorphine waiver qualification: https://www.samhsa.gov/medication-assisted-treatment/buprenorphine-waiver-management/qualify-for-physician-waiver.

72. Wesson DR, Ling W. The Clinical Opiate Withdrawal Scale (COWS). *J Psychoact Drugs*. 2003;35(2):253–259; also see https://www.drugabuse.gov/sites/default/files/files/ClinicalOpiateWithdrawalScale.pdf.

Chapter 20

Non-Pharmacological Therapies for Substance Use Disorders

MICHAEL F. WEAVER, M.D., DFASAM

Psychosocial and other non-pharmacological interventions are an essential component of treatment of substance use disorder (SUD). Such interventions can be used alone or in conjunction with medications; in fact, many studies show that the combination of pharmacological and non-pharmacological interventions may be more effective than either approach used alone [1]. When medication management and addiction treatment services are being delivered by separate providers, close coordination and integration of services is essential. All treatment personnel, including addiction medicine and addiction psychiatry specialists, who have special training and experience in evaluating patients and prescribing pharmacotherapies, need to establish close linkages and open communications [2].

Many different types of non-pharmacological treatments are in use today. The principal evidence-based non-pharmacological approaches are briefly described here.

12-Step Programs and Facilitation

12-Step programs such as Alcoholics Anonymous (AA) and Narcotics Anonymous (NA) are fellowships of men and women who offer their hope, strength, and experience to anyone desiring to abstain from drinking or drug use. Fellowship meetings are held at various times throughout the day and evening and in multiple formats, such as speaker meetings, Step discussion meetings, women's meetings, and the like. Participation is anonymous, there is no cost, and questions are not asked of newcomers. Participants are not told what to do, but learn from experienced members what worked for them. No cost is incurred by the patient beyond the expenditure of time. Participation in a 12-Step program does not conflict with or replace other clinical interventions such as medications, psychotherapy, or commitment to a religious preference.

Physicians and other clinicians have an obligation to inform patients with alcohol or other SUDs of the existence, format, and benefits of participating in a 12-Step program. This obligation is based on empirical evidence that participation in AA (and by extension, other 12-Step programs) and engagement in and commitment to AA are consistent predictors of positive patient outcomes [3]. Even attendance at AA meetings without "commitment" produces modest yet positive results [4]. Resistance and objections to 12-Step programs are to be expected, and a calm, encouraging stance usually overcomes patients' initial fears or concerns.

To help the patient with an SUD find a 12-Step meeting, it is worthwhile to have a schedule of local meetings available to give to such a patient. Alternatively, patients can be educated about how to find meetings online at www.aa.org. Clinicians familiar with 12-Step programs are well aware that members are generous with their time and efforts in assisting newcomers. Putting a patient in touch with a willing group member to provide a personal introduction to 12-Step programs can go a long way toward assuaging any initial uncertainty on the part of the patient.

12-Step programs do not diagnose or offer medical advice, nor are they opposed to members using prescribed medications (although individual members may hold such beliefs). The pamphlet titled "The AA Member: Medications and Other Drugs" (available from Alcoholics Anonymous World Services, Inc., 475 Riverside Drive, New York, NY 10115) explains the AA position and emphasizes to AA members that they must be honest with their physicians about their use of alcohol and/or drugs, as well as how medications may be affecting them.

Occasionally, an AA member may advise another not to take some or all medications. As an organization, AA offers no opinion on medical matters, so it may be necessary to review with the patient the rationale for the course of treatment that an AA member (not AA itself) finds objectionable. Obviously, this requires tact and patience. It is important for the patient to understand that he or she can benefit from medical input as well as what the 12-Step program has to offer.

SUDs are widely recognized as chronic illnesses that require patient monitoring over time to assess outcomes. The number of 12-Step meetings attended can be used to examine the dose–response relationship. For example, a one-year follow-up study found that individuals who attended 50 or more AA meetings in months 9 through 12 of treatment had higher rates of abstinence (about 60%) than those who attended only one to 19 meetings (30%) [5]. Overall, research shows that attending AA (and presumably other 12-Step meetings) on a regular basis for at least 27 weeks in a given year correlates with 70% abstinence by year 16 of follow-up.

Motivational Enhancement Therapy

Motivational enhancement therapy (MET), also known as motivational interviewing (MI), is a patient-centered counseling approach that is designed to initiate behavior change by helping patients resolve their ambivalence about engaging in treatment and stopping substance use. MET employs strategies to evoke rapid and internally motivated change in the patient, rather than guiding the patient stepwise through the recovery process. The techniques used are designed to highlight and help resolve ambivalence about becoming abstinent, and to help move patients along the "stages of change" toward the goal of abstinence.

MET typically consists of an initial assessment session, followed by two to four individual treatment sessions with a therapist. The first treatment session focuses on providing feedback based on the assessment battery to stimulate discussion regarding personal substance use and to elicit self-motivating statements. Motivational interviewing principles are used to strengthen motivation and create a plan for change. Coping strategies for high-risk situations are suggested and discussed with the patient.

In subsequent sessions, the therapist monitors change, reviews the cessation strategies being employed, and continues to encourage commitment to change or sustained abstinence.

Cognitive-Behavioral Therapy

Cognitive-behavioral therapy (CBT) is among the most well-studied and empirically supported non-pharmacological treatments for SUD. Cognitive-behavioral strategies are based on the theory that learning processes play a critical role in the development of maladaptive behavioral patterns.

Through CBT, individuals learn to identify and correct problematic behaviors. Specifically, CBT focuses on identifying and changing thoughts and behaviors that contribute to compulsive alcohol or drug use and/or place the individual at high risk of relapse. CBT helps patients identify triggers for alcohol or drug use, such as persons (e.g., drinking friends, irritating co-workers), places (particular bars, clubs, or restaurants), or emotions (sadness or anger).

Patients are taught how to avoid high-risk situations or triggers whenever they can, and to cope effectively with situations or triggers that are unavoidable. Relapse prevention encompasses several cognitive-behavioral strategies that facilitate abstinence as well as provide help for persons who experience relapse.

Psychotherapy

Individual and/or group psychotherapy can help patients reduce the frequency of their substance use and the amount of alcohol or drug consumed.

Group therapy is one of the most common non-pharmacological interventions for SUDs. The primary advantages of group therapy are that it is economical and allows one health care provider to meet with multiple patients in a given session. Therefore, it usually costs less than individual therapy and offers the added benefit of peer support.

Group therapy affords patients the opportunity to hear from other persons dealing with the same issues, and the acceptance received from peers in group therapy can help patients combat the social stigma associated with SUDs. Moreover, peer modeling allows patients to learn from others who have succeeded in achieving abstinence and maintaining sobriety.

Finally, the public nature of groups can be a powerful motivator. Secrecy is a common feature of SUDs, and the group helps to combat secrecy while assisting patients in becoming more accountable for their progress in treatment.

Individual therapy can be provided in many types of treatment settings (inpatient, outpatient, or a criminal justice institution). It affords privacy, which encourages some patients to disclose information more freely, and it allows for more one-on-one time between patient and therapist than would be possible in a group setting.

In addition, if comorbid conditions (such as depression or an eating disorder) are found, individual therapy can be tailored to address the patient's particular needs.

Although individual therapy can vary widely because of different therapeutic orientations, a few common characteristics are found. Typically, individual therapy is focused on working toward and achieving clearly defined goals (such as abstinence from all substances, quitting smoking, enhanced medication compliance, or reliable attendance at medical appointments). In addition, other areas of life that have been affected by an SUD are addressed, such as issues in the workplace, with interpersonal relationships, with physical health, or legal problems.

Contingency Management

Contingency management programs work in various ways, but their key element is identifying a group of behaviors that are likely to lead to lasting recovery, then rewarding participants for exhibiting those behaviors [6]. For example, patients can be rewarded for negative urine drug tests, attending group or individual therapy sessions, or completing therapy homework assignments. They also can be rewarded for consistency (e.g., after several successive negative urine drug screens, the amount of the reward increases). On the other hand, if a urine drug sample contains illicit drugs, the amount of the reward is reset to the lower starting amount.

The rewards themselves usually are not cash, but prizes such as gift cards or lottery tickets. Research has shown that the chance of winning a large reward tends to be just as motivating as actually receiving a reward—hence the use of lottery tickets in programs.

Contingency management is a way to enhance the outcome of substance use treatment, but it can be expensive to implement. However, lottery tickets or small-denomination gift cards are less expensive and still work as motivational incentives, so contingency management can add value when used as a component of a comprehensive treatment program. Although the rewards are not large, they are more tangible than an abstract goal such as abstinence, and they provide participants with an external motivation to keep them engaged in treatment. Participants learn to apply CBT skills in day-to-day life so that they can remain abstinent and earn prizes. Eventually, the prizes become less important than the achievement of abstinence, and patients begin to see the other benefits—their life rewards—as more important than the prizes.

Community Reinforcement Approach

An intensive outpatient therapy, the Community Reinforcement Approach (CRA) initially was used in the treatment of cocaine use disorder. The goal of this therapy is to achieve abstinence long enough for the patient to learn new life skills that will help him or her sustain abstinence.

Patients typically attend one or two individual counseling sessions each week, where they focus on improving family relations, learn a variety of skills to minimize their substance use, receive vocational counseling, and develop new recreational activities and social networks. Patients submit urine samples two or three times a week. This approach facilitates patients' engagement in treatment and systematically aids them in gaining substantial periods of abstinence.

Family and Couples Therapy

The effects of SUDs are far-reaching, affecting family members and loved ones as well as the patient. Family members and partners who are involved in the treatment process can be educated about factors that are important to the patient's recovery (such as establishing a substance-free environment). Family members and partners also can provide social support to the patient and can help motivate them to remain in treatment.

Preventing and Responding to Relapse

Relapse has been defined as "a breakdown or setback in a person's attempt to change or modify any target behavior" [7]. The risk of relapse is highest in the first 6–12 months after initiating abstinence, then diminishes gradually over a period of years. Therefore, it is reasonable to continue treatment for a year or longer if the patient responds well. Relapse can be fatal, as evidenced by the rising number of deaths attributed to opioid overdose.

Not all relapses are alike. The term *lapse* (sometimes referred to as a *slip*) refers to an episode of alcohol or other drug use after a period of abstinence. A lapse usually is impulsive and involves a brief period of use. Most lapses are of short duration, with relatively minor consequences, and are marked by the patient's desire to return to abstinence. However, a lapse also can progress to a full-blown relapse (marked by loss of control) of varying proportions.

Relapse rarely is caused by a single factor and often is the result of a confluence of physiological and environmental factors [8,9]. Although some individuals in relapse return to pretreatment levels of active drug use, others use alcohol or other drugs problematically but do not return to previous levels of abuse and thus suffer fewer harmful effects. Patients in relapse vary in the quantity and frequency of their substance use, as well as the accompanying medical and psychosocial sequelae. It is recommended that providers and patients jointly develop a relapse prevention plan that includes strategies to reduce the risk of overdose if relapse should occur [11].

Whenever the best clinical course is unclear, consultation with another practitioner can be helpful. The results of the consultation should be discussed with the patient and any written consultation reports added to the patient's record [12].

Adherence to both medication regimens and session appointments is associated with better treatment outcomes, and regular therapy or counseling can help patients plan for possible obstacles and teach them ways to handle them should they occur [13]. Nevertheless, lack of adherence to pharmacological regimens occurs in a substantial proportion of patients (depending on the medication, its side effect profile, and the length of the treatment regimen), with some studies reporting that up to 73% of patients fail to follow their treatment plan. However, engaging in behaviors that violate the treatment agreement does not constitute grounds for automatic termination of treatment. Rather, such behaviors should be taken as a signal to reassess the patient's status, to implement changes in the treatment plan (such as by intensifying the treatment structure or intensity of services), and to document such changes in the patient's medical record [14].

Patients with more serious or persistent problems may benefit from referral to a specialist for additional evaluation and treatment. For example, the treatment of SUD in a patient with a comorbid psychiatric disorder may be best managed through consultation with or referral to a specialist in psychiatry or addiction psychiatry [15]. In other instances, aberrant or dysfunctional behaviors may indicate the need for more vigorous engagement in peer support, counseling, or psychotherapies, or possibly referral to a more structured treatment setting [16].

How Long Should Treatment Last?

Because SUDs have so many dimensions and disrupt so many aspects of an individual's life, treatment is never simple, nor is the decision to stop treatment. The optimal duration of treatment differs from one patient to the next, and any decision about how long to treat a patient with non-pharmacological approaches should take into account lifestyle changes, environmental risk factors, and intensity of craving [17].

It is widely recognized that treatment of SUDs is a long-term process, with a substantial risk of relapse during the first two to three years [17]. For most patients, treatment should continue over the long term or even throughout their lives [18]. Such long-term treatment, which is common to many chronic medical conditions, should not be seen as a treatment failure, but rather as a cost-effective way of prolonging life and improving the patient's quality of life by supporting the natural and ongoing process of change and recovery.

Nevertheless, continuation of treatment should be driven by evidence of progress, with frequent examination of outcomes. Such evidence may include monitoring treatment adherence and progress toward treatment goals, as well as monitoring the patient's continuing substance use (if any) and any symptoms of mental disorders. Measurements should be taken in as close to "real time" as practical—in some cases, at every treatment session. Assessing the quality of the patient's engagement and the strength of the therapeutic alliance allows for modification of the treatment plan and level of care in response to the patient's progress or lack thereof [19].

Conclusion

Many different types of non-pharmacological therapies are available to treat opioid use disorders. These include 12-Step programs, MET, CBT, contingency management, and family therapy. Each of these approaches helps to prevent and treat relapse to substance use.

The duration of non-pharmacological treatment should reflect the needs of the individual patient. It is particularly helpful for physicians to be aware of these treatment modalities for cases involving patients with pain management issues.

For More Information on the Topics Discussed:

American Society of Addiction Medicine (ASAM):

See Chapters 55 to 66,on non-pharmacological therapies, in RK Ries, DA Fiellin, SC Miller, R Saitz, eds. *The ASAM Principles of Addiction Medicine, Fifth Edition.* Philadelphia, PA: Wolters Kluwer; 2014.

National Institute on Drug Abuse (NIDA):

Principles of Drug Addiction Treatment: A Research-Based Guide (Third Edition). NIH Publication No. 12–4180. Bethesda, MD: NIDA, National Institutes of Health; 2012. (Access at: https://www.drugabuse.gov/publications/principles-drug-addiction-treatment-research-based-guide-third-edition/preface.)

In the Literature:

Donovan DM, Ingalsbe MH, Benbow J, Daley DC. 12-Step interventions and mutual support programs for substance use disorders: An overview. *Soc Work Public Health.* 2013;28(3–4):313–32.

References

1. Fishman MJ, Mee-Lee D, Shulman GD, et al., eds. *Supplement to the ASAM Patient Placement Criteria on Pharmacotherapies for the Management of Alcohol Use Disorders.* Philadelphia, PA: Lippincott, Williams & Wilkins, Inc.; 2010.
2. Fiellin DA, for the Physician Clinical Support System for Buprenorphine (PCSS-B). *PCSS-B Guidance on Treatment of Acute Pain in Patients Receiving Buprenorphine/Naloxone.* East Providence, RI: American Academy of Addiction Psychiatry; Nov. 10, 2005.
3. Weiss R, Griffin M, Gallop R, et al. Self-help group attendance and participation among cocaine dependent patients. *Drug Alcohol Depend* 2000;60(2):169–177.

4. Forcehimes A, Tonigan J. Self efficacy as a factor in abstinence from alcohol/ other drug abuse: A meta-analysis. *Alcohol Treat Q.* 2008;26(4):480–489.
5. Moos R, Moos B. Paths of entry into Alcoholics Anonymous: A 16-year follow-up of initially untreated individuals. *J Clin Psychol.* 2006;62:735–750.
6. McKay JR, Lynch KG, Coviello D, et al. Randomized trial of continuing care enhancements for cocaine-dependent patients following initial engagement. *J Consult Clin Psychol.* 2010;78:111–120.
7. Marlatt GA, JR Gordon. *Relapse Prevention: Maintenance Strategies in Addictive Behavior Change.* New York: Guilford; 1985.
8. Kraus ML, Alford DP, Kotz MM, et al. Statement of the American Society of Addiction Medicine Consensus Panel on the use of buprenorphine in office-based treatment of opioid addiction. *J Addict Med.* 2011 Dec;5(4):254–263.
9. National Institute on Drug Abuse (NIDA). *Principles of Drug Addiction Treatment, Third Edition.* NIH Publication No. 12–4180. Rockville, MD: NIDA, National Institutes of Health; 2012.
10. Fiellin DA, for the Physician Clinical Support System for Buprenorphine (PCSS-B). *PCSS-B Guidance on Treatment of Acute Pain in Patients Receiving Buprenorphine/Naloxone.* East Providence, RI: American Academy of Addiction Psychiatry; Nov. 10, 2005.
11. Gibson AE, Degenhardt L. Mortality related to pharmacotherapies for opioid dependence: A comparative analysis of coronial records. *Drug Alcohol Rev.* 2007;26:405–410.
12. McNicholas L. Clinical guidelines for the use of buprenorphine in the treatment of opioid addiction. *A Tool for Buprenorphine Care.* 2008 May;1(12):12–20.
13. Anton RF, O'Malley SS, Ciraulo DA, et al. Combined pharmacotherapies and behavioral interventions for alcohol dependence: The COMBINE study: A randomized controlled trial. *JAMA.* 2006;295:2003–2017.
14. Finch JW, Kamien JB, Amass L. Two-year experience with buprenorphine/naloxone (Suboxone) for maintenance treatment of opioid dependence within a private practice setting. *J Addict Med.* 2007 Jun;1(2):104–110.
15. Rastegar DA, Kunins HV, Tetrault JM, et al., for the U.S. Society of General Internal Medicine's Substance Abuse Interest Group. 2012 update in addiction medicine for the generalist. *Addict Sci Clin Pract.* 2013 Mar 13;8:6. (Review)
16. O'Brien CP. Toward a rational selection of treatment for addiction. *Curr Psychiatry Rep.* 2007 Dec;9(6):441–442.
17. Weiss R, Griffin M, Gallop R, et al. Self-help group attendance and participation among cocaine dependent patients. *Drug Alcohol Depend.* 2000;60(2):169–177.
18. World Health Organization (WHO). *Guidelines for the Psychosocially Assisted Pharmacological Treatment of Opioid Dependence.* Geneva, Switzerland: WHO; 2009.
19. American Society of Addiction Medicine (ASAM). *Public Policy Statement on Office-Based Opioid Agonist Treatment (OBOT).* Chevy Chase, MD: The Society; 2010.

Chapter 21

Mindfulness as a Component of Addiction Treatment

SHARONE ABRAMOWITZ, M.D., FASAM

Encounters between health care professionals and chronic pain patients who also have substance use disorders (SUDs) often are marked by anxiety and frustration on all sides. Typically involving arguments over whether continued use of opioids is helpful, these tense encounters ignore the true mind–body nature of such complex syndromes.

Integrating mindfulness-informed approaches into the treatment plan for such patients has the potential to reduce their focus on the prescription pad and replace it with active engagement in a framework of mind–body healing.

General Principles of Mindfulness

The goal of mindfulness practice is reflective engagement with the whole experience of pain and addiction. As the prescription pad is replaced with a focus on breathing, both the clinician and the patient relax [1].

Similar to focusing a spotlight on the here-and-now, mindfulness practices intentionally attend—in an open and discerning way—to whatever is arising in the present moment. During mindfulness meditation (MM), all experiences ("good" or "bad") are observed and accepted without judgment, regardless of whether they involve drug cravings or freedom from drug cravings, physical pain or being pain free, pessimism or optimism [2]. Ancient spiritual traditions—such as Buddhist meditation, yoga, tai chi, and prayer—promote mindful presence. As a result, modern society's distractions and chronic ills are inspiring many people to learn mindfulness practices through venues as diverse as meditation and yoga centers, smartphone apps, schools, and courses within medical settings.

Developed by Jon Kabat-Zinn and described in his 1990 book *Full Catastrophe Living* [3], mindfulness-based stress reduction (MBSR) is an eight-week, well-studied, complementary medicine course that is offered in more than 200 medical settings. The course teaches a Theravada-style Buddhist mindfulness meditation practice, body scanning (attention is sequentially guided throughout the body to observe the sensations in each region without judgment), and Hatha yoga postures (which cultivate awareness of the mind–body experience and a non-harming attitude toward the body) [3].

Because it promotes a non-judgmental uncoupling of pain's sensory aspects from its evaluative and emotional dimensions, MBSR long has been studied in chronic pain patients [1]. Other mindfulness-based interventions (MBIs), which address behaviors related to SUDs, have incorporated elements of MBSR, including mindfulness-based relapse prevention (MBRP), other cognitive therapy and relapse prevention strategies, and mindfulness-oriented recovery enhancement (MORE) [4,5].

A review of mechanisms that mediate MBIs found strong evidence for MBI's effectiveness in reducing cognitive and emotional reactivity, and moderate evidence for MBI's ability to improve mindfulness and reduce rumination and worry [6]. An early study found that more than half of chronic pain patients who completed MBSR training experienced at least a 33% reduction in their current pain and general body problems [7]. Research also shows that MBSR may improve an individual's ability to cope with stress and pain, with gains lasting up to four years [6].

Even though it promotes daily practice, rates of compliance with MBSR are surprisingly strong, and compare favorably with behavioral pain management approaches [7].

Although additional well-designed controlled trials are needed, available evidence suggests that also MBSR may be useful for fibromyalgia and low back pain—two conditions that not infrequently lead to the misuse of opioid analgesics [8,9].

Most of the research into the effectiveness of MBIs designed specifically for patients with SUDs—such as MBRP and MORE—has been conducted by the researchers who developed those interventions. For example, a randomized controlled trial (RCT) that compared MBRP to conventional relapse prevention approaches or treatment as usual found, at 12-month follow-up, that the benefits of MBRP exceeded those of either of the other two interventions in terms of reducing drug use and heavy drinking in patients enrolled in SUD aftercare [10].

MORE, which integrates mindfulness with cognitive-behavioral therapy (CBT) reappraisal techniques and positive psychology savoring approaches, was tested as an intervention for patients with co-occurring chronic pain who were assessed as at risk for opioid misuse [11]. The intervention included three minutes of mindful breathing before the patient ingested an opioid analgesic, with the goal of separating craving from a legitimate need for pain relief. The study found that MORE led to significant reductions in pain severity and pain-related functional interference, and that these changes were maintained for three months following the intervention [11].

Further studies are planned to test the ability of MORE to improve pain management while reducing opioid intake.

Other MBIs integrate some elements of 12-Step meetings with mindfulness practices. An example is Refuge Recovery, as described in Noah Levine's 2014 book, *Refuge Recovery: A Buddhist Path to Recovering from Addiction* [12]. These meetings include meditation, a Buddhist-informed reading, and group sharing.

Clinical Presentation

"My pain is always ten-plus and it's 24/7!" "I can't live without my Oxy." "Drinking is the only time when I can forget about my pain."

Chronic pain patients who are engaged in problematic substance use often make statements like these. Such comments reflect their struggles with poor cognitive and emotional regulation because of their addiction-mediated states (involving craving, use of alcohol and other drugs to reduce unpleasant feelings or avoid withdrawal-mediated anxiety, and poor impulse control), as well as pain-mediated states that involve selective attention to pain-related stimuli (known as *pain attentional bias*), and catastrophizing (examples of which include magnifying pain's negative effects, rumination about pain, and feelings of helplessness).

MBIs can lower anxiety and help chronic pain patients learn much-needed self-regulation because they focus on how to uncouple craving triggers from behaviors, and pain sensations from catastrophizing [13].

Both physical pain and addictive craving hijack attention, causing the individual's mind to "put on blinders." Such hyper-focus leads to catastrophizing and pain attentional bias [11]. This, in turn, cycles into aversive behavior to try to escape the intensified pain experience through (for example) overuse of opioid analgesics and other prescribed medications, as well as use of habit-forming, non-prescribed substances (such as alcohol, stimulants, and marijuana) and avoidance of physical treatment modalities like physical therapy and stretching. The resulting cycle, which alternates between hyper-focus and aversion, parallels the nature of all human suffering, which is explained in Buddhist philosophy as one of holding on too tightly (grasping) and then turning away (aversion) [13].

Mindfulness meditation can interrupt this cycle of suffering. One variation is a daily practice of sitting quietly and anchoring one's attention to inhalations and exhalations, while non-judgmentally reviewing the mind's natural thought, feeling, and sensation distractions. This type of practice can train the mind to be aware of the changing nature of painful physical and emotional states, including craving, without having to act on them or react to them [14].

Treatment Using Mindfulness

As noted earlier, clinical encounters with chronic pain patients who exhibit problematic substance use can be tense for both the clinician and the patient. Mindfulness can be practiced even during these challenging clinical encounters. When a clinician mindfully listens to and experiences a patient's report without distraction and judgment (accepting both the patient's negative cognitive biases and the clinician's own frustrations), the patient's tensions may resolve so that he or she becomes less defensive, distressed, and demanding [1].

When, in turn, a patient practices experiencing physical discomfort and cravings during the clinical encounter (noticing where it is and is not felt in the body, what feelings it evokes, and its changing nature), the patient's reactive behaviors decline, which then lowers the clinician's frustrations [1,6].

There may be further psychological and neurobiological benefits to MBIs for chronic pain and addiction. Meditatively watching mind–body states come forward and retreat may diminish the natural negativity bias of the brain [15]. It is likely that evolution wired the human brain to focus intently on danger, and this may be especially true of chronic pain patients [16]. An RCT of an eight-week MBI with chronic pain patients provided evidence that MBI may reduce such a bias [17].

Slow breathing from the diaphragm—alone or as part of MBIs such as meditation, yoga, or body scanning—triggers the vagus nerve and, in turn, the parasympathetic nervous system's "rest and relax" neurochemicals. This can lead to quiet, suffering-free relaxation, even if only for a few moments. The goal of mindfulness practice is for the patient to learn how to engage in this process more effectively and thus achieve longer periods free of pain and suffering [14].

Patients who have a history of trauma and depression are particularly likely to be found in populations suffering from chronic pain and SUDs [15,17]. MBIs can help patients recognize previously unrecognized triggers of pain and addictive behavior, such as past traumatic events. For example, meditation may allow a female patient who is experiencing a pain flare-up to recognize emotions linked to a relative who once molested her, particularly if she recently heard some news about her molester.

A longitudinal controlled study of an eight-week course of MBSR training found an increase in gray matter concentration in patients' left hippocampus [5]. Both major depression and post-traumatic stress disorder (PTSD) are associated with reduced volume of the hippocampus [17]. The hippocampus may play a central role in mediating some of the benefits of meditation because of its involvement in the modulation of cortical arousal and responsiveness, as well as its role in regulating emotion. A recent review of neuroimaging studies associated with mindfulness shows that in addition to the hippocampus, the medial cortex, insula, amygdala, frontal regions (including the prefrontal cortex), and basal ganglia all may be positively affected by mindfulness [5]. Some of these regions, especially the prefrontal cortex, also play a role in the neurophysiological mechanisms underlying SUDs [13].

Conclusion

The principal clinical message of this chapter is that MBIs promote healthy self-regulation for patients who have either chronic pain or SUDs, as well as co-occurring pain and SUDs [11]. While some patients will not accept mindfulness-based practices, most should be introduced to these low-harm, non-pharmacological interventions, because many will find them beneficial [4].

For More Information on the Topics Discussed:

In the Literature:

Black DS. Mindfulness-based interventions: An antidote to suffering in the context of substance use, misuse, and addiction. *Subst Use Misuse.* 2014 Apr;49(5):487–491.

Shonin E, Van Gordon W. The mechanisms of mindfulness in the treatment of mental illness and addiction. *Int J Ment Health Addict.* 2016;14(5):844–849.

Witkiewitz K, Bowen S, Harrop EN, et al. Mindfulness-based treatment to prevent addictive behavior relapse: Theoretical models and hypothesized mechanisms of change. *Subst Use Misuse.* 2014 Apr;49(5):513–524.

References

1. Gu J, Strauss C, Bond R, et al. How do mindfulness-based cognitive therapy and mindfulness-based stress reduction improve mental health and well-being? A systematic review and meta-analysis of mediation studies. *Clin Psychol Rev.* 2015 Jan 31;37C:1–12.
2. Garland EL, Manusov EG, Froeliger B, et al. Mindfulness-oriented recovery enhancement for chronic pain and prescription opioid misuse: Results from an early-stage randomized controlled trial. *J Consult Clin Psychol.* 2014 Jun;82(3):448–459.

3. Kabat-Zinn J. *Full Catastrophe Living*. New York: Random House; 1990.
4. Sturgeon JA. Psychological therapies for the management of chronic pain. *Psychology Res Behav Manag*. 2014;7:115–124.
5. Hölzel BK, Carmody J, Vangel M, et al. Mindfulness practice leads to increases in regional brain gray matter density. *Psychiatry Res*. 2011 Jan 30;191(1):36–43.
6. Kabat-Zinn J. An outpatient program in behavioral medicine for chronic pain patients based on the practice of mindfulness meditation: Theoretical considerations and preliminary results. *Gen Hosp Psychiatry*. 1982 Apr;4(1):33–47.
7. Kabat-Zinn J, Lipworth L, Burney R, et al. Four-year follow-up of a meditation-based program for the self-regulation of chronic pain: Treatment outcomes and compliance. *Clin J Pain*. 1986;2(3):159–173.
8. Lauche R, Cramer H, Dobos G, et al. A systematic review and meta-analysis of mindfulness-based stress reduction for the fibromyalgia syndrome. *J Psychosom Res*. 2013 Dec;75(6):500–510.
9. Cramer H, Haller H, Lauche R, et al. Mindfulness-based stress reduction for low back pain. A systematic review. *BMC Complement Altern Med*. 2012 Sep 25;12:162.
10. Bowen S, Witkiewitz K, Clifasefi SL, et al. Relative efficacy of mindfulness-based relapse prevention, standard relapse prevention, and treatment as usual for substance use disorders: A randomized clinical trial. *JAMA Psychiatry*. 2014;71(5):547–556.
11. Garland EL, Howard MO. Mindfulness-oriented recovery enhancement reduces pain-attentional bias in chronic pain patients. *Psychother Psychosom*. 2013;82(5):311–318.
12. Levine N. *Refuge Recovery: A Buddhist Path to Recovering from Addiction*. New York: Harper Collins; 2014.
13. Cheetham A, Allen NB, Yücel M, et al. The role of affective dysregulation in drug addiction. *Clin Psychol Rev*. 2010 Aug;30(6):621–634.
14. Busch V, Magerl W, Kern U, et al. The effect of deepened slow breathing on pain perception, autonomic activity, and mood processing—An experimental study. *Pain Med*. 2012 Feb;13(2):215–228.
15. Kasai K, Yamasue H, Gilbertson MW, et al. Evidence for acquired pregenual anterior cingulate gray matter loss from a twin study of combat-related post-traumatic stress disorder. *Biol Psychiatry*. 2008 Mar 15;63(6):550–556.
16. Marchand WR. Neural mechanisms of mindfulness and meditation: Evidence from neuroimaging studies. *World J Radiol*. 2014 Jul 28;6(7):471–479.
17. Sheline YI. 3D MRI studies of neuroanatomic changes in unipolar major depression: The role of stress and medical comorbidity. *Biol Psychiatry*. 2000 Oct 15;48(8):791–800.

Chapter 22

Preventing Avoidable Work Disability

MARIANNE CLOEREN, M.D., M.P.H., FACOEM,
FACP AND STEPHEN COLAMECO, M.D.,
M.ED., DFASAM

Addiction professionals often are asked to provide opinions or coordinate the treatment of patients experiencing substance abuse, dependence, or addiction who also are enmeshed in complicated benefit or compensation systems, including Workers' Compensation. In such patients, recovery from the substance use disorder (SUD) can be compromised by system hurdles (such as insurer resistance to covering addiction treatment) as well as issues with secondary gains (such as attorney advice for maximum benefit based on profound disability).

Beliefs about disability and other potentially modifiable risk factors for unnecessary work disability are common in patients with chronic pain and addiction. These risk factors include fear and avoidance, pain catastrophization, perceived injustice, childhood trauma, and psychiatric illness. Excessive and inappropriate medical care, often including unnecessary procedures and medications, contributes to disability beliefs, which usually are entrenched by the time a patient presents to an addiction professional.

This chapter provides information about recognizing risk factors for disability, assessing work capacity, and developing treatment strategies that promote optimal return to function.

How Is Work Disability Created?

The U.S. system for managing painful medical conditions tends to emphasize identification of underlying biological factors rather than a more comprehensive approach to pain that encompasses social, psychological, and behavioral contributors to the pain experience. This often leads to overuse of diagnostic tests that uncover minor pathology (such as disc bulges), which then is added to the patient's problem list [1–4].

Once there is a diagnosis, the focus is on reducing or eradicating symptoms (that is, pain score management). However, suggesting to patients that eradication of symptoms and full participation in life activities are contingent on symptom improvement may inadvertently increase disability behavior. In reality, limitations on participation in life and work activities are largely unrelated to the actual diagnosis, but more often are attributable to beliefs and attitudes on the part of the patient, the employer, the benefits system, and the health care system.

This "medicalization" of symptoms leads to overuse of diagnostic testing, procedures, and medications, and may lead patients to adopt unreasonable expectations that there will be a diagnostic test to explain all their symptoms, as well as a procedure or medication to relieve each of those symptoms.

When a patient is involved in one of the many systems that offer benefits contingent on the diagnosis and degree of disability, additional incentives are introduced, which may lead to worse outcomes [5–8]. These systems include Workers' Compensation, Social Security Disability, Veterans Administration (VA) benefits for service-connected conditions, military disability benefits, and other disability insurance systems. In these systems, the greater the disability or degree of impairment, the greater the chance of receiving benefits.

In the Workers' Compensation, military, and VA systems, the amount of financial compensation increases with the level of impairment. While it seems reasonable that a person should receive more compensation if he or she is more severely injured, such policies also incentivize the patient to appear or become as impaired as possible. This, of course, is counter to the actual goals of care, which is for the patient to participate fully in recovery and become as functional and productive as possible. The use of opioids and other mood-altering medications often complicates the picture.

Causes of Work Disability

Although a diagnosis always is attached to a decision that an employee is unable to work, research has shown that the medical facts are the *least* important determinants of return-to-work prognosis. Factors that contribute to unnecessary work disability include:

- Employer practices (such as not offering limited duty) [9];
- Physician practices (including overuse of diagnostic tests and treatments or inappropriate prescribing of potentially addicting medications);

- Job factors (such as low autonomy or limited job satisfaction) [10];
- Patient attitudes, behaviors, and history (for example, a history of psychiatric disorder or adverse childhood experiences, pain catastrophization, fearful or avoidant behavior, disability mindset, low self-efficacy, and perceived injustice) [11–14]; and
- The adversarial nature of the benefits system.

The Role of the Physician

Physicians play an important role in treating individuals who have sustained a compensable injury by: (a) establishing a diagnosis, (b) providing treatment, (c) assessing the degree of impairment, and (d) communicating with third parties. According to the American College of Occupational and Environmental Medicine (ACOEM), the role of the physician also should include understanding and promoting the important role of work in the health of patients [15]. This role serves the fundamental purpose of restoring health, optimizing functional capacity, and minimizing the destructive impact of injury or illness on the patient's life.

Clinical Presentation

Patients who are seeking compensation or other benefits may be sent by an employer or insurer to an addiction professional for an independent medical evaluation when excessive substance use or addiction is suspected. In this type of evaluation, no physician–patient treatment relationship is established. Instead, the role of the physician is to review the records provided, interview the patient, perform a physical examination, and answer the questions posed by the referral source in a detailed and objective report.

In contrast, if the patient is referred by a health care professional involved in the treatment of a patient in a Workers' Compensation case, the addiction professional also may have the role of a treating provider, with all the usual implications of a therapeutic relationship.

Patients may be referred for treatment of SUDs by a claims adjustor or case manager for the Workers' Compensation insurer, but the threshold for this type of referral is set fairly high. Typically, the following must be true for such a referral to occur:

- The treating (usually the prescribing) physician must recognize that the patient has an SUD and agree with the need for treatment.
- The patient must accept the recommendation for treatment.

- The insurer must agree that the SUD was causally related to the work injury, and that its treatment is likely to result in a better vocational or cost outcome.
- The patient's attorney must not oppose treatment.

Patients also may come to an addiction professional through referral from their primary care physician or on their own. If their condition is complicating recovery from a work injury but was not actually *caused* by the work injury or its treatment, it may be appropriate to work with the patient's personal medical insurer or the patient directly to help the patient access treatment. (This is more likely to occur when the substance in question is not one prescribed to treat a work-related injury; for example, alcohol rather than opioid analgesics.)

In performing a clinical evaluation of a patient whose chronic pain is complicated by an SUD, the addiction professional should recognize that the original painful condition has most likely been exhaustively evaluated by many other professionals, using a multitude of diagnostic tests. Unless it is likely that the cause of the pain is an easily treatable condition that was missed, there is no reason to perform additional diagnostic tests related to the pain. In fact, doing so can become counterproductive by distracting attention from the SUD. It also is possible that the original painful condition is not a significant factor in the patient's ongoing pain, as chronic pain can persist long after tissue injury has resolved.

Obtaining a history of the evolution of the painful condition is important in engaging the patient, but the clinical history should quickly move to the use of medications and other substances, following the guidelines discussed in other chapters of this Handbook.

Pain scales are widely used in clinical practice, and patients treated in pain clinics may come to expect them. The addiction professional should recognize that such scales provide a subjective numerical expression of how a patient describes his or her pain experience. However, these scales have been shown to be of little value in measuring the effectiveness of treatment in restoring a patient to optimal function. Many patients continue to report high levels of pain even as they are improving in other measures of health, such as participation in family and work activities.

In contrast, it can be helpful to address several elements of a functional examination that are not often documented in clinical encounters. These include:

- Evidence for or against sedation or other impairment;
- Evidence of withdrawal symptoms (such as tremor or scratching);
- Physiological signs of substance use (for example, pupillary constriction);
- Pain behavior and movement during the office visit;

- Gait and station;
- Need for assistive devices, as well as any discrepancy between physical findings and the use of such devices;
- Tests or other demonstration of ability to use the affected body part (such as by gripping an object, reaching or squatting);
- Ability to rise from a chair, as well as the patient's use of his or her arms to assist in such movements; and
- The patient's level of cooperation with the physician's requests.

Tests related to the area of pain are worth performing, in part to detect pain-catastrophizing behavior, if any, although they have not been shown to have much diagnostic value. The tests described in 1987 by Dr. Gordon Waddell, since named the "Waddell signs," have been used, inaccurately, to "diagnose" malingering. In fact, such tests cannot show whether a patient is deliberately feigning low back pain, but they can be very useful in identifying patients whose pain has a large emotional (non-mechanical) component.

Diagnostic Testing

By the time patients with chronic pain arrive at the office of an addiction professional, most have had myriad diagnostic tests. To establish an accurate base of information, it is advisable for the addiction professional to obtain the original report of each relevant diagnostic test, rather than relying on notes or summaries of test results (which may be incomplete or inaccurate). Depending on the system and how the patient was referred, authorization may be needed to perform any additional diagnostic tests. In most cases, performing urine toxicology tests is appropriate, as is checking the state's Prescription Drug Monitoring Program (PDMP). (Note that states vary in the restrictions they impose on access to their PDMPs. Some allow access only for the purpose of delivering health care services; therefore, PDMPs in those states should not be consulted for medicolegal purposes.)

Assessing Patient Coping and Reaction Styles

Several tools are useful in identifying and measuring the impact of personal coping and reaction styles, which have been shown to contribute to avoidable disability. They include:

- *The Pain Catastrophizing Scale:* Multiple research studies have validated the tendency to catastrophize pain as a significant risk factor for work disability. Individuals who catastrophize ruminate about their pain, magnify their pain, and feel helpless to manage their pain [16].

- *The Injustice Experience Questionnaire:* Patients with chronic pain often feel wronged or victimized —a perception that can interfere with recovery when patients dwell on the harm they believe has been done to them [17].
- *The Fear-Avoidance Beliefs Questionnaire (FABQ) for Patients with Low Back Pain:* The FABQ identifies fear-avoidance beliefs in patients with low back pain. It helps predict the level of pain avoidance behavior, because such avoidance can interfere with recovery and return to function [18].
- *The Adverse Childhood Experiences Questionnaire (ACEQ):* Developed by the Centers for Disease Control and Prevention in partnership with Kaiser Permanente, the ACEQ is used to identify adults who are at risk for negative health outcomes—including chronic pain and addiction—as the result of adverse experiences in childhood. Such experiences include physical or sexual abuse, neglect, domestic violence, and addiction or mental illness in family members [19].

Identification of specific disability risk factors may point toward particular therapeutic approaches (such as cognitive behavioral therapy, acceptance and commitment therapy, and trauma-informed therapy), which can be helpful in developing more effective coping strategies and resilience.

Evaluating Patient Work Capacity

In evaluating work capacity in a patient with pain, it can be helpful to use a screening tool to measure the impact of the painful condition on the patient's participation in activities. Note that such screening generally does not reflect the patient's *actual* physical abilities, because most patients engage in self-limiting behavior. However, it can be helpful to use such measurements in determining when the patient is not fully participating in life and how the patient is experiencing or coping with pain, as well as in setting goals and measuring progress. Available tools include the following:

- *The Oswestry Low Back Pain Disability Questionnaire and Index:* This questionnaire provides a score that indicates the degree to which the patient's back pain experience is limiting his or her involvement in life. While the score cannot be used to determine the actual severity of the clinical pathology, it is very useful in determining how well (or poorly) the patient is functioning in the presence of pain [20].
- *The Orebro Musculoskeletal Pain Screening Questionnaire (Short Form):* This brief tool measures the impact of a painful musculoskeletal condition on the patient's ability to function, and also addresses the patient's anxiety, depression, and beliefs about disability [21].
- *The Linton Activity Screening Questionnaire:* This somewhat longer tool is not specific to any particular type or area of pain. It measures pain

levels, functional impact, fear/avoidance behavior, and beliefs about disability [22].

- *The American Chronic Pain Association Quality of Life Scale:* This simple 10-point scale is designed to measure the patient's current level of functioning. It is meant to be used to track progress over time [23].

Treatment

The role of addiction professionals may involve directing the care of a patient or providing an opinion to the treating professional, an attorney, or an insurer. For patients with SUDs, treatment options include medication-assisted treatment in outpatient settings; intensive outpatient programs (which include individual counseling and group therapy); outpatient functional restoration programs (which typically combine detoxification with physical reconditioning and cognitive-behavioral therapy); and inpatient treatment in programs that employ medication-assisted treatment and other therapies for SUDs, as well as a chronic pain track that includes functional restoration [15].

A strong rationale may be needed to obtain authorization for admission to an inpatient program. Such a rationale may include the patient's need for a large daily dose of opioids, or his or her need for multiple medications that have abuse potential (such as benzodiazepines given in combination with opioids), a history or indications of prescription drug abuse complicated by an alcohol use disorder or psychiatric disorder, or severe physical deconditioning [24].

In patients with chronic pain who are at risk for unnecessary work disability, treatment must include approaches to help the patient learn to manage his or her pain. This usually involves a comprehensive treatment plan that gives attention to maladaptive behaviors, physical reconditioning, mental health (co-occurring psychiatric disorders are common in these patients), and spiritual health (which may include faith communities, meditation, and gratitude or forgiveness exercises) [5].

In addition to providing an opinion about the presence of a condition requiring addiction treatment, the addiction professional should make explicit recommendations about the type and duration of treatment needed. An opinion about the causal relationship to the work injury (e.g., did the condition predate the work injury, or did it arise during treatment for the work injury?) and the impact of the condition on recovery from the work injury also may be required.

The patient's vocational goals and plans should be included in the treatment plan and explicitly addressed with the patient. Case management conferences with the insurance case manager can be helpful in reporting progress and developing plans for return to work or vocational rehabilitation.

Pain psychologists can be valuable resources in the long-term management of patients with chronic pain who are recovering from addiction. A new model of treatment, referred to as "work-focused cognitive-behavioral therapy," places the goal of occupational recovery at the center of the treatment plan [25].

Conclusion

Long-term absence from the workplace on the part of individuals experiencing both pain and addiction often is not attributable to medical factors, but instead results from the interplay of various factors, some external (such as legal or system incentives) and some internal to the patient.

Addiction professionals should be alert to the psychosocial factors that may contribute to unnecessary work disability, and avoid compounding such problems by reinforcing patients' maladaptive beliefs. These include pain catastrophization, disability beliefs, fear and avoidance, and perceived injustice. Screening tools are available to identify such tendencies, and various interventions are available to help address them.

By focusing on improving a patient's ability to cope, and by measuring progress toward functional goals rather than focusing on symptoms, addiction professionals can help patients with chronic pain recover from addiction while preserving or reclaiming their life roles.

For More Information on the Topics Discussed:

American College of Occupational and Environmental Medicine (ACOEM):

The Personal Physician's Role in Helping Patients with Medical Conditions Stay at Work or Return to Work. Elk Grove Village, IL: ACOEM; 2017.

In the Literature:

Dewa CS, Hees H, Trojanowski L, et al. Clinician experiences assessing work disability related to mental disorders. *PLoS One.* 2015 Mar 19;10(3):e0119009.

Meshberg-Cohen S, Reid-Quiñones K, Black AC, et al. Veterans' attitudes toward work and disability compensation: Associations with substance abuse. *Addict Behav.* 2014 Feb;39(2):445–448.

Robinson JP, Dansie EJ, Wilson HD, et al. Attitudes and beliefs of working and work-disabled people with chronic pain prescribed long-term opioids. *Pain Med.* 2015 Jul;16(7):1311–1324.

References

1. Deyo RA, Mirza SK, Turner JA, et al. Overtreating chronic back pain: Time to back off? *J Am Board Fam Med*. 2009;22(1):62–68.
2. Jarvik JG, Deyo RA. Diagnostic evaluation of low back pain with emphasis on imaging. *Ann Intern Med*. 2002;137(7):586–597.
3. Hadler NM. MRI for back pain; Need for less imaging, better understanding. *JAMA*. 2003;289:2863–2865.
4. Jarvik JG, Hollingworth W, Martin B, et al. Rapid magnetic resonance imaging vs. radiographs for patients with low back pain: A randomized controlled trial. *JAMA*. 2003;289(21):2810–2818.
5. Turk DC, Okifuji A. Perception of traumatic onset, compensation status and physical findings: Impact on pain severity, emotional distress, and disability in chronic pain patients. *J Behav Med*. 1996;19(5):435–453.
6. Cassidy JD, Carroll LJ, Côté P, et al. Effect of eliminating compensation for pain and suffering on the outcome of insurance claims for whiplash injury. *NEJM*. 2000;20(16):1179–1186.
7. Lysgaard A, Fonager K, Nielsen C. Effect of financial compensation on vocational rehabilitation. *J Rehabil Med*. 2005;37(6):388–391.
8. Koljonen P, Chong C, Yip D. Difference in outcome of shoulder surgery between workers' compensation and nonworkers' compensation populations. *Int Orthop*. 2007;33(2):315–320.
9. Mitchell K. Top 10 return-to-work myths—and the realities behind them. *Workforce Magazine*. 07 Aug 2002. http://www.workforce.com/2002/08/07/top-10-return-to-work-myths-and-the-realities-behind-them/
10. Gice J. The relationship between job satisfaction and workers' compensation claims. *CPCU Journal*. 1996;48(3):178–183.
11. Sullivan MJL. Toward a biopsychomotor conceptualization of pain: Implications for research and intervention. *Clin J Pain*. 2008;24:281–290.
12. Dersh J, Gatchel RJ, Polatin P, et al. Prevalence of psychiatric disorders in patients with chronic work-related musculoskeletal pain disability. *Occup Environ Med*. 2002;44:459–468.
13. Sullivan MJ, Thorn B, Haythornthwaite JA, et al. Theoretical perspectives on the relation between catastrophizing and pain. *Clin J Pain*. 2001;17:52–64.
14. Ayre M, Tyson GA. The role of self-efficacy and fear-avoidance beliefs in the prediction of disability. *Aust Psychol*. 2001;36:250–253.
15. American College of Occupational and Environmental Medicine (ACOEM). *The Personal Physician's Role in Helping Patients with Medical Conditions Stay at Work or Return to Work*. Elk Grove Village, IL: ACOEM; 2017.
16. Sullivan MJL. *The Pain Catastrophizing Scale*. Montreal, Quebec, Canada: McGill University; 2009.
17. Sullivan MJL. *The Injustice Experience Questionnaire*. Montreal, Quebec, Canada: McGill University; 2008.
18. Waddell G, Newton M, Henderson I, et al. A Fear-Avoidance Beliefs Questionnaire (FABQ) and the role of fear-avoidance beliefs in chronic low back pain and disability. *Pain*. 1993;52:157–168.

19. World Health Organization (WHO). *Preventing Child Maltreatment: A Guide to Taking Action and Generating Evidence*. Geneva, Switzerland: WHO; 2006.
20. Fairbank JC, Pynsent PB. The Oswestry Disability Index. *Spine*. 2000 Nov 15;25(22):2940–2953.
21. Linton SJ, Nicholas M, MacDonald S. Development of a short form of the Örebro Musculoskeletal Pain Screening Questionnaire. *Spine*. 2011 Oct 15;36(22):1891–1895.
22. Linton SJ, Hallden BA. *The Linton Activity Screening Questionnaire*. Department of Occupational and Environmental Medicine, Orebro Medical Centre, Orebro, Sweden: 2005. http://www.rdehospital.nhs.uk/docs/patients/services/spinal%20unit/LintonQuestionnaire1.pdf
23. American Chronic Pain Association (ACPA). *Quality of Life Scale: A Measure of Function for People with Pain*. Rocklin, CA: ACPA; 2003.
24. Horgan CM, Reif S, Ritter GA, et al. Organizational and financial issues in the delivery of substance abuse treatment services. *Recent Dev Alcohol*. 2001;15:9–26.
25. Reme SE, Grasdal AL, Løvvik C, et al. Work-focused cognitive-behavioural therapy and individual job support to increase work participation in common mental disorders: A randomised controlled multicentre trial. *BMJ*. 2014;72:10.

Chapter 23

Revising the Treatment Plan and/or Ending Addiction Treatment

JOHN A. HOPPER, M.D. AND
THEODORE V. PARRAN, JR., M.D.

Outcomes of treatment for substance use disorders (SUDs) typically are positive for patients who remain in treatment for a reasonable length of time [1]. However, some patients struggle to discontinue their misuse of opioids or other drugs, are inconsistent in their adherence to treatment plans, or succeed in achieving some therapeutic goals while not doing well with others [2]. Regular assessment of the patient's level of engagement in treatment and the strength of the therapeutic alliance allows for modification of the treatment plan and level of care in response to the patient's progress or lack thereof (see Chapter 11 of this Handbook).

Reasons for Revising the Treatment Plan

Certain medical factors may cause a patient's dose requirements to change. These include (but are not limited to) starting, stopping, or changing the dose of other prescription medications; the onset and progression of pregnancy; the onset of menopause; the progression of liver disease; and a significant increase or decrease in weight [3]. An increase in the dose of the drug(s) used in treatment may help to suppress drug cravings. Coordination with other prescribing physicians to limit the number of short-acting opioids obtained by prescription generally is recommended [3].

Behaviors that are not consistent with the treatment agreement should be taken seriously and used as an opportunity to further assess the patient and make necessary revisions in the treatment plan. In some cases, such as when a patient's behavior raises concerns about staff safety or diversion of controlled medications, it may be best to refer the patient to a more structured treatment environment, such as an opioid treatment program (OTP), or even for medically managed withdrawal [2].

Patients who have more serious or persistent problems should be referred to a pain or addiction specialist (or both) for additional evaluation and treatment. For example, the treatment of addiction in a patient with a comorbid mental disorder may be best managed through consultation with or referral to a specialist in addiction psychiatry. In other instances, aberrant or dysfunctional behaviors may indicate the need for more vigorous engagement in peer support, counseling or psychotherapy, or possibly referral to a more structured treatment setting, such as a residential setting, partial hospitalization, or intensive outpatient program.

Patient Relapse

Relapse always should be ruled out as the reason for a patient's loss of stability [4]. However, relapse *does not* constitute grounds for automatic termination of treatment. Rather, it should be taken as a signal to reassess the patient's status, to implement changes in the treatment plan (such as by intensifying the treatment structure or intensity of services), and to document any changes in the patient's medical record [5].

Relapse has been described as "a breakdown or setback in a person's attempt to change or modify any target behavior" [6] and as "an unfolding process in which the resumption of substance abuse is the last event in a long series of maladaptive responses to internal or external stressors or stimuli" [7]. Rarely is it caused by any single factor; instead, it is a dynamic process in which the patient's readiness to change interacts with other external and internal factors [6,8].

In fact, rates of relapse in the treatment of SUDs are comparable to relapse rates seen in other chronic medical disorders, such as diabetes and hypertension [9]. For this reason, comparable long-term adjustment of the treatment plan is appropriate.

Precipitants of Relapse

Specific precipitants of relapse vary substantially from time to time, even in the same individual [10]. Attributing causality is even more complex in patients who have co-occurring medical or mental disorders. In a survey [11], investigators asked more than 100 patients to identify the factors that contributed to their relapse. Factors identified most often were inability to manage stress or negative emotional states (69%); interpersonal conflicts with family or others

(29%); poor adherence to the treatment regimen (25%); negative thinking (11%); and insufficient motivation to change (10%).

Severity of Relapse

Not all relapses are alike. The term *lapse* refers to an initial episode of drug use after a period of abstinence. A lapse usually is impulsive and involves a brief period of use. Most lapses are of short duration, with relatively minor consequences, and are marked by the patient's desire to return to abstinence. However, a lapse also can progress to a full-blown relapse (marked by loss of control) of varying proportions. The effects of the initial lapse are mediated by the individual's affective and cognitive state, as well as the response of caregivers and others [6].

Continued use implies just that: continued use of non-prescribed psychoactive substances, including alcohol, without having first achieved a period of stability or abstinence, regardless of whether an intervention has taken place. Abstinence in a protected environment (e.g., a residential treatment program or incarceration), followed by a return to drinking or drug use, is more appropriately considered "continued use" than "relapse." The same is true of continued use while in outpatient treatment (e.g., drinking or drug use between outpatient therapy sessions).

Continued problem potential addresses the issues of co-occurring physical or mental health problems that are related to substance use. For example, a psychotic, paranoid individual who is fearful of being poisoned and thus fails to take his or her medication would be described as having a "high relapse or continued problem potential" and is at high risk for becoming acutely psychotic and/or increasingly paranoid. By the nature of his or her mental health disorder, such an individual is at high risk of relapse to substance use.

Adjusting the Treatment Plan to Prevent Relapse

A number of clinical strategies have been developed to help patients address relapse risk [6,8,11–13]. The following principles are common to many models of relapse prevention:

- *Help the patient identify environmental cues and stressors that act as relapse triggers.* Identifying environmental cues can lead to the development of a relapse prevention plan through the use of techniques such as cue avoidance, cue desensitization, and stimulus control. Patients may be familiar with the recovery concept of "people, places, and things" as a framework for thinking about external triggers.

- *Teach the patient how to identify and manage negative emotional states.* Interventions that help patients develop skills to cope with or manage negative emotional states can reduce the risk of relapse, but these must be tailored to each patient's situation and needs. The recovery term "HALT" (hungry, angry, lonely, tired) can be a used to help patients explore internal triggers.
- *Encourage the patient to work toward a more balanced lifestyle.* Lifestyle can be assessed by evaluating patterns of daily activities; sources of stress and stressful life events; the balance between "wants" (activities engaged in for pleasure or self-fulfillment) and "shoulds" (external demands); health, exercise, sleep and relaxation patterns; interpersonal activities; and religious beliefs [6].
- *Help the patient understand and manage craving.* Volkow and Fowler [14] hypothesize that dopamine stimulation that occurs with long-term alcohol or drug use leads to disruption of brain circuitry involved in regulating drives. This disruption, in turn, leads to a conditioned response to the stimulus (craving), which leads to compulsive use of the substance. Behavioral interventions include avoiding, leaving, or changing situations that trigger or worsen craving; attending support group meetings; and using anti-craving medications.
- *Teach the patient how to identify and interrupt lapses and relapses.* Patients should have an emergency plan to address a lapse so that a full-blown relapse can be avoided. However, if relapse does occur, the patient needs strategies to interrupt it. Intervention strategies should be based on the severity of the patient's lapse or relapse, the presence of coping mechanisms, and his or her history of relapse [11].
- *Encourage the patient to develop a recovery support system.* Positive family and social supports generally enhance recovery. Families are more likely to provide such support if they are engaged in the treatment process and have an opportunity to ask questions, share their concerns and experiences, and learn practical coping strategies as well as behaviors to avoid. Use of peers (or "sponsors") in long-term recovery is strongly encouraged in most mutual support recovery programs.

Adjusting the Treatment Plan in Response to Relapse

Rather than discharging the patient from treatment, intensified care management may be the most appropriate way to manage patients whose response to treatment is persistently sub-optimal.

Guidelines issued by the Department of Defense DoD and the Department of Veterans Affairs (VA) [15] suggest that "relapse can be used as a signal to re-evaluate the treatment plan, rather than evidence that the patient cannot succeed or was not sufficiently motivated." The DoD-VA guidelines recommend that care providers consider:

- Adding or substituting another medication or psychosocial intervention to the treatment plan;
- Altering the intensity of treatment by increasing the level of care, the frequency of visits, or the dose of medication; or
- Making an effort to re-engage the patient in treatment.

Patients who continue to misuse opioids after sufficient exposure to treatment (including psychosocial services) or who experience continued symptoms of withdrawal or craving should be evaluated for potential transfer to a more structured treatment environment, such as an OTP [7,16–18].

When the best clinical course is not clear, consultation with another health care professional may be helpful. The results of the consultation should be discussed with the patient and any written consultation reports added to the patient's medical record [5].

Reasons for Ending Treatment

The physician and patient may, at mutually agreed-upon intervals, weigh the potential benefits and risks of continuing treatment and discuss whether the current therapy continues to be appropriate or whether it should be discontinued.

Voluntary Termination of Treatment

Ideally, voluntary termination of treatment occurs only when a patient has achieved maximum benefit from the treatment regimen. However, patients sometimes leave addiction treatment for non-therapeutic reasons, including incarceration, hospitalization, loss of insurance benefits, inability to afford treatment, and transportation problems. In many of these situations, discharge is not preceded by planned withdrawal of the treatment medication. If treatment is continued, boundaries should be adjusted to support safe and appropriate medication use. If it is discontinued, the patient should be tapered off the medication through use of a safe, carefully structured regimen [18].

Factors to be considered in determining a patient's suitability for long-term medication-free status include the presence of stable housing and income, the availability of adequate psychosocial supports, and the absence of legal problems. For patients who have not achieved these indices of stabilization, a period of maintenance—during which the patient addresses such barriers—usually is advised [12].

For patients who are being treated for opioid use disorder, medically supervised withdrawal should be followed by a period of drug-free treatment in order to minimize the risk of relapse to opioid abuse. Supervised use of oral, injected, or depot naltrexone (an opioid antagonist) for a period of several months to two years following tapering off of opioid agonist therapy often is recommended. Both the patient and physician should accept as a possible outcome that the patient will need or want to return to opioid maintenance treatment on a long-term basis.

The process of tapering the patient off the opioid and the risk of overdose attendant on subsequent use of opioids by a patient who has lost his or her tolerance are important topics for patient counseling. Such tapers should be done without imparting any sense of failure, shame, or guilt [4] (also see the sidebar on opioid tapers that accompanies this chapter).

Involuntary Termination of Treatment

A patient may become a candidate for involuntary or administrative discharge because the treating physician concludes that the patient is not progressing satisfactorily. For example, if many days of dosing are missed and repeated attempts to help a patient comply with daily dosing requirements have failed, it may not be safe to continue maintenance therapy [18]. Or a patient may be out of compliance with the treatment plan or with office procedures. Administrative discharge for non-payment of fees may be part of the structure to which a patient agreed at the time of admission. (In addiction treatment, a patient's sudden lack of funds also may be an indicator of relapse [17].)

Under any of these circumstances, the physician may consider involuntary termination of treatment as a last resort, but with care not to abandon the patient [5]. Before reaching a final decision to discharge a patient, the physician ought to review and adjust the psychosocial services being provided to the patient and consider the use of alternative medications [4].

Conditions that will result in termination of treatment, as well as contingencies for alternative care, should be outlined in some detail in the informed consent or treatment agreement [20]. Such conditions generally include:

- *Nonadherence with the treatment plan*: The patient does not or will not follow the treatment regimen outlined in the plan.
- *Nonadherence with follow-up activities*: The patient repeatedly cancels scheduled visits.
- *Nonadherence with office policies*: The patient uses weekend on-call physicians or multiple health care providers to obtain prescription refills, even though office policy limits the number of refills between visits.

- *Inappropriate behavior*: The patient is rude and uses improper language with office personnel, exhibits violent behavior, makes threats of physical harm, or uses anger to jeopardize the safety and well-being of office personnel or other patients.
- *Nonpayment for services:* The patient owes a backlog of bills and has made no effort to arrange a payment plan or access public resources for payment. The office should avoid discriminatory practices and follow the same policies for nonpayment regardless of the patient's underlying medical problems.

Special Considerations

Certain factors may require additional arrangements or a delay in terminating a patient who is being treated for an opioid use disorder. For example [20]:

- If the patient is in an acute phase of treatment, termination must be delayed until the acute phase has passed, unless further treatment poses a risk to staff, other patients, or the treatment milieu.
- If the clinician is the only source of treatment for opioid addiction within a reasonable driving distance, he or she may need to continue care until other arrangements can be made.
- If the clinician is the only source of a particular type of specialized medical care, he or she is ethically obligated to continue care until the patient can be safely transferred to another practitioner who is able to provide treatment and follow-up or medically supervised withdrawal from the treatment medication.
- If the clinician is a member of a prepaid health plan, the patient cannot be discharged until the practitioner has communicated with the third-party payer to request that the patient be transferred to another practitioner or program.

Steps in Ending Treatment

When it is appropriate to terminate treatment and none of the foregoing special considerations is present, termination of the physician–patient relationship should be formally documented. The patient should be given a written notice that he or she must find another health care provider within a stipulated period of time. The written notice should be mailed to the patient by both regular and certified mail, return receipt requested. Copies of the letter should be filed in the patient's medical record, along with the original certified mail receipt and the original certified mail return receipt, even if the patient refuses to sign for the certified letter [5]. As noted above, if the patient participates in a managed care insurance program, the provider should contact the insurance company to review provider obligations in terminating treatment.

If a maintenance medication (e.g., methadone, buprenorphine, or naltrexone) is to be discontinued, the patient should be tapered off the medication through use of a safely structured regimen, and followed closely [21,22]. He or she also should be advised to continue nonpharmacological therapies. It may be necessary to reinstate pharmacotherapy or other treatment services if relapse appears imminent or actually occurs [21]. Such relapse poses a significant risk of overdose, which should be carefully explained to the patient [4]. Patients also should be assured that relapse need not occur in order for medication-assisted therapy to be reinstated [22].

Conclusion

When prescribing opioids for chronic pain or addiction, providers should recognize that adjustments to the treatment plan are a common and expected step. As with any chronic condition, the physician must monitor the course of the disease along with the patient's response to treatment. A comprehensive treatment plan may *include* opioids, but it rarely is based *solely* on opioid treatment. Balancing empathy for the patient's suffering with a clinical focus on maximizing function is the physician's best guide to delivering effective treatment of chronic pain.

If a patient is diagnosed with a co-occurring SUD and chronic pain, the treatment options must be altered to reflect the imperative of preserving patient safety. One of three approaches typically is employed in such a situation:

- Medically supervised withdrawal from controlled drugs, followed by aggressive bio-psycho-social-spiritual-familial treatment of the SUD, along with use of non-controlled drugs for comprehensive pain management;
- Opioid agonist treatment with buprenorphine in an office setting, accompanied by appropriate selections from the SUD and chronic pain treatments described previously; or
- Admission to an OTP for treatment with methadone, combined with the types of addiction and chronic pain treatment described previously.

Simply ignoring the patient's SUD and continuing to prescribe opioids for his or her pain endangers the health and safety of the patient, his or her family, and the community. This is likely to result in doing harm and thus is inconsistent with the basic ethical principles of medical care.

For More Information on the Topics Discussed:

American Society of Addiction Medicine:

Parran TV Jr., McCormick RA, Delos Reyes CM. Assessment (Chapter 20). In RK Ries, DA Fiellin, SC Miller, R Saitz, eds. *The ASAM Principles of Addiction Medicine, Fifth Edition*. Philadelphia, PA: Wolters Kluwer; 2014.

Saxon AJ. Special issues in office-based opioid treatment (Chapter 51). In RK Ries, DA Fiellin, SC Miller, R Saitz, eds. *The ASAM Principles of Addiction Medicine, Fifth Edition*. Philadelphia, PA: Wolters Kluwer; 2014.

Finch JW, Parran TV Jr., Wilford BB, et al. Clinical, ethical, and legal considerations in prescribing drugs with abuse potential (Chapter 111). In RK Ries, DA Fiellin, SC Miller, R Saitz, eds. *The ASAM Principles of Addiction Medicine, Fifth Edition*. Philadelphia, PA: Wolters Kluwer; 2014.

Prescriber's Clinical Support System for Opioids, www.pcss-o.org. Sponsored by the American Academy of Addiction Psychiatry (AAAP) in collaboration with other specialty societies and with support from SAMHSA, the Prescriber's Clinical Support System for Opioids (PCSS-0) offers multiple resources—including live and recorded webinars—related to opioid prescribing and the diagnosis and management of opioid use disorders.

References

1. Fiellin DA, Kleber H, Trumble-Hejduk JG, et al. Consensus statement on office-based treatment of opioid dependence using buprenorphine. *J Subst Abuse Treat*. 2004;27(2):153–159.
2. Fiellin DA, Friedland GH, Gourevitch MN. Opioid dependence: Rationale for and efficacy of existing and new treatments. *Clin Infect Dis*. 2006;43:S173–S177.
3. Baxter LE, chair, for the ASAM Methadone Action Group. Clinical guidance on methadone induction and stabilization. *J Addict Med*. 2013 Nov-Dec;7(6):377–386.
4. Stephenson DK, for the CSAM Committee on Treatment of Opioid Dependence. *Draft Guidelines for Physicians Working in California Opioid Treatment Programs*. San Francisco, CA: California Society of Addiction Medicine; 2008.
5. Federation of State Medical Boards (FSMB). *Model Policy on Opioid Addiction Treatment in the Medical Office*. Dallas, TX: The Federation; 2013.
6. Marlatt G, Gordon JR, eds. *Relapse Prevention: Maintenance Strategies in the Treatment of Addictive Behaviors*. New York: Guilford Press, 1985.
7. National Institute on Drug Abuse (NIDA). *Topics in Brief: Medication-Assisted Treatment for Opioid Addiction*. Washington, DC: National Institutes of Health, April 2012. (Accessed at: www.drugabuse.gov.)
8. Dimeff LA, Marlatt GA. Relapse prevention. In R Hester, W Miller, eds. *Handbook of Alcoholism Treatment Approaches, 2nd Edition*. Boston, MA: Allyn, Bacon; 1995:176–194.

9. Vollkow ND, Koob G. Brain disease model of addiction: Why is it so controversial? *Lancet Psychiatry*. 2015 Aug;2(8):677–679.

10. Connors GJ, Longabaugh R, Miller WR. Looking forward and back to relapse: Implications for research and practice. *Addiction*. 1996 Dec;91(Suppl):S191–S196.

11. Daley DC, Marlatt GA, Spotts CE. Relapse prevention: Clinical models and intervention strategies. In AW Graham, TK Schultz, MF Mayo-Smith, RK Ries, BB Wilford, eds. *The ASAM Principles of Addiction Medicine, Third Edition*. Chevy Chase, MD: American Society of Addiction Medicine; 2003:467–485.

12. Fishman MJ, Mee-Lee D, Shulman GD, Kolodner G, Wilford BB, eds. *Supplement to the ASAM Patient Placement Criteria on Pharmacotherapies for the Management of Alcohol Use Disorders*. Philadelphia, PA: Lippincott, Williams & Wilkins, Inc.; 2010.

13. Tims F, Leukefeld C, eds. *Relapse and Recovery in Drug Abuse*. NIDA Research Monograph 72. Rockville, MD: National Institute on Drug Abuse (NIDA), National Institutes of Health, 1987.

14. Volkow ND, Fowler JS. Addiction, a disease of compulsion and drive: Involvement of the orbitofrontal cortex. *Cereb Cortex*. 2000 Mar;10(3):318–325. Review.

15. Veterans Health Administration (VHA), Department of Veteran Affairs. *Clinical Practice Guidelines for Management of Substance Use Disorders (SUD), Version 2.0*. Washington, DC: Department of Veterans Affairs; 2009.

16. Alford DP, LaBelle CT, Kretsch N, et al. Collaborative care of opioid-addicted patient in primary care using buprenorphine. *Arch Intern Med*. 2011;171(5):425–431.

17. Center for Substance Abuse Treatment (CSAT). *Substance Abuse Treatment: Group Therapy*. (Treatment Improvement Protocol [TIP] Series 41. DHHS Publication No. [SMA] 05-3991.) Rockville, MD: CSAT, Substance Abuse and Mental Health Services Administration; 2005.

18. Center for Substance Abuse Treatment (CSAT). *Clinical Guidelines for the Use of Buprenorphine in the Treatment of Opioid Addiction*. (Treatment Improvement Protocol [TIP] Series 40. DHHS Publication No. [SMA] 04-3939.) Rockville, MD: CSAT, Substance Abuse and Mental Health Services Administration; 2004.

19. Center for Substance Abuse Treatment (CSAT). *Detoxification and Substance Abuse Treatment*. (Treatment Improvement Protocol [TIP] Series 45. DHHS Publication No. (SMA) 06-4131.) Rockville, MD: CSAT, Substance Abuse and Mental Health Services Administration; 2006.

20. Institute for Research, Education and Training in Addiction (IRETA). *Best Practices in the Use of Buprenorphine. Final Expert Panel Report*. Pittsburgh, PA: Community Care Behavioral Health Organizations; October 18, 2011.

21. McNicholas L. Clinical guidelines for the use of buprenorphine in the treatment of opioid addiction. *A Tool for Buprenorphine Care*. 2008 May;1(12):12. https://www.mirecc.va.gov/visn4/Bulletins/May08BP.pdf

22. Finch JW, Kamien JB, Amass L. Two-year experience with buprenorphine-naloxone (Suboxone) for maintenance treatment of opioid dependence within a private practice setting. *J Addict Med*. 2007 Jun;1(2):104–110.

ADAPTING TREATMENT TO THE NEEDS OF SPECIFIC PATIENT POPULATIONS

The chapters in **Section V** address the treatment needs of patients in specific population groups.

- The author of **Chapter 24** describes the management of pain and addiction in patients who also are diagnosed with a co-occurring psychiatric disorder. The author of the **Sidebar to Chapter 24** provides an example of such a situation in his discussion of post-traumatic stress disorder and how the presence of such a disorder affects patient management.
- In **Chapter 25,** the authors review the management of pain and addiction in patients who also have a co-occurring medical disorder, while the author of the **Sidebar to Chapter 25** describes the effects of traumatic brain injury and how its presence can affect the overall treatment plan.
- The authors of **Chapter 26** review the management of patients whose chronic pain is caused by fibromyalgia and how the presence of this little-understood condition affects the treatment of chronic pain and the patient's risk for opioid addiction.
- Smoking cigarettes is a documented risk factor for chronic pain. Because this particular risk associated with smoking is not widely recognized, the author of **Chapter 27** reviews the current research and its implications for patient care.
- The author of **Chapter 28** describes the risks for development of chronic pain and addiction in adolescents and young adults, which differ from those typically seen in the adult population and thus require different interventions.
- In **Chapter 29,** the authors discuss the physiological and psychological factors common to older adults that are significant in the diagnosis of chronic pain and addiction and the development of an appropriate treatment plan.

- As described by the author of **Chapter 30**, women have special vulnerabilities to pain and addiction and benefit from treatment plans tailored to their needs. Use of opioids by pregnant women has significant implications for their offspring, many of whom manifest the symptoms of opioid neonatal abstinence syndrome at birth.
- The authors of **Chapter 31** discuss the special vulnerabilities of military personnel and veterans as a result of their exposure to the demands of military training and service in combat situations. Such individuals have been shown to benefit from care for pain and addiction that takes their special circumstances into account.

Chapter 24

Pain and Addiction in Patients with Co-Occurring Psychiatric Disorders

PENELOPE P. ZIEGLER, M.D., FASAM

It is often said that pain makes all of life's other problems worse, and other life problems make pain worse. Understandably, patients with psychiatric disorders or symptoms present a variety of challenges to the clinician who is attempting to treat their pain condition. Therefore, an integrated, comprehensive approach is especially important in this population.

Evaluating Pain in Patients with a Psychiatric Disorder

The first step in evaluating a patient with a known or suspected psychiatric diagnosis who presents with a complaint of pain is to obtain a clear psychiatric history from the patient. Determining when the patient first experienced psychiatric symptoms, who else has provided psychiatric treatment and for how long, and the current psychiatric treatment plan is essential. The following questions are useful in eliciting this information:

- When did you first notice the symptoms of your psychiatric disorder?
- When did you first see a medical or mental health professional for help with these symptoms?
- What treatment strategies have been recommended and/or implemented?

- What medications have been prescribed?
- What medications are you taking now?
- Have you received psychotherapy? When and by whom?
- Are you in therapy now? With whom?
- Have you ever been hospitalized for psychiatric care? Where and for how long?
- Have you ever had any legal issues related to your psychiatric problems?
- Does anyone else in your family have psychiatric illness or mental health issues?
- Has anyone in your family committed suicide?
- How do you think your psychiatric condition is affecting your pain?
- How is your pain affecting your psychiatric condition?

It is important to obtain releases of information for telephone or email communications with, and records from, all current treatment provider(s) and any important past providers or institutions. The state Prescription Drug Monitoring Program (PDMP) is useful in verifying that the patient has provided accurate information about current psychotropic medications.

A mental status evaluation that includes a brief cognitive screening—such as the Mini-Cog [1], The Mini-Mental Status Exam [2], or the Modified Mini-Mental Exam [3]—also is useful. If current symptoms of depression are a concern, a standardized screening tool such as the Beck Depression Inventory (BDI) [4] is recommended. If possible, the clinician should review relevant medical records, particularly any records of psychiatric admissions.

Mood disorders, especially depression, are common in patients with chronic pain, and they may precede or appear at the same time as the onset of the painful condition. Many other psychiatric disorders also are common in persons with chronic pain, and their presence may increase patients' risk of developing certain chronic pain conditions. This is especially true in patients with trauma-related disorders, including post-traumatic stress disorder (PTSD), whether that trauma occurred as a result of combat exposure during military service, exposure to terrorism, or trauma related to childhood emotional, physical, and/or sexual abuse [5]. (Some patients have a history of multiple exposures to trauma.) In addition, many patients with a diagnosis and history of treatment for depression have undiagnosed and untreated trauma-related symptoms. Therefore, taking a careful trauma history is essential.

Personality disorders, especially borderline personality disorder (BPD), also are associated with a higher than average incidence of chronic pain. Studies show that patients with a diagnosis of BPD have higher pain scores on screening instruments than patients who do not have such a diagnosis. BPD patients also are more likely to be referred to specialized pain management programs and more likely to misuse pain medications (in fact, abuse of substances is a diagnostic criterion for BPD) [6].

These patients can be among the most complex and challenging to manage, especially when other substance use, overeating, and/or over-exercising (extremely common in BPD) also are involved [7]. It is extremely important that a coordinated team approach be adopted, involving ongoing communication among team members, including the psychiatrist, psychotherapist, pain specialist, physical therapist, and others.

Anxiety disorders are among the most frequently diagnosed psychiatric issues and can be associated with chronic pain conditions, especially when the symptoms of generalized anxiety or panic disorder render pain symptoms more intense or more frequent. This occurs through a combination of mechanisms. For example, in patients with recurrent headaches and generalized anxiety, the anxiety and worry can lead to muscle tension and teeth-grinding or jaw-clenching, which increase the frequency and severity of the headaches. In patients with panic disorder with avoidant behavior, low back pain can be exacerbated by fear of a panic attack. This can lead the patient to avoid potentially helpful therapies, such as physical therapy appointments or water-walking classes that could be helpful in relieving pain and strengthening core musculature.

Assessing Suicidality and Suicide Risk

Suicide always should be a concern in caring for patients with chronic pain, especially if the patient has a history of depression, suicidal ideation, or previous suicide attempts. Numerous studies have demonstrated a high prevalence of suicidal ideation in the population of patients with chronic pain, with or without a history of diagnosed mood disorder [8,9]. Moreover, patients with pain and a psychiatric diagnosis are even more likely to report suicidal ideation [10].

Therefore, every patient who presents with a complaint of chronic pain should be screened for suicide risk, beginning with questions about passive ideation and "life weariness" and moving to more specific suicidal fantasies, plans, or intentions. Potentially lethal methods and access to such methods always should be explored. For many pain patients, lethal means of suicide are available on their bedside table in the form of potent opioid and sedative medications.

Several large studies indicate that the single factor most consistently predictive of suicidal ideation, intent, and suicide attempts in chronic pain patients is sleep disturbance. The thinking pattern known as *catastrophization*, which often is accompanied by a sense of entrapment, can aggravate suicidality. Many patients with psychiatric illness experience sleep disturbance, and some also are prone to catastrophization, so it is critical to question such patients thoroughly about their sleep patterns, their experience of non-restful sleep, and their experience of being sleep-deprived [11].

Psychiatric Medications with the Potential to Influence Patients' Perception of Pain

Studies show that treatment with selective serotonin reuptake inhibitors (SSRI) antidepressants is associated with an increase in suicidal ideation, particularly in the first few months of therapy and especially in persons under age 25. However, the overall suicide rate has declined since SSRIs have been in wide use. Other classes of antidepressant medications have not been associated with an increase in suicidal ideation. Some antidepressants, especially serotonin-norepinephrine reuptake inhibitors (SNRIs) and tricyclics, have been shown to be helpful to selected patients in terms of reducing their pain scores and improving their sleep, while also improving symptoms of depression.

If a patient is taking an SSRI that appears to be helpful in reducing the patient's symptoms of depression, and the patient reports that the medication has not increased the severity or frequency of his or her pain, the SSRI can be continued. Alternatively, consideration can be given to switching the patient to an SNRI, with the goal of continuing to treat the depression while improving the patient's pain.

Anxiolytic medications can be problematic in pain patients, particularly when combined with opioids. As discussed earlier, SSRIs can be very effective for the treatment of generalized anxiety. However, when benzodiazepines or similar sedating medications are prescribed, they can work in combination with opioids to depress respiration and exaggerate sedative effects. Many cases of intentional or accidental opioid overdoses would not have had fatal outcomes if a benzodiazepine had not been on board. Therefore, extreme caution should be exercised in prescribing sedating medications to patients who are taking opioids for pain, including efforts to address the anxiety symptoms with alternative medications (such as SSRIs or anticonvulsants), with cognitive-behavioral therapy or desensitization therapy, and other approaches.

Mood stabilizers—including lithium carbonate, various anticonvulsants, and atypical antipsychotic drugs—can work well in combination with opioids and other pain medications in patients diagnosed with bipolar disorder. In fact, some anticonvulsants have been shown to reduce pain levels and to work well as preventative strategies. Such agents include to primate or valproate to prevent migraine; carbamazepine, gabapentin, and pregabalin for neuropathic pain; and pregabalin for fibromyalgia.

However, topiramate, gabapentin, and pregabalin have not been demonstrated to be effective as mood stabilizers. Therefore, patients who need mood stabilization should be prescribed an alternative anticonvulsant such as valproate or carbamazepine, either of which is an appropriate choice for the treatment of co-occurring mood disorder and pain.

Other drugs with sedative effects should be used with caution in patients taking opioid medications because of the risk that they will contribute to death from overdose. Such drugs include the non-benzodiazepine sleep medications known as Z-drugs (zolpidem, eszopiclone, and zaleplon), barbiturates, carisoprodol and other muscle relaxants and antispasmodics, and antihistamines. In patients with co-occurring addiction, these drugs also are very reinforcing.

Alternative approaches to treat insomnia include:

- Addressing sleep hygiene issues and careful evaluation of the type of sleep disturbance;
- Adding (or adjusting the dose of) an antidepressant medication in the event of early morning waking, which is a symptom of unrelieved depression;
- Use of a low-dose tricyclic antidepressant (such as amitriptyline or trazadone) at bedtime;
- Use of gabapentin or topiramate at bedtime;
- Consideration of an atypical antipsychotic such as quetiapine at bedtime.

Barbiturates, carisoprodol, and most muscle relaxant medications should be avoided in patients with chronic pain who are at risk of developing a substance use disorder (SUD) because of their abuse potential and because they potentiate opioids and thus increase the risk of overdose. Moreover, in controlled studies, most of these medications have not been found to be superior to placebos.

Drugs with stimulant effects also can be problematic for patients who are being treated for psychiatric disorders as well as pain. Since many of the stimulants prescribed to treat attention-deficit hyperactivity disorder (ADHD)—such as dextroamphetamine, mixed amphetamine salts (Adderall®), lisdexamfetamine (Vyvanse®), and methylphenidate preparations—have strong reinforcing effects, they can contribute to the development or worsening of SUDs, especially in persons taking opioid medications.

Many persons diagnosed with ADHD have not been adequately evaluated to determine whether their diagnosis is accurate, nor have they been given an alternative, less reinforcing medication or a non-pharmacological treatment such as neuro-feedback and cognitive-behavioral therapy. An additional concern in pain patients is the increasingly common practice of prescribing stimulants for daytime sleepiness secondary to high-dose opioids. This practice demonstrably increases the risk of addiction.

Avoiding Drug–Drug Interactions When Treating Comorbid Pain and Psychiatric Conditions

The additive sedative effects of opioids and other sedating drugs and the risks they pose in overdose situations were discussed earlier. However, it is also worth noting that, in some cases, the dose of opioid medications being used to treat severe pain is so high that adding *any* medication that further depresses the respiratory system can be extremely dangerous. This is a particular risk in a patient whose respiratory system is compromised by even mild chronic obstructive or restrictive pulmonary disease, sleep apnea, or other chronic respiratory disorder.

Drugs that interfere with opioid pharmacokinetics usually affect their elimination from the body, either by metabolism or excretion. Opioid metabolism usually relies on Phase I metabolism through the CYP450 system, primarily CYP3A and CYP2D6 (this includes codeine, hydrocodone, oxycodone, methadone, tramadol, and fentanyl, with CYP2B6 also contributing to methadone metabolism); and Phase II metabolism via conjugation by the enzyme UDP-glucuronosyltransferase-2B7 (UGT2B7) which metabolizes morphine, hydromorphone, and oxymorphone. Therefore, other drugs that rely on these enzyme systems—or that inhibit or induce them—can alter the metabolism of opioids. Many psychiatric medications fall into this category, including SSRIs, SNRIs, tricyclic antidepressants, anticonvulsants, atypical antipsychotics, barbiturates, and some benzodiazepines. The interaction of such drugs with certain opioids can lead to reduced opioid efficacy and increased toxicity of opioids, increased serotonin-enhancing drugs with serotonin syndrome, and greater toxicity of the anticonvulsant [12].

Methadone is an opioid that is especially prone to drug–drug interactions (DDIs) with psychotropics and other prescription medications, over-the-counter agents, and dietary supplements; accordingly, special caution is warranted in prescribing any of these medications for patients who use methadone.

Genetic variability from patient to patient in the metabolic pathways also is a factor in some drug interactions. Buprenorphine is a CYP3A4 substrate, and increased levels occur following its administration in a patient taking ketoconazole, which is a strong CYP3A4 inhibitor. Drug interactions with other strong CYP3A4 inhibitors (such as clarithromycin, telithromycin, itraconazole, and the HIV antiretroviral medications indinavir, tazanavir, nefazodone, nelfinavir, ritonavir, lopinavir/ritonavir, and saquinavir/ritonavir) also can cause an increase in the systemic levels or pharmacodynamic effects of buprenorphine. Extensive tables of drug–drug interactions are available and should be consulted whenever patients are prescribed multiple medications [13,14].

The Impact of Emotions and Psychiatric Symptoms on Patients' Experience of Pain

Anxiety is a symptom commonly associated with chronic pain. Individuals with anxiety often experience *catastrophization*, which can be accompanied by feelings of desperation and hopelessness, and which definitely makes the perception of pain more severe. Many patients with generalized anxiety disorder engage in worrying or projecting about feared negative future occurrences. For example, when pain intensifies slightly, such a patient thinks, "This is bad, but what if it gets worse? What if the pain lasts all night and I can't get any sleep? How am I going to get up for work and take care of the kids if I don't get any sleep?"

This type of thinking pattern becomes a self-fulfilling prophecy because, when the mind is racing with fear, falling asleep becomes almost impossible. Fears can grow to irrational proportions: "That's it, I just know I'm going to be in such pain that I won't sleep all night, will be late to work, will get fired, won't be able to support my kids, and we'll all end up living on the street eating out of a dumpster!" Sedative medication can break the cycle temporarily, but worrying will return when the drug wears off. Opioids also offer temporary relief, which helps to explain why some patients with pain and anxiety take pain medications to ease their fears even when the pain is not severe. This can result in a cycle of increased dosing, the development of tolerance, and the emergence of drug-seeking behavior [15,16].

Such patients often are helped by working individually with a cognitive-behavioral therapist to address the pattern of catastrophization, escalating fear, and resulting hopelessness. These therapies can be very effective in reducing the patient's level of anxiety and perceived need for higher doses of pain medication or the addition of sedating medications. For some patients, it is even more effective to participate in group therapy with other patients who are experiencing chronic pain and anxiety. Adding community-based support groups such as *Emotions Anonymous (EA)*, a 12-Step program for persons with anxiety or depression, or *Pills Anonymous*, a 12-Step program for patients experiencing problems with prescription medications, can be very beneficial. Patients also can benefit from reading books and articles about anxiety and its impact on pain (see the accompanying text box for suggested readings).

Panic disorder involves recurrent episodes of unexpected panic attacks or surges of intense fear accompanied by somatic experiences, including palpitations, sweating, trembling, shortness of breath, feelings of choking, chest pain, nausea, dizziness, a sensation of being cold or hot, paresthesias, and psychological experiences of derealization, depersonalization, "going crazy," or dying. Patients report sudden onset of symptoms and peaking within minutes, after which the panic attack subsides spontaneously. Individuals with panic disorder develop a "second fear" of having additional attacks that can lead to multiple avoidant behaviors. In severe cases, this can progress to agoraphobia.

Panic attacks and fear of panic attacks lead to an increased risk of suicide. When chronic pain also is present, both the acute panic episodes and fear of repeated episodes makes the pain more severe and more difficult to treat. Also, avoidant behaviors can prevent patients from engaging in activities that could help reduce their pain, such as physical therapy, exercise, yoga, and meditation. Studies have suggested that panic disorder is especially common in patients with episodic migraine [17].

Symptoms of *depression* often include negative, pessimistic thinking patterns that can definitely affect the individual's perception of pain. For some patients, the diagnosis of a chronic pain disorder for which there is no quick and easy solution is accompanied by a cognitive and emotional process not unlike the grief process associated with loss of a loved one. In the earliest stage, denial and minimization are prominent, accompanied by a search for alternative opinions and magical thinking about simple ways to correct the problem.

This stage usually is followed by a period of anger and blaming of other people, institutions, or realities. Depression itself often has strong anger components, which may be associated with passive-aggressive behavior; a desire to retaliate; and a feeling of being victimized by caregivers and other professionals, insurance companies, the driver of the other car, the spouse or significant other who must be at work in order to earn a living for the family and thus is not at home to care for the sufferer, and the like.

The bargaining stage is characterized by "what ifs" and "if onlys," with the patient "negotiating" with the pain and the circumstances that led to the painful condition, as well as ruminating about how things could have turned out differently. Most such individuals move back and forth between anger, bargaining, and denial as the reality of the situation becomes increasingly clear.

This interwoven anger, blaming, resentment, bargaining, discouragement, and sense of being thwarted at every turn combine to create feelings of helplessness, hopelessness, despair, and self-pity: in short, the very essence of anger turned inward that we call depression. When these are added to all the specific losses involved, including the loss of certain physical abilities, loss of the sense of mastery and self-confidence, and sometimes the loss of physical attractiveness, life looks bleak. Therefore it is no surprise that suicidal ideation is so frequently associated with chronic pain [18].

Reaching a stage of *acceptance* does not mean that the individual accepts being in constant or intermittent pain, or is at peace with the way things are. Rather, acceptance involves understanding the reality of the situation and an evolving definition of a "new normal." Most individuals never completely accept living in pain, but many resolve to go on living anyway, seeking support from others and making an effort to find meaning in life as it is. However, reaching this stage is extremely difficult for persons who are severely depressed, anxious, and fearful or avoidant, or who do not have the skills to self-regulate emotional responses and behavior. Therefore, competent, intensive psychiatric and psychological treatment for these co-occurring psychiatric conditions is essential to maximize outcomes in treating the chronic pain condition.

Conclusion

When psychiatric and substance use disorders co-occur, the combination can be very challenging for both patient and physician [19]. In fact, studies show that untreated or inadequately treated mental disorders can interfere with the effective treatment of addiction [19,20]. The two disorders may have a separate etiology, or one disorder may play a role in initiating the other. Typically, they become intertwined, thus complicating the treatment plan and process.

Therefore, whenever a patient enters treatment for either an SUD or a mental disorder, especially in the presence of pain, he or she should be assessed for the presence of the other problem [21]. Many patients with co-occurring disorders do well with simultaneous interventions for pain and psychiatric or substance use disorders. For this reason, the presence of a co-occurring disorder should not automatically exclude a patient from any avenue of treatment [22].

For More Information on the Topics Discussed:

American Society of Addiction Medicine (ASAM):

See Chapters 85 to 92 in Section 11, Co-Occurring Addiction and Psychiatric Disorders. In RK Ries, DA Fiellin, SC Miller, R Saitz, eds. *The ASAM Principles of Addiction Medicine, Fifth Edition.* Philadelphia, PA: Wolters Kluwer; 2014.

American Psychiatric Association (APA):

Patients and Families: Help with Anxiety Disorders. (Access at: http://www.psychiatry.org/.)

Mayo Clinic Patient Care and Health Information:

Generalized Anxiety Disorder. (Access at: http://www.mayoclinic.org/diseases-conditions/generalized-anxiety-disorder/basics/definition/con-20024562.)

National Institute of Mental Health (NIMH):

Information for patients and health care professionals, available in English and Spanish. (Access at: http://www.nimh.nih.gov/.)

References

1. Borson S, Scanlan J, Brush M, et al. The Mini-Cog: A cognitive "vital signs" measure for dementia screening in multi-lingual elderly. *Int J Geriatr Psychiatry.* 2000;15(11):1021–1027.

2. Folstein MF, Folstein SE, McHugh PR. Mini-mental state: A practical method for grading the cognitive state of patients for the clinician. *J Psychiatr Res.* 1975;12:189–198.

3. Teng EL, Chui HC. The Modified Mini-Mental State (3MS) examination. *J Clin Psychiatry.* 1987;48(8):314–318.

4. Steer RA, Ball R, Ranieri RA, et al. Dimensions of the Beck Depression Inventory–II in clinically depressed outpatients. *J Clin Psychol.* 1999;55(1):117–128.

5. Villano CL, Rosenblum A, Magura C, et al. Prevalence and correlates of post-traumatic stress disorder and chronic severe pain in psychiatric outpatients. *J Rehab Res Dev.* 2007;44(2):167–177.

6. Sansone RE, Sonsone LA. Chronic pain syndromes and borderline personality disorder. *Innov Clin Neurosci.* 2012;9(1):10–14.

7. Kalira V, Treisman GJ, Clark MR. Borderline personality disorder and chronic pain: A practical approach to evaluation and treatment. *Curr Pain Headache Rep.* 2013;17(8):350.

8. Cheatle MD, Wasser T, Foster C, et al. Prevalence of suicidal ideation in patients with chronic non-cancer pain referred to a behaviorally based pain program. *Pain Physician.* 2014;17:E359–E367.

9. Cheatle MD. Depression, chronic pain and suicide by overdose: On the edge. *Pain Med.* 2011;12(Suppl 2):S43–S48.

10. Kowal J, Wilson KG, Henderson PR, et al. Change in suicidal ideation following interdisciplinary treatment of chronic pain. *Clin J Pain.* 2014;30(6):463–471.

11. Winsper C, Tang NK. Linkages between insomnia and suicidality: Prospective associations, high-risk subgroups and possible psychological mechanisms. *Int Rev Psychiatry.* 2014 Apr;26(2):189–204.

12. Overholser BR, Foster DR. Opioid pharmacokinetic drug–drug interactions. *Am J Manag Care.* 2011;17(Suppl 11):S276–S287.

13. Pergolizzi JV, Raffa RB. Common opioid-drug interactions: What clinicians need to know. (Accessed at: http://www.practicalpainmanagement.com.)

14. McCance-Katz EF, Sullivan L, Nallani S. Drug interactions of clinical importance among the opioids, methadone and buprenorphine, and other frequently prescribed medications: A review. *Am J Addict.* 2010;19(1):4–16.

15. Turk DC, Wilson HD. Fear of pain as a prognostic factor in chronic pain: Conceptual models, assessment and treatment implications. *Curr Pain Headache Rep.* 2010;14(2):88–95.

16. Quartana PJ, Campbell CM, Edwards RR. Pain catastrophizing: A critical review. *Expert Rev Neurother.* 2009;9(5):745–758.

17. Smitherman TA, Kolivas ED, Bailey JR. Panic disorder and migraine: Comorbidity, mechanisms, and clinical implications. *Headache.* 2013;53(1):23–45.

18. Furnes B, Dysvik E. Dealing with grief related to loss by death and chronic pain: An integrated theoretical framework. Part I. *Patient Prefer Adherence.* 2010 Jun 24;4:135–140. (https://www.ncbi.nlm.nih.gov/pmc/articles/PMC2898114/)

19. McCance-Katz E, Moody D, Prathikanti S, et al. Rifampin, but not rifabutin, may produce opiate withdrawal in buprenorphine-maintained patients. *Drug Alc Depend.* 2011 Nov 1;118(2–3):326–334.

20. Ziedonis D, Steinberg ML, Smelson D, et al. Co-occurring addictive and psychotic disorders. In AW Graham, TK Schultz, MF Mayo-Smith, RK Ries, BB Wilford, eds. *The ASAM Principles of Addiction Medicine, Third Edition.* Chevy Chase, MD: American Society of Addiction Medicine; 2003:1297–1319.

21. National Institute on Drug Abuse (NIDA). *Principles of Drug Addiction Treatment: A Research-Based Guide (3rd Edition).* NIH Publication No. 12–4180. Bethesda, MD: NIDA, National Institutes of Health; 2012.

22. Substance Abuse and Mental Health Services Administration (SAMHSA). *Pharmacologic Guidelines for Treating Individuals with Post-Traumatic Stress Disorder and Co-Occurring Opioid Use Disorders.* HHS Publication No. (SMA) 12-4688. Rockville, MD: SAMHSA; 2012.

Sidebar 24a

Pain and Addiction in Patients with Post-Traumatic Stress Disorder

STEVEN A. ERAKER, M.D.

Post-traumatic stress disorder (PTSD) has been described as the "complex somatic, cognitive, affective and behavioral effects of psychological trauma." It occurs in some individuals after they experience, witness, or learn about a traumatic event that involves actual or threatened harm to themselves or others.

The link between PTSD, pain, and addiction is well established. Patients with more significant symptoms of PTSD tend to have higher rates of substance use disorder (SUD), as well as anxiety, depression, and physical health problems, including pain. Indeed, it is possible that some individuals use drugs or alcohol to cope with distressing symptoms of pain and PTSD [1].

Prevalence of PTSD

In the United States, lifetime prevalence of PTSD is 3.5% among men and 9.7% among women, for a total of 6.8% among all adults. (There is no difference in prevalence between urban and rural residents.) Among military veterans, lifetime prevalence of PTSD ranges from 10.1% in Gulf War veterans to 30.9% among Vietnam War veterans. Between 13.8% and 68.2% of personnel who served in Operation Iraqi Freedom and Operation Enduring Freedom report PTSD [2].

Up to 80% of patients with PTSD report chronic pain, and up to half of all patients diagnosed with chronic pain have PTSD. By definition, *chronic* pain persists for at least three months, which is beyond the amount of time required for most injuries to heal; thus, it may have no medical explanation. Approximately one in three Americans suffers from chronic pain and one in four has a significant impairment of functional activity as a result. PTSD occurs more often when the onset of pain corresponds with a traumatic event [3].

Causes of PTSD

PTSD is more likely to occur following interpersonal violence than after motor vehicle accidents or natural disasters. Also, the duration of stress is more important than the severity of physical injury. Higher levels of perceived pain are associated with greater affective distress and disability. Neuroanatomical, neurotransmitter, and physiological alterations contribute to PTSD, chronic pain, and addiction. Negative beliefs about self, self-management, and treatment efficacy also are factors [4].

Diagnosing PTSD

Clinical Presentation

Symptoms of PTSD include nightmares, intrusive thoughts, flashbacks of prior trauma, avoidance of trauma and/or associated reminders, hypervigilance, and negative cognitive or mood change. Such symptoms may continue for more than a month immediately following the traumatic event or be delayed in their onset. During this period, isolation, emotional numbness, and irritability contribute to distress, as the individual's social, occupational, and interpersonal functioning declines [5].

Patient History

When patients are screened for PTSD and chronic pain, the results are considered "positive" if a patient answers "yes" to any three of the following items [6]:

Question: In your life, have you ever had an experience that was so frightening, horrible, or upsetting that in the past month you:

1. Had nightmares about it or thought about it when you did not want to?
2. Tried hard not to think about it or went out of your way to avoid situations that reminded you of it?

3. Were constantly on guard, watchful, or easily startled?
4. Felt numb or detached from others, activities, or your surroundings?

Assessment of the patient's functional capacity, pain level, and psychosocial factors is equally important in evaluating and treating chronic pain and PTSD. Therefore, it is important to ask the patient to describe how his or her pain affects their daily or desired activities. In addition, a number of validated instruments for evaluating pain, functional capacity, and psychosocial status can be helpful [7].

Physical Examination and Targeted Diagnostic Testing

Every patient should be evaluated for physical factors that may be contributing to the presenting symptoms, including [8]:

- Traumatic brain injury;
- Metabolic or endocrine factors (such as hypothyroidism, vitamin D or B12 deficiency, low testosterone level, and exposure to infectious agents);
- Exposure to environmental agents (as occurs in Gulf War syndrome and with exposure to lead or Agent Orange); and
- Substance use disorder (SUD).

Reaching a Diagnosis

Once information from the patient's history, physical examination, and relevant screening instruments has been collected and evaluated, a differential diagnosis can be reached. Possibilities include:

- Adjustment disorders;
- Acute stress disorder (with a typical duration of 48 hours to four weeks post-trauma);
- Anxiety disorder;
- Obsessive-compulsive disorder;
- Major depressive disorder;
- Personality disorders;
- Dissociative disorders;
- Conversion disorder;
- Psychosis; and
- Traumatic brain injury.

Diagnostic criteria for PTSD, as outlined in the *Diagnostic and Statistical Manual of Mental Disorders* (DSM-5) [9], include the following:

1. Exposure to actual or threatened death, serious injury, sexual violence, military combat, natural disasters, and h hospitalization in an intensive care unit (ICU), through one or more of the following: direct experience, personal witness, trauma involving a close family member or friend, and repeated or extreme exposure to aversive details.
2. Re-experiencing one or more of the following: memories, dreams, dissociative reactions, flashbacks, physiological reactions, or psychological distress in response to reminders.
3. Avoidance of stimuli associated with the traumatic event.
4. Internal memories, thoughts, or feelings.
5. External activities, places, people, conversations, objects, or situations.
6. Negative alterations in cognition and mood.
7. Memory loss, negative beliefs, self-blame, negative emotions, anhedonia, detachment, or lack of positive emotions.
8. Hyper-arousal.
9. Irritability and anger; reckless, self-destructive behavior; hypervigilance; exaggerated startle response; impaired concentration; clinically significant distress or impairment in social, occupational, or other areas; sleep difficulties.

Treating PTSD

Interdisciplinary pain treatment is recommended for patients diagnosed with pain and PTSD, as both conditions need to be addressed simultaneously. A biopsychosocial, evidence-based approach is recommended. Because early intervention has been shown to improve outcomes, a concurrent stepped-care approach should be adopted, including referral to a mental health specialist as soon as the PTSD diagnosis is made. Essential steps include the following [10]:

Step 1: Self-care, with a support network.
Lifestyle modifications, including exercise and social networking.
Step 2: Primary care for the pain and PTSD, with support from mental health professionals.
- Cognitive-behavioral therapy, which is evidence-based and shown to be the most effective therapy for PTSD and chronic pain;
- Group and/or family therapy;
- Exposure therapy (PTSD);

- Treatment by a pain/PTSD team, including specialists in mental health, physical therapy, recreational therapy, pharmacy, social work, and community resources (social, church, Veterans of Foreign Wars [VFW], etc.);
- Complementary integrative medicine (acupuncture, chiropractic, mindfulness, tai-chi, yoga, etc.);
- Pharmacotherapy to treat core symptoms such as depression, anxiety, and nightmares (note that benzodiazepines should be avoided whenever possible):
  - SSRIs: Sertraline and paroxetine (only FDA-approved), fluoxetine;
  - SNRI: venlafaxine, duloxetine;
  - Other: mirtazapine, nefazodone;
  - Mood stabilizers: Topiramate (effective in some studies);
  - Guanfacine (may help with arousal symptoms);
  - Prazosin (may reduce the occurrence of distressing dreams and improve sleep quality); or
  - Beta blockers (may be helpful if given within one hour after trauma to disrupt physiological stress response).

Step 3: Specialty mental health and pain care.
EMDR (eye movement desensitization and reprocessing), which alters how the patient reacts to memories of trauma;
Specialists in psychiatry and psychology;
Specialists in pain medicine, physiatry, and orthopedics/neurosurgery.
Step 4: Functional restoration (outpatient or inpatient).

Recovery rates are highest in the first 12 months after onset of symptoms. The average duration of symptoms is 36 months with treatment and 64 months without. Even with treatment, there is a 50% chance of relapse at two years, while half of patients develop chronic symptoms. (Predictors of chronicity include previous trauma, premorbid psychiatric function, panic reaction at time of event, prolonged terror, dissociation at time of event, and/or SUD.) [11]

PTSD and Opioids

In a review of military veterans with mental health disorders and chronic pain who were prescribed opioids, investigators found that patients with PTSD were more likely than those without PTSD to receive higher doses of opioids and concurrent prescriptions for sedative-hypnotics, and to obtain early refills of their prescribed opioids [12].

A retrospective analysis of veterans diagnosed with PTSD and opioid use disorder found that those treated with buprenorphine showed significant improvement in PTSD symptoms at eight months, with increasing improvement up to 24 months [13].

Conclusion

Traumatic life events—including earthquakes, war, and interpersonal conflicts—can trigger a cascade of psychological and biological changes known as post-traumatic stress disorder (PTSD).

PTSD is a major public health concern in both civilian and military populations, as well as across race, age, and gender, as well as socioeconomic status. While PTSD has been recognized for centuries, its definition and description continue to evolve. For example, the fifth edition of the American Psychiatric Association's DSM includes some major changes in the diagnostic criteria for PTSD [14].

For More Information on the Topics Discussed:

American Society of Addiction Medicine (ASAM):

Saladin ME, Back SE, Payne RA, et al. Posttraumatic stress disorder and substance use disorder comorbidity (Chapter 91). In RK Ries, DA Fiellin, SC Miller, R Saitz, eds. *The ASAM Principles of Addiction Medicine, Fifth Edition.* Philadelphia, PA: Wolters Kluwer; 2014.

National Center for PTSD:

The National Center for PTSD, part of the U.S. Department of Veterans Affairs, has a website with targeted information for anyone interested in PTSD (including veterans, family, and friends), as well as for professional researchers and health care professionals. The site also offers videos and information about an online app called PTSD Coach. (Access at: http://www.ptsd.va.gov.)

The Clinician's Guide to Medications for PTSD was developed for researchers, providers, and helpers by the U.S. Department for Veterans Affairs. (Access at: http://www.ptsd.va.gov.)

National Institute of Mental Health:

Science News About Post-Traumatic Stress Disorder. (Access at: https://www.nimh.nih.gov/health/topics/post-traumatic-stress-disorder-ptsd/index.shtml.)

References

1. National Center for PTSD. (Accessed at: http://www.ptsd.va.gov).
2. Ciechanowski P. Posttraumatic stress disorder in adults: Epidemiology, pathophysiology, clinical manifestations, course and diagnosis. *Up to Date*; 2015. (Accessed at: www.uptodate.com.)
3. Stewart MO, Karlin BE, Murphy JL, et al. National dissemination of cognitive-behavioral therapy for chronic pain in veterans. *Clin J Pain*. 2015;31:8:722–729.
4. Phifer J, Skelton K, Weiss T, et al. Pain symptomatology and pain medication use in civilian PTSD. *Pain*. 2011;152:2233–2240.
5. Vieweg WV, Julius DA, Fernandez A, et al. Posttraumatic stress disorder: Clinical features, pathophysiology, and treatment. *Am J Med*. 2006;119:383.
6. Yehuda R. Post-traumatic stress disorder. *NEJM*. 2002;346:108.
7. Monson CM, Fredman SJ, Macdonald A, et al. Effect of cognitive-behavioral therapy for PTSD. A randomized controlled trial. *JAMA*. 2012;308:700.
8. Kroenke K, Bair MJ, Damush TM, et al. Optimized antidepressant therapy and pain self-management in primary care patients with depression and musculoskeletal pain: A randomized controlled trial. *JAMA*. 2009; 301(20): 2099–2110.
9. Otis JD, Keane T, Kerns RD, et al. The development of an integrated treatment for veterans with comorbid chronic pain and posttraumatic stress disorder. *Pain Med*. 2009;10:1300–1311.
10. Fareed A, Eilender P, Haber M, et al. Comorbid posttraumatic stress disorder and opiate addiction: A literature review. *J Addict Dis*. 2013;32:2.
11. Outcalt S, Yu Z, Hoen MS, et al. Health care utilization among veterans with pain and posttraumatic stress symptoms. *Pain Med*. 2013;15:1872–1879.
12. Seal et al. Association of mental health disorders with prescription opioids and high risk opioid use in U.S. veterans of Iraq and Afghanistan. JAMA. 2012 Mar 7;307(9):940–947.
13. Seal KH, Maguen S, Bertenthal D, et al. Observational evidence for buprenorphine's impact on PTSD symptoms in veterans with chronic pain and opioid use disorder. *J Clin Psych*. 2016 Sep;77(9):1182–1188.
14. Difede J, Olden M, Cukor J. Evidence-based treatment of post-traumatic stress disorder. *Annu Rev Med*. 2014;65:319–332.

Chapter 25

Pain and Addiction in Patients with Co-Occurring Medical Disorders

STEPHEN COLAMECO, M.D., M.ED., DFASAM,
AND MELVIN I. POHL, M.D., DFASAM

This chapter addresses pain control in patients who have co-occurring pain and substance use disorder (SUD), as well as one or more other significant medical problems (see Table 25.1). Such patients pose unique challenges in pain management.

Patients with chronic painful conditions, regardless of the fact that they also suffer from an SUD, must be treated promptly and effectively, according to guidelines set forth by the World Health Organization [1], the American Academy of Pain Medicine [2] and the American Pain Society [3], the Joint Commission on Accreditation of Healthcare Organizations [4], and the Agency for Health Care Policy Research of the U.S. Department of Health and Human Services [5].

Issues confronting clinicians who treat such patients include concerns over the possibility that a patient with an SUD might exaggerate his or her symptoms in order to gain access to opioid analgesics [6]. However, such a patient's "drug-seeking behaviors" might reflect inadequately treated, uncontrolled pain (pseudoaddiction) rather than true addiction. Genuine untreated addiction is characterized by aberrant and potentially manipulative behaviors, which may involve selling drugs, forging prescriptions, injecting oral formulations, reporting multiple episodes of prescription "loss," repeated episodes of intoxication, and the like, all with the goal of obtaining and using drugs for their mood-enhancing effects. In treating patients with a history of addiction, the clinician should provide explicit written rules about expected behaviors (as well as unacceptable behaviors), specifying the consequences for violations of the rules (see Chapter 8 of this Handbook) [6].

TABLE 25.1 Complex Medical Disorders Seen in Patients with Co-Occurring Pain and Addiction

1. Opioids and Respiratory Function

- Opioids activate receptors in the respiratory centers, most of which are located in the brainstem and midbrain.
- Respiratory drive is generated in the brainstem and is modulated by the cortex and peripheral chemoreceptors.
- Opioids cause respiration to slow and become irregular, and can result in hypercapnia and hypoxemia.
- Respiratory suppression is seen more often at higher opioid doses.
- Underlying pulmonary conditions and sedating medications can increase the incidence of opioid-induced respiratory depression.
- Severe opioid-induced respiratory depression can be fatal.
- Severe opioid-induced respiratory depression can be reversed by naloxone, which is an opioid receptor antagonist.

2. Severe Dyspnea

- Opioids are used in the palliation of severe dyspnea in advanced pulmonary disease and end-of-life care.
- Medical literature supporting effectiveness of this treatment is good.
- Oral and parenteral opioids can be used in addition to bronchodilators, oxygen and pulmonary rehabilitation.
- Nebulized opioids are not beneficial in treating dyspnea.
- Opioids should be started at a low dose and titrated slowly, with close monitoring.
- Lower-dose opioids (up to 30 MED) are unlikely to increase mortality risk.

3. Pulmonary Diseases

- The risk of significant respiratory depression by opioids is increased in patients with pulmonary disease.
- In severe COPD, opioids above 30 MED show a linear dose-response association with increased mortality.
- Lower-dose opioids (up to 30 MED) are unlikely to increase mortality.
- Lower-dose opioids are unlikely to significantly increase hypercapnia or hypoxemia.
- Lower-dose opioids given concurrently with low-dose benzodiazepines are unlikely to increase mortality.
- Extra caution is warranted in patients with hypercapnia ($PCO2 > 45$) or hypoxemia (on oxygen).

TABLE 25.1 Continued

4. Cardiopulmonary Diseases

• Opioids such as morphine can reduce cardiac pain in acute myocardial infarction. Doses should be titrated to pain relief.
• Opioids may be helpful in acute pulmonary edema by reducing anxiety associated with dyspnea.
• Opioids may act as venodialators, reducing cardiac filling pressures, preload and sympathetic drive.

5. Medical Conditions That Cause Hypoventilation

• Obesity Hypoventilation Syndrome—BMI > 30, awake chronic hypercapnea, and sleep- disordered breathing.
• Chest wall deformities such as kyphoscoliosis, fibrothorax, and those occurring post-thoracoplasty.
• Neuromuscular diseases, including myasthenia gravis, amyotrophic lateral sclerosis, Guillain-Barré syndrome, and muscular dystrophy.

6. Use of Sedating Medications

• Oral and IV benzodiazepines can cause respiratory depression, which is potentiated by opioids.
• Death as a result of high-dose benzodiazepines alone is uncommon.

Source: Authors.

Chronic Low Back Pain

Chronic low back pain is among the presenting complaints most frequently reported by patients and one of the reasons for which opioids are most often prescribed. For this reason, there has been a rapid increase in the variety and number of surgical and interventional procedures employed to treat back pain in recent years [7].

As a result, over-reliance on medical interventions has caused many patients to become "medically focused"—a situation in which the patient assumes that the sole cause of pain and disability is biological, so the only potential solution lies in medical intervention.

Many patients with chronic back pain present to addiction specialists for evaluation or treatment of SUD, having already failed "medical" treatments. Such patients often are deconditioned, angry, depressed, or anxious. Some present with "failed back surgery syndrome," at which point they are no longer candidates for further surgery. Such patients typically have varying degrees of pathology, including disc degeneration, spinal stenosis, foraminal narrowing, and facet arthropathy.

Having exhausted medical treatments, such patients may feel hopeless. Shifting care from passive, medically focused approaches to active participation in a functional restoration program and ongoing self-care often is a challenge. Many patients present in the pre-contemplation stage of change, and are not yet ready to actively participate in their own recovery. The clinician who provides care to such an individual faces the challenge of helping the patient move through the process of change, choosing among non-interventional treatments, and evaluating the patient for psychiatric comorbidity.

Opioid Withdrawal or Induction onto Agonist Treatment

The first step in treating individuals being prescribed opioids for chronic back pain is to determine whether the patient has an active opioid use disorder (OUD) or other SUD and, if so, the relative severity of that disorder. This determination guides treatment.

Psychological and Behavioral Therapies

For patients with OUDs or SUDs, cognitive-behavioral interventions may be an important first step in helping the individual move from pre-contemplation to an active stage of change. A Cochrane Review reported that "small to moderate benefits, more for disability, mood and catastrophic thinking than for pain, were found in trials which compared CBT with no treatment" [8].

Other approaches with demonstrated utility include mindfulness-based therapy and acceptance and commitment therapy [9].

Multidisciplinary Biopsychosocial Rehabilitation

A 2015 Cochrane Systems Review and meta-analysis [10] concluded that "Multidisciplinary biopsychosocial rehabilitation interventions were more effective than usual care (moderate quality evidence) and physical treatments (low quality evidence) in decreasing pain and disability in people with chronic low back pain."

In the past, insurers were unlikely to cover participation in multidisciplinary pain programs that offer cognitive-behavioral and functional-restorative treatments for chronic low back pain. Increasingly, however, insurers recognize that addiction may have developed as a result of treatment for a work-related injury and so may authorize treatment in outpatient or inpatient pain programs that address both addiction and chronic pain. Based on the current evidence, commercial insurers may consider multidisciplinary pain management appropriate in selected cases [11,12].

Self-Care

Self-care approaches—including gratitude work, self-directed cognitive-behavioral interventions, trans-epidermal nerve stimulation (TENS), acupressure, exercise, movement therapies, and nutrition—are covered in Chapter 17 of this Handbook.

Medications

Non-steroidal anti-inflammatory drugs (NSAIDs) often are used for the management of chronic low back pain, but the potential benefits of treatment must be weighed against known cardiovascular, renal, hepatic, and gastrointestinal adverse effects. According to a Cochrane Review, "There was low quality evidence that NSAIDs are slightly more effective than placebo in chronic low back pain. The magnitude of the difference was small, and when we only accounted for trials of higher quality, these differences [were] reduced" [13].

Opioids are relatively contraindicated in the treatment of chronic low back pain, even in patients with no history of addiction. While opioids can relieve acute back pain or exacerbations of chronic pain, their long-term effectiveness has not been demonstrated, while the risk of developing addiction is well known [14].

Muscle relaxants often are prescribed for low back pain. While these medications may be effective for short-term symptomatic relief, there is a lack of data to support their long-term effectiveness, so the approved indications are for short-term use only. Muscle relaxants often produce side effects that include drowsiness and dizziness, and they may interact negatively with opioids, benzodiazepines, or other sedating medications. While some benzodiazepines have muscle relaxant properties, this effect lasts only a few weeks. Benzodiazepines are relatively contraindicated in patients who have SUDs and, in general, long-term use of muscle relaxants is not advised.

Medications for neuropathic pain may be appropriate when there is evidence of radiculopathy or peripheral neuropathy. As noted earlier, caution should be used when choosing anticonvulsant agents that have a known potential for abuse.

Sleep Apnea

Obstructive sleep apnea increasingly is recognized as an important cause of medical morbidity and mortality. Yet it is an under-diagnosed problem, even though estimates suggest that one in five adults has mild obstructive sleep apnea and one in 15 has moderate or severe sleep apnea [15]. Medical disorders linked to sleep apnea include hypertension, obesity, congestive heart failure, diabetes, and disorders related to atherosclerosis, such as stroke, angina, and acute myocardial infarction [16].

Sleep-disordered breathing is associated with a threefold increase in mortality [17]. Diminished longevity in patients with untreated or inadequately treated sleep apnea may be the result of cardiovascular events, cardiac arrhythmia during sleep (induced by hypoxia), or fatalities from sleep-related vehicle crashes. (Persons with untreated moderate to severe sleep apnea have a 15-fold increase in risk of involvement in a traffic accident [18].)

The economic cost associated with undiagnosed sleep disorder also appears high. For example, one study found that, prior to receiving a diagnosis of sleep apnea, patients used 23–50% more medical resources than the population as a whole [19].

Risk Factors for Sleep Apnea

Risk factors for sleep apnea include obesity, hypertension (HTN), snoring, excessive use of alcohol or sedatives, diabetes, tobacco use, male gender, large neck circumference, and age over 40.

Up to 70% of patients who take opioids suffer from sleep-disordered breathing [20]. Patients on opioids typically show ataxic breathing patterns (irregular respiratory pauses) during sleep, with prolonged obstructive apnea/hypopneas, a mixture of obstructive and central apneas, or an ataxic breathing pattern [21].

Opioids cause most of the central apneas that are not effectively treated with continuous positive airway pressure (CPAP) therapy. More sophisticated modes of ventilation may be required, such as bi-level ventilation with a backup rate, or adaptive servoventilation. Opioids increase both central and obstructive apneic events in a dose-related fashion. Tapering patients to lower doses of opioids is prudent and presumably provides some margin of safety.

Diagnosing and Treating Sleep Apnea

Diagnosing sleep apnea and initiating treatment is a safety issue, and it also can help to treat pain by improving sleep and reducing daytime fatigue (which permits mobilization, another important component of a multidisciplinary approach to pain management).

The risk of developing sleep apnea should be addressed with any patient to whom opioids are prescribed. It is important to ask such patients about their history or symptoms of sleep apnea, such as snoring, daytime fatigue, witnessed apnea, morning headaches, nighttime gasping for air, choking, coughing, excessive daytime sleepiness, and restless leg syndrome.

Chronic Pancreatitis

Chronic pancreatitis, which also is a challenging condition to treat, typically is caused by heavy alcohol consumption. Less common but nevertheless important causes include ductal obstruction, adverse effects of medications, hypercalcemia, and hyperlipidemia.

Pain associated with chronic pancreatitis may be severe and disabling. Unfortunately, there is limited objective information to guide treatment, with most recommendations based on expert opinion rather than clinical evidence.

The first principle in treating pancreatitis is to completely avoid alcohol consumption; which may involve treatment for an alcohol use disorder. It also is prudent to instruct patients to avoid high-fat meals and to be consistent in consuming any pancreatic supplement medications that are prescribed.

Medications Used in Treatment

There are few published studies on the effectiveness of NSAIDs in the management of pain caused by pancreatitis. Of particular concern is gastrointestinal (GI) toxicity, with the potential for development of peptic ulcers, which further complicate the evaluation and management of abdominal pain. Acetaminophen is a low-potency analgesic that usually is inadequate for the treatment of chronic pancreatitis pain. Opioids often are prescribed, but there are few studies of their long-term effectiveness in treating pancreatitis pain. Another concern is that, because of their spasmogenic effects, opioids increase pressure in the sphincter of Oddi, thereby increasing pain.

Unlike most other opioids, buprenorphine does not increase pressure in the sphincter of Oddi and thus may be a safer option in terms of avoiding pain exacerbation and the potential for abuse [22,23]. Many clinicians prescribe antioxidants along with analgesics, but there are conflicting data about the effectiveness of antioxidant therapy [24].

Several interventional procedures have been used to treat chronic pancreatitis. If the pancreatic duct is dilated, endoscopic or surgical decompression can be considered. Procedures other than pancreatic duct decompression include nerve blocks, partial pancreatic resection, pancreatic resection with islet cell transplantation, and surgical denervation. Unfortunately, most clinical studies involving these and other interventional techniques involve small numbers of subjects and only short-term follow-up.

As is the case with many complex pain syndromes, especially in the context of addiction, the best care for chronic pancreatitis often is multi-modal, addressing psychological, behavioral, environmental, spiritual, and biological factors that interact to influence pain and function.

Cirrhosis

Cirrhosis of the liver often is caused by or overlaps with alcohol use disorder (AUD). Pain management in cirrhotic patients is a difficult clinical challenge, especially when AUD also is present. Moreover, there is a paucity of evidence-based guidelines for the treatment of such patients.

Many analgesics are known to cause adverse (and potentially fatal) effects, including hepatic encephalopathy, hepatorenal syndrome, and gastrointestinal bleeding, as well as toxic effects related to inappropriate dosing. Acetaminophen and NSAIDs, anticonvulsants, antidepressants, and opioids are largely metabolized in the liver, but there are no endogenous markers for hepatic clearance that can be used as a guide for drug dosing, nor are there readily available tests to accurately estimate the extent of residual liver function. Moreover, there are few high-quality studies that examine the pharmacology and adverse effects produced by analgesics in patients with advanced liver dysfunction [25].

Recommendations regarding the use of over-the-counter (OTC) medications are varied. Chandok [25] reports that no prospective, long-term studies have assessed the safety of long-term use of acetaminophen in patients with cirrhosis, and that, in such patients, the half-life of oral acetaminophen is double the half-life seen in healthy controls. Given the facts that (a) many individuals fail to heed the clinician's advice to abstain from alcohol, and (b) there is a longer half-life of acetaminophen in patients with cirrhosis, reducing the maximum dose to 2 gm/day is recommended [25].

Some clinicians, especially non-gastroenterologists, prescribe NSAIDs rather than acetaminophen, but Chandok [25] advises that NSAIDs should be avoided in this population. The reason is that, in patients with portal hypertension, use of NSAIDs is associated with renal impairment, in particular the hepatorenal syndrome, which is potentially fatal. Also, NSAIDs can cause bleeding in patients who already are at increased risk as a result of thrombocytopenia and coagulopathy. Of particular concern is the elevated risk of GI bleeding due to esophageal or gastric varices, portal hypertensive gastropathy, or gastric antral vascular ectasias.

Opioids and sedative-hypnotic medications are a major cause of hepatic encephalopathy in patients with cirrhosis and generally should be avoided. Most of these drugs are metabolized in the liver, which dictates lowered doses and longer dosing intervals. When opioids *are* prescribed, low-dose buprenorphine may be the most appropriate option for patients with a history of SUDs, but dose adjustments will be necessary. In a study that examined the pharmacokinetics of sublingual 2.0 mg buprenorphine/0.5 naloxone in patients with severe liver failure as well as healthy controls, peak buprenorphine exposures increased to 281.4% in subjects with liver failure, compared to 171.8% in controls [26].

Pain Related to HIV/AIDS

Based on a systematic review of 61 studies, Parker and collelagues [27] esti-mated that the prevalence of moderate to severe pain in patients diagnosed with human immunodeficiency virus/acquired immune deficiency syndrome (HIV/AIDS) ranges from 54–83%, based on a three-month recall period. All nine studies that reviewed the adequacy of pain management found marked under-treatment of pain related to HIV/AIDS [27].

According to the International Association for the Study of Pain (IASP), nearly half the pain seen in patients with HIV/AIDS is neuropathic, caused by injury to the central or peripheral nervous systems by direct viral infection, infection with secondary pathogens, or the neurotoxic effects of drug therapy. According to the IASP, nociceptive pain may be caused by a tumor (such as Kaposi's sarcoma), oral pain, pancreatitis, myopathy, arthralgia, HIV-related headache, headache not related to HIV, and other conditions. Factors interact-ing with or associated with such pain may include anxiety, depression, fatigue, anorexia, and pruritus [28].

The general approach to managing HIV/AIDS-related pain is the same as in managing any complex pain condition. First, establish a diagnosis by assessing underlying biological/medical conditions that may be causative. When manag-ing an individual with HIV/AIDS, this requires collaboration with the treating infectious disease specialist. As causes (such as infection) are identified, they should be promptly treated. In most situations, there will be no easily identified cause, so the clinicians are likely to find themselves dealing with chronic pain syndromes such as neuropathy.

Given the frequency of interactions between a range of drugs and antiviral medications, it is important to assess the potential for such interactions before prescribing. The treatment goal is to reduce pain to a manageable level and to facilitate functional improvement to the greatest extent possible. When the pain is caused by HIV/AIDS, this often requires a multimodal approach.

While some guidelines recommend the use of anticonvulsant medications to treat HIV-associated sensory neuropathy, questions remain as to the safety and efficacy of this approach, particularly in patients with co-occurring SUDs. Abuse of pregabalin and gabapentin has been reported. Moreover, a systematic review of pharmacological treatment of painful HIV-associated sensory neu-ropathy did not find support for the use of gabapentin, pregabalin, lamotrigine, amitriptyline, or mexilitine in managing this condition [29]. The authors did find randomized control trial evidence of analgesic efficacy superior to placebo for smoked cannabis and high dose (8%) topical capsaicin, but they did not recommend cannabis use. In the study, serotonin-norepinephrine reuptake inhibitors (SNRIs; such as duloxetine) were not examined, but given the effec-tiveness of that class of medication in treating anxiety and depression, they may represent a better treatment option than anticonvulsants, especially when there is a psychiatric treatment indication for SNRIs.

Opioids are effective in managing moderate-to-severe nociceptive and neuropathic pain, at least in the short to intermediate term. When treating patients with SUDs, opioids should be avoided in managing HIV pain except in palliative or hospice care. When other analgesic treatment options have failed, buprenorphine is a safer option than other opioids. Unless the patient requires treatment for an opioid use disorder, it is best to initiate treatment with a low-dose buprenorphine formulation (such as a transdermal patch or low-dose buccal film).

Conclusion

The complex medical conditions discussed in this chapter, although disparate in their presentations and clinical manifestations, suggest similar clinical principles in patient management. In each condition, pain is known to be under-treated in patients with a history of SUD. Treatment of pain in the presence of addiction further complicates an already complex treatment course, often requiring the chronic use of opioid medications. If this occurs, strict enforcement of a set of rules understood by the patient, the clinician, and the treatment team is essential to diminish the possibility of drug misuse while providing appropriate analgesia.

In every case, adequate assessment of the pain and its possible underlying causes, as well as adoption of a multidisciplinary team approach to pain control, is most appropriate. Ideally, such a team would include specialists in pain management and addiction medicine or addiction psychiatry, as well as clinicians who are expert in the medical condition giving rise to the pain.

For More Information on the Topics Discussed:

American Society of Addiction Medicine (ASAM):

See Chapters 72–84 in the Section on Medical Disorders and Complications of Addiction. In RK Ries, DA Fiellin, SC Miller, R Saitz, eds. *The ASAM Principles of Addiction Medicine, Fifth Edition*. Philadelphia, PA: Wolters Kluwer; 2014.

National Center for Complementary and Integrative Health (NCCIH):

Complementary Health Approaches for Chronic Pain. *NCCIH Clinical Digest for Health Professionals*. Sep 2016. (Access at: https://nccih.nih.gov/health/providers/digest/chronic-pain.)

Pain Related to Cirrhosis:

Chandok N, Watt KDS. Pain management in the cirrhotic patient: The clinical challenge. *Mayo Clin Proc.* 2010 May;85(5):451–458. Access at: https://www.ncbi.nlm.nih.gov/pmc/articles/PMC2861975/.)

Pain Related to HIV/AIDS:

HIV-Related Pain. The Well Project. May 11, 2016. (Access at: http://www.thewellproject.org/hiv-information/hiv-related-pain.)

Pain Related to Sleep Apnea:

Lettieri CJ. The association of obstructive sleep apnea and chronic pain. *Medscape Pulm Med.* 2013 May 24. (Access at: http://www.medscape.com/viewarticle/804588.)

References

1. World Health Organization (WHO). *Cancer Pain Relief: With a Guide to Opioid Availability, 2nd Edition.* Geneva, Switzerland: WHO; 1996.
2. American Academy of Pain Medicine (AAPM) and American Pain Society (APS). *The Use of Opioids for the Treatment of Chronic Pain (Consensus Statement).* Glenview, IL: The Societies; 1993.
3. American Pain Society (APS). *Principles of Analgesic Use in the Treatment of Acute Pain and Cancer Pain, 4th Edition.* Glenview, IL: American Pain Society; 1993.
4. Joint Commission on Accreditation of Healthcare Organizations (JCAHO). *Joint Commission Statement on Pain Management.* April 8, 2016. (Accessed at: https://www.jointcommission.org/joint_commission_statement_on_pain_management/)
5. Agency for Health Care Policy Research (AHCPR). *Clinical Practice Guideline No. 9: Management of Cancer Pain.* Rockville, MD: AHCPR, Department of Health and Human Services; 1994.
6. Portenoy RK, Dole V, Joseph H, et al. Pain management and chemical dependency: Evolving perspectives. *JAMA.* 1997;276(7):592–593.
7. Deyo RA, Mirza SK, Turner JA, et al. Overtreating chronic back pain: Time to back off? *J Am Board Fam Med.* 2009 Jan–Feb;22(1):62–68.
8. William AC. *Psychological Therapy for Adults with Longstanding Distressing Pain and Disability.* Cochrane Library 2016. (Accessed at: http://www.cochrane.org/CD007407/SYMPT_psychological-therapy-adults-longstanding-distressing-pain-and-disability/.)
9. McCraken LM, Vowles KE. Acceptance and commitment therapy and mindfulness for chronic pain. *Am Psychologist.* 2014;69(2):178–187.
10. Kamper SJ. Multidisciplinary biopsychosocial rehabilitation for chronic low back pain: Cochrane systematic review and meta-analysis. *BMJ.* 2015;350:444.

11. Aetna, Inc. *Policy on Chronic Pain Programs* (Policy No. 037). Last reviewed April 14, 2017. (Accessed at: http://www.aetna.com/cpb/medical/data/200_299/0237.html.)
12. Cigna, Inc. *Pain Management Clinic.* (Accessed at: http://www.cigna.com/healthwellness/hw/medical-topics/pain-management-clinic-tr3230.)
13. Enthoven WTM. *Non-Steroidal Anti-Inflammatory Drugs for Chronic Low Back Pain.* Cochrane Library, 2016. (Accessed at: http://www.cochrane.org/CD012087/BACK_non-steroidal-anti-inflammatory-drugs-chronic-low-back-pain.)
14. Shaheed CA, Maher CG, Williams KA, et al. Efficacy, tolerability, and dose-dependent effects of opioid analgesics for low back pain: A systematic review and meta-analysis. *JAMA Intern Med.* 2016;176(7):958–968.
15. Bresnitz EA, Goldberg R, Kosinski RM. Epidemiology of obstructive sleep apnea. *Epidemiol Rev.* 1994;16(2):210–227. Review.
16. Heatley EM, Harris M, Battersby M, et al. Obstructive sleep apnoea in adults: A common chronic condition in need of a comprehensive chronic condition management approach. *Sleep Med Rev.* 2013 Oct;17(5):349–355.
17. Horstmann S, Hess CW, Bassetti C, et al. Sleepiness-related accidents in sleep apnea patients. *Sleep.* 2000 May 1;23(3):383–389.
18. Karimi M, Hedner J, Lombardi C, et al., for the Esada Study Group. Driving habits and risk factors for traffic accidents among sleep apnea patients—A European multi-centre cohort study. *J Sleep Res.* 2014 Dec;23(6):689–699.
19. Marshall NS, Wong KK, Liu PY, et al. Sleep apnea as an independent risk factor for all-cause mortality: The Busselton Health Study. *Sleep.* 2008 Aug;31(8):1079–1085.
20. Rose AR, Catcheside PG, McEvoy RD, et al. Sleep disordered breathing and chronic respiratory failure in patients with chronic pain on long term opioid therapy. *J Clin Sleep Med.* 2014 Aug 15;10(8):847–852.
21. Correa D, Farney RJ, Chung F, et al. Chronic opioid use and central sleep apnea: A review of the prevalence, mechanisms, and perioperative considerations. *Anesth Analg.* 2015 Jun;120(6):1273–1285.
22. Staritz M, Poralla T, Manns M, et al. Effect of modern analgesic drugs (tramadol, pentazocine and buprenorphine) on the bile duct sphincter in man. *Gut.* 1986;27:567–569.
23. Cuer JC, Dapoigny M, Ajmi S, et al. Effects of buprenorphine on motor activity of the sphincter of Oddi in man. *Eur J Clin Pharmacol.* 1989;36:203–204.
24. Gachago C, Draganov PV. Pain management in chronic pancreatitis. *World J Gastroenterol.* 2008;28:14(20):3137–3148.
25. Chandok N, Watt KDS. Pain management in the cirrhotic patient: The clinical challenge. *Mayo Clin Proc.* 2010 May;85(5):451–458.
26. Nasser AF, Heidbreder C, Liu Y, et al. Pharmacokinetics of sublingual buprenorphine and naloxone in subjects with mild to severe hepatic impairment (Child-Pugh classes A, B, and C) in hepatitis C virus-seropositive subjects, and in healthy volunteers. *Clin Pharmacokinet.* 2015 Aug;54(8):837–849.
27. Parker R, Stein DJ, Jelsma J. Pain in people living with HIV/AIDS: A systematic review. *J Int AIDS Soc.* 2014;17:18719.

28. Uebelacker LA, Weisberg RB, Herman DS, et al. Chronic pain in HIV-infected patients: Relationship to depression, substance use, and mental health and pain treatment. *Pain Med*. Available in PMC 2016 Oct 1.
29. Phillips TJC, Brown M, Ramirez JD, et al. Sensory, psychological, and metabolic dysfunction in HIV-associated peripheral neuropathy: A cross-sectional deep profiling study. *Pain*. 2014 Sep;155(9):1846–1860.

Pain and Addiction in Patients with Traumatic Brain Injury

SANJOG S. PANGARKAR, M.D.

Formally defined "as an alteration in brain function, or other evidence of brain pathology, caused by an external force" [1], traumatic brain injury (TBI) is a major cause of death and disability in the United States.

Causes of Traumatic Brain Injury

The most common cause of TBI is impact and acceleration or deceleration forces, such as those caused by a bump, blow, or jolt to the head that disrupts the normal function of the brain (for example, blows that occur in motor vehicle crashes). However, not all blows or jolts to the head result in a TBI.

The severity of a TBI may range from "mild" (a brief change in mental status or consciousness) to "severe" (an extended period of unconsciousness or memory loss after the injury). Most TBIs that occur each year are categorized as mild [2].

According to data collected by the Centers for Disease Control and Prevention (CDC) in 2013 [2], falls were the leading cause of TBI in that year, accounting for 47% of all TBI-related emergency department (ED) visits, hospitalizations, and deaths in the United States. Falls disproportionately affect the youngest and oldest age groups.

Being struck by or against an object was the second leading cause of TBI, accounting for about 15% of TBI-related ED visits, hospitalizations, and deaths in the United States in 2013. Of these, more than 1 in 5 (22%)

TBI-related ED visits, hospitalizations, and deaths in children less than 15 years of age were caused by being struck by or against an object [2].

Among all age groups, motor vehicle crashes were the third overall leading cause of TBI-related ED visits, hospitalizations, and deaths (14%). When looking at just TBI-related deaths, motor vehicle crashes also were the third leading cause (19%) in 2013 [3].

TBIs contribute to about a third of all injury deaths [2]. Survivors of TBI suffer effects that can persist for as little as a few days or as long as the rest of their lives. Typical effects include impaired thinking or memory, movement, sensation (e.g., vision or hearing), or emotional functioning (e.g., personality changes, depression) [2]. Penetrating head injuries present a greater risk of post-traumatic seizures and epilepsy than do closed head injuries [4].

Clinical Presentation

Cognitive abilities that are affected by TBI include attention, abstract thinking, memory/learning, processing speed, planning/reasoning, and tinnitus/vertigo. The pain symptoms most often associated with TBI are headache, chest pain, spine pain, and limb pain.

In addition, several behavioral symptoms are associated with TBI and pain. Patients may present with these symptoms without mentioning TBI, so a careful history is helpful in eliciting information about any previous head injury that may be complicating the patient's clinical situation. Behavioral symptoms include depression, anxiety, aggression, agitation and irritability, substance use, sleep disturbance, apathy, and impulsivity [5,6].

Reaching a Diagnosis

The diagnosis of TBI is made clinically. Information needed to diagnose (or exclude) TBI includes:

- Medical history and physical examination;
- A CT scan without contrast;
- An MRI of the brain with diffusion tensor imaging (DTI), if needed;
- An electroencephalogram (EEG), if a seizure disorder is suspected;
- Diagnostic imaging of the painful area (if indicated);
- Neuropsychological testing (when clarification is needed); and
- Electrodiagnostic testing (when the diagnosis is not clear).

Treatment of Traumatic Brain Injury

To date, no pharmacological agents have been shown to improve outcomes from TBI. A number of promising neuroprotective treatment options have emerged from preclinical studies. Most of these treatments target the lesion. However, translation of preclinical effective neuroprotective drugs to clinical trials has proven challenging. Thus, there is a compelling need to develop treatments for TBI.

Accumulating evidence indicates that the mammalian brain has a significant, albeit limited, capacity for both structural and functional plasticity, as well as the type of regeneration that is essential for spontaneous functional recovery after injury. A new therapeutic approach is to stimulate neurovascular remodeling by enhancing angiogenesis, neurogenesis, oligodendrogenesis, and axonal sprouting, which in concert may improve neurological functional recovery after TBI [7].

Patients referred to chronic pain programs who have problems with memory and concentration, confusion about their medical diagnosis, headaches, neck and arm pain, and a history of extensive medical work-ups and numerous unsuccessful treatments may be suffering from an undiagnosed TBI.

Treatment outcomes in patients with the dual diagnosis of TBI and chronic pain are similar to those of patients with chronic pain alone, although the duration of treatment typically is longer for patients with co-occurring TBI and chronic pain [8].

Conclusion

Further study is needed to clarify diagnostic and treatment issues associated with TBI. First and foremost, there is a clear need for the research community to come to a consensus about defining and measuring TBI, and then to apply these practices consistently across studies. Also, in order to provide better evidence on the prevalence and outcomes of TBI in military and veteran populations, large, prospective epidemiological studies are needed that recruit and retain the most representative samples possible and employ standard definitions and measures [9].

Such research should be based on methods of collecting the information necessary for assessing the occurrence and severity of TBI near the time of injury, without relying on subject recall or hospital records. If this level of standardization and consistency is achieved in all future studies of TBI, our ability to synthesize data and draw meaningful conclusions from results would be greatly enhanced [9].

For More Information on the Topics Discussed:

American Society of Addiction Medicine (ASAM):

Blow FC, Barry KL. Traumatic injuries related to alcohol and other drug use: Epidemiology, screening and prevention (Chapter 81). In RK Ries, DA Fiellin, SC Miller, R Saitz, eds. *The ASAM Principles of Addiction Medicine, Fifth Edition.* Philadelphia, PA: Wolters Kluwer; 2014.

Veterans Administration (VA), U.S. Department of Defense (DoD):

Recently Updated Clinical Practice Guidelines for the Management of Traumatic Brain Injury. (Access at: http://www.healthquality.va.gov/guidelines/Rehab/mtbi/.)

The Department of Veterans Affairs also maintains a website on traumatic brain injury, containing information for clinicians, patients and family members. (Access at: http://www.publichealth.va.gov/exposures/traumatic-brain-injury.asp.)

In the Literature:

Marshall S, Bayley M, McCullagh S, et al., for the TBI Expert Consensus Group. Updated clinical practice guidelines for concussion/mild traumatic brain injury and persistent symptoms. *Brain Inj.* 2015;29(6):688–700.

References

1. Menon DK, Schwab K, Wright DW, et al. Position statement: Definition of traumatic brain injury. *Arch Phys Med Rehabil.* 2010 Nov;91(11):1637–1640.
2. Centers for Disease Control and Prevention (CDC). *Traumatic Brain Injury and Concussion.* Atlanta, GA: CDC; 2017. (Accessed at: https://www.cdc.gov/traumaticbraininjury/get_the_facts.html.)
3. Kotapka MJ, Gennarelli TA, Graham DI, et al. Selective vulnerability of hippocampal neurons in acceleration-induced experimental head injury. *J Neurotrauma.* 1991 Winter;8(4):247–258.
4. Temkin NR. Preventing and treating posttraumatic seizures: The human experience. *Epilepsia.* 2009 Feb;50(Suppl 2):10–13.
5. Cifu DX, Taylor BC, Carne WF, et al. Traumatic brain injury, posttraumatic stress disorder, and pain diagnoses in OIF/OEF/OND veterans. *J Rehabil Res Dev.* 2013;50:1169–1176.
6. Higgins DM, Kerns RD, Brandt CA, et al. Persistent pain and comorbidity among Operation Enduring Freedom/Operation Iraqi Freedom/Operation New Dawn veterans. *Pain Med.* 2014;15(5):782–790.

7. Xiong Y, Zhang Y, Mahmood A, et al. Investigational agents for treatment of traumatic brain injury. *Expert Opin Investig Drugs*. 2015 Jun;24(6):743–760.
8. Moore DF, Jaffee MS. Military traumatic brain injury and blast. *NeuroRehab*. 2010;26:179–181.
9. Carlson KF, Kehle SM, Meis LA, et al. Prevalence, assessment, and treatment of mild traumatic brain injury and posttraumatic stress disorder: A systematic review of the evidence. *J Head Trauma Rehab*. 2011 Mar–Apr;26(2):13–15.

Chapter 26

Pain and Addiction in Patients with Fibromyalgia

KAREN MUCHOWSKI, M.D., FAAFP,
AND STEVEN R. HANLING, M.D.

Fibromyalgia is a chronic pain syndrome. Current data point to abnormal central pain processing as the etiology of the syndrome. Evidence supports an imbalance in inhibitory neurotransmitters (serotonin, norepinephrine) and excitatory neurotransmitters (Substance P, glutamate) [1]. Functional MRI studies show increased blood flow in areas of the brain that involve pain processing, and reduced blood flow in areas associated with pain inhibition [2]. In some patients, Substance P levels in the cerebral spinal fluid are elevated, while levels of serotonin, norepinephrine, and dopamine are depressed [3].

New evidence shows that abnormal peripheral pain processing also may play a role. Small studies have found reduced blood flow and abnormal cytokine markers in muscle tissue following exercise [4,5]. Because of abnormal pain processing, hyperalgesia (increased sensitivity to painful stimuli) as well as allodynia (sensitivity to normally non-painful stimuli) are commonly seen in patients with fibromyalgia. Growth hormone and cortisol abnormalities are seen in some patients [6]. Therefore, dysfunction in the hypothalamic-pituitary-adrenal (HPA) axis may play a role.

In the United States, fibromyalgia occurs in 2–5% of the population [7], with older studies identifying fibromyalgia in more women than men (i.e., a 7:1 ratio of women to men) [8]. However, more recent studies, which employed the 2010 American College of Rheumatology (ACR) diagnostic criteria, found a 2:1 ratio of women to men, which is consistent with prevalence data on other chronic pain disorders [9,10].

The incidence of fibromyalgia increases with age, with the highest rates of incidence in patients over 45 years of age [11]. Compared to patients with other chronic diseases, patients with fibromyalgia have higher levels of psychological distress, lower scores for health-related quality of life, and incur health care costs three times higher than those of matched controls [12].

Fibromyalgia also carries the potential for significant occupational disability [13,14], with up to half of patients experiencing disruption in their employment because of the disorder [15].

Clinical Presentation

Patient History

Patients with fibromyalgia experience widespread pain. Other common symptoms include fatigue (reported by up to 90% of patients), sleep disturbance (reported by up to 75%), headaches, morning stiffness, and cognitive issues. Comorbidities are common, with higher rates of depression, anxiety, headache syndromes, and irritable bowel syndrome than are seen in the general population [4]. Post-traumatic stress disorder (PTSD) and physical or sexual abuse also are reported with some frequency [16,17]. A recent cohort study found that 45% of patients with fibromyalgia (versus 3% of controls) met the criteria for PTSD [18]. A meta-analysis found that patients with fibromyalgia were twice as likely as controls to have a history that includes physical or sexual abuse [19].

In most patients, the onset of fibromyalgia is insidious, but in 20–45% of patients, symptoms appeared following a traumatic event (either physical or emotional) [20]. Having a first-degree family member with fibromyalgia greatly increases the risk of developing this syndrome [3,21]. Twin studies show that the risk of developing fibromyalgia is attributable to both genetic and environmental factors in equal proportions [4]. Secondary fibromyalgia is present in 10–30% of patients with other rheumatological disorders (such as osteoarthritis, rheumatoid arthritis, and systemic lupus erythematosus) [7].

Physical Examination

A full physical examination, focusing on the musculoskeletal system, is necessary to rule out other conditions. Patients with fibromyalgia should have a normal physical examination, without evidence of synovitis or inflammatory disease. "Tender points" have been removed from the diagnostic criteria because 25% of patients with fibromyalgia did not evidence 11 tender points on examination [10].

Diagnostic Testing

The American College of Rheumatology (ACR) revised its diagnostic criteria for fibromyalgia in 2010. The criteria are meant to facilitate research, but can also assist in clinical diagnosis and management. Using the available criteria, primary care professionals can confidently diagnose fibromyalgia without specialty consultation for confirmation [22,23].

Useful tools include the Widespread Pain Index (WPI) ≥7 and Symptom Severity (SS) scale ≥5 OR WPI 3–6, as well as the SS scale ≥9 (see Figure 26.1) [22]). Diagnosis of fibromyalgia requires that symptoms be present at a similar

New Clinical Fibromyalgia Diagnostic Criteria – Part 1.

To answer the following questions, patients should take into consideration
• how you felt the past week,
• While taking your current therapies and treatments, and
• exclude your pain or symptoms from other known illnesses such as arthritis, Lupus, Sjogren's, etc.

Determing Your Widespread Pain Index (WPI)
The WPI Index score from Part 1 is between 0 and 19.

Check each area you have felt pain in over the past week.

☐ Shoulder girdle, left
☐ Shoulder girdle, right
☐ Upper arm, left
☐ Upper arm, right
☐ Lower arm, left
☐ Lower arm, right
☐ Hip (buttock) left
☐ Hip (buttock) right
☐ Upper leg left
☐ Upper leg right

☐ Lower leg left
☐ Lower leg right
☐ Jaw left
☐ Jaw right
☐ Chest
☐ Abdomen
☐ Neck
☐ Upper back
☐ Lower back
☐ None of these areas

Neck
Upper Back
Shoulder girdle
Jaw
Chest
Upper Arm
Lower Back
Lower Arm
Hip (Buttock)
Upper Leg
Abdomen
Lower Leg
Back Side
Front Side

Count up the number of areas checked and enter your Widespread Pain Index or WPI score score here _____.

Symptom Severity Score (SS score) – Part 2a.

Indicate your level of symptom severity over the past week using the following scale.

Fatigue

☐ 0 = No problem
☐ 1 = Slight or mild problems; generally mild or intermittent
☐ 2 = Moderate; considerable problems; often present and/or at a moderate level
☐ 3 = Severe: pervasive, continuous, life disturbing problems

Walking unrefreshed

☐ 0 = No problem
☐ 1 = Slight or mild problems; generally mild or intermittent
☐ 2 = Moderate; considerable problems; often present and/or at a moderate level
☐ 3 = Severe: pervasive, continuous, life disturbing problems

Cognitive symptoms

☐ 0 = No problem
☐ 1 = Slight or mild problems; generally mild or intermittent
☐ 2 = Moderate; considerable problems; often present and/or at a moderate level
☐ 3 = Severe: pervasive, continuous, life disturbing problems

Tally your score for Part 2a (not the number of checkmarks) and enter it here_____.

Figure 26.1 *Clinical Diagnostic Criteria for Fibromyalgia*

Source: Guy Jr. GP, Zhang K, Bohm MK, et al. Vital Signs: Changes in opioid prescribing in the United States, 2006–2015, Figure 1. MMWR. 2017 Jul 7;66(26):699.

Symptom Severity Score (SS score)- *Part 2b*

Check each of the following OTHER SYMPTOMS that you have experienced over the past week?

☐ Muscle pain	☐ Nervousness	☐ Loss/change in taste
☐ Irritable bowel syndrome	☐ Chest pain	☐ Seizures.
☐ Fatigue/tiredness	☐ Blurred vision	☐ Dry eyes
☐ Thinking or remembering problem	☐ Fever	☐ Shortness of breath
	☐ Diarrhea	☐ Loss of appetite
☐ Muscle Weakness	☐ Dry mouth	☐ Rash
☐ Headache	☐ Itching	☐ Sun sensitivity
☐ Pain cramps in abdomen	☐ Wheezing	☐ Hearing difficulties
	☐ Raynauld's	☐ Easy bruising
☐ Numbness/tingling	☐ Hives/welts	☐ Hair loss
☐ Dizziness	☐ Ringing in ears	☐ Frequent urination
☐ Insomnia	☐ Vomiting	☐ Painful urination
☐ Depression	☐ Heartburn	☐ Bladder spasms
☐ Constipation	☐ Oral ulcers	
☐ Pain in upper abdomen		
☐ Nausea		

Count up the number of symptoms checked above. *If you tallied:	Enter your score for Part 2b here
0 symptoms Give yourself a score of 0	Now add Part 2a AND 2b scores, and enter
1 to 10 Give yourself a score of 1	This is your Symptom Severity Score (SS score), which can range from 0 to 12.
11 to 24 Give yourselfa score of 2	
25 or more Give yourself a score of 3	

What Your Scores Mean

A patient meets the diagnostic criteria for fibromyalgia if the following three conditions are met:

la. The WPI score (Part 1) is greater than or equal to 7 AND the SS score (Part 2a & b) is greater than or equal to 5; OR

lb. The WPI score (Part 1) is from 3 to 6 AND the SS score (Part 2a & b) is greater than or equal to 9

2 Symptoms have been present at a similar level for at least 3 months.

3 You do not have a disorder that would otherwise explain the pain

For example:

If your WPI (Part 1) was 9 and your SS score (Parts 2a & 2 b) was 6, then you would meet the new FM diagnostic criteria.

If your WPI (Part 1) was 5 and your SS score (Parts 2a & 2b) was 7, then you would NOT meet the new FM diagnostic criteria

*The new FM diagnostic criteria did not specify the number of "Other Symptoms" required to score the point rankings from 0 to 3. Therefore, we estimated the number of symptoms needed to meet the authors' descriptive categories of:

0 =No symptoms
1 = Few symptoms
2 =A moderate number
3 =A great many symptoms

• Wolfe F. et al. 2010 Arthritis Care Research 62(5), 600-610.

For information about Fibromyalgia Network, call our office Monday through Friday, 9: 00 a.m to 5:00 p.m. (PST) at (800) 853-2929 or visit us online at www.fainetnews.com

This survey is not meant to substitute fora diagnosis by a medical professional. Patients should not diagnose themselves. Patients should always consult their medical professional for advice and treatment. This survey is intended to give you insight into research on the diagnostic criteria and measurement of symptom severity for fibromyalgia.

Source: Fibromyalgia Network (www.fmnetnews.com).

Figure 26.1 *Continued*

level for at least three months, in the absence of any disorder that otherwise would explain the patient's pain. (This diagnostic criterion is more consistent with our current understanding of the syndrome and may be more inclusive than the ACR research-based criteria.)

Laboratory testing is not required for the diagnosis of fibromyalgia, but is useful in excluding other disorders. Erythrocyte sedimentation rate, C-reactive protein, complete blood count, electrolyte panel, and liver function testing may be useful, depending on the patient's clinical presentation. Higher rates of fibromyalgia are seen in patients with HIV, hepatitis B and C infections, so testing for those infections may be appropriate in selected patients.

Non-Pharmacological Therapies for Fibromyalgia

Non-pharmacological therapies should be used as an initial approach, because many are more effective than pharmacological treatments [24]. Simply establishing the diagnosis of fibromyalgia can improve satisfaction with health and reduce health care utilization [25–26].

Patient education about fibromyalgia increases self-efficacy, reduces pain and depression, and increases function. Education should include the facts that fibromyalgia is a chronic disease with a waxing and waning course; that it is not a precursor to other diseases; that there are effective therapies, and that self-management of the disease is crucial [27].

Cognitive behavioral therapy (CBT) is beneficial for many patients with chronic pain. In patients with fibromyalgia, CBT has been shown to reduce pain and improve quality of life [24] and self-efficacy [28]. Goals of CBT include increasing self-efficacy, changing the locus of control from external to internal, and overcoming learned helplessness. Strong evidence exists that multicomponent therapy (a combination of patient education, exercise, and CBT) offers short-term benefits in terms of reduced pain, fatigue, and depression, and improved quality of life [29].

Diminished aerobic fitness is common in patients with fibromyalgia, so *exercise programs* are effective in reducing many symptoms of fibromyalgia and have few adverse effects. Low- to moderate-intensity aerobic exercise improves pain and well-being [30]. Benefits also are seen with strength training. Studies involving lower-intensity exercise, or a goal of achieving 50% of the maximum heart rate. found lower rates of attrition and greater symptom improvement [24,31] than no exercise. Both land- and water-based exercises are effective in improving fitness and reducing common symptoms of fibromyalgia [32]. Exercise prescriptions for patients should be individualized and focus on minimizing pain (low intensity first, avoiding activities that hurt), while slowly increasing exercise time [33]. Meditative movement therapies (qi jong, tai chi, yoga) improve overall function, sleep, depression, and fatigue [34,35], with some of these effects lasting for up to six months after the intervention.

Patients with fibromyalgia often seek relief from *complementary and alternative medicine* modalities. A recent meta-analysis found that acupuncture (especially electrical acupuncture) increased pain relief and reduced morning stiffness [36]. Small studies evaluating balneotherapy showed promise for improving pain [24]. Meta-analyses of *hydrotherapy and hypnosis/guided imagery* also showed improvement in pain scores [37,38]. There is weak evidence to support *chiropractic manipulation, massage, ultrasound or electrotherapy* [10], and more studies are needed to further evaluate these modalities.

Pharmacological Therapies for Fibromyalgia

Pharmacological treatments are available for patients who do not achieve the desired improvement with non-pharmacological interventions. However, the effect sizes of many medications are modest, with a small number of patients achieving a 30% reduction in pain. Physicians need to set realistic expectations for patients before prescribing analgesic medications.

Cyclobenzaprine is a muscle relaxant with a chemical structure similar to that of tricyclic antidepressants (TCAs). It produces a modest improvement in global functioning [39] (with an odds ratio [OR] of 3.0 [at a 95% confidence interval (CI) 1.6–5.60], and an number needed to treat (NNT) of 4.8 [95% CI 3.0–11]). It is a good first choice for patients who also suffer from sleep disturbance.

Tricyclic antidepressants (TCAs) offer effective treatment for many pain disorders, including fibromyalgia. Three meta-analyses have found that TCAs produce a moderate to large effect in reducing pain [29,40,41]. Among patients taking TCAs, 30% reported a reduction in pain, compared to 27.8% of patients taking a placebo (NNT 4.9 [95% CI 3.5–8.0]). Smaller effects were seen in improvements of sleep, fatigue, mood, and health-related quality of life.

Selective serotonin reuptake inhibitors (SSRIs) and *selective norepinephrine reuptake inhibitors (SNRIs)* improve pain by increasing the levels of inhibitory neurotransmitters (serotonin or norepinephrine). Older SSRIs (such as fluoxetine, paroxetine, sertraline) used at higher doses improve pain, fatigue, and depression scores [4,42]. However, the effect size is smaller than that seen with the TCAs [40]. The SNRIs duloxetine and milnacipran have a small to moderate effect on pain reduction [24,43]. Patients taking SNRIs reported a 30% reduction in pain, compared to a 32% reduction reported by those taking a placebo (NNT 10 [95% CI 8.00–13.40]). Duloxetine (but not milnacipran) improved sleep and depression scores [43].

Antiepileptics such as glutamate affect neurotransmitters involved in pain activation; gabapentin and pregabalin reduce glutamate transmission. Only one study with gabapentin has been reported, and it showed a 30% reduction in pain (RR 1.01–2.53) [44]. A systematic review of five studies found that pregabalin reduced pain more than did placebo (relative risk [RR] 1.59, 95% CI 1.33–1.90, number needed to benefit [NNTB] 12 [95% CI 9–21]) [45] and had a small effect on sleep improvement.

Opioids such as tramadol bind opioid mu-receptors and weakly inhibit uptake of serotonin and norepinephrine. One randomized control trial of tramadol versus placebo showed improved pain control [46]. Although stronger opioids sometimes are prescribed for fibromyalgia (32% of patients referred to a specialty pain clinic were given opioids [47]), no studies of stronger opioids have been published [7]. However, one recent study showed that opioids may worsen fibromyalgia pain [48]. Because of their high risk profile and unproven efficacy in the treatment of this disorder, opioids are not recommended for the treatment of fibromyalgia.

Other medications that have been used to treat fibromyalgia include sodium oxybate, which is the sodium salt of gamma hydroxybutyrate and has central nervous system (CNS) depressant properties. Two randomized controlled trials involving 14 weeks of therapy with sodium oxybate showed reduced pain as well as improved sleep and function [49,50]. An open-label extension study for an additional 38 weeks showed that the improvements continued over that period of time [51].

Small studies with naltrexone have shown promise in reducing symptoms of fibromyalgia, but further research is needed [52,53].

Conclusion

Research suggests that fibromyalgia is caused by a problem in how the body processes pain or, more precisely, a hypersensitivity to stimuli that normally are not painful. Therefore, several researchers supported by the National Institutes of Health (NIH) are focusing on ways the body processes pain in an effort to better understand why individuals with fibromyalgia have increased sensitivity to pain. Examples of such studies include [54]:

- Establishment of a tissue bank of brain and spinal cord tissue to study fibromyalgia and to determine the extent to which chronic pain in fibromyalgia patients is associated with the activation of cells in the nervous system and the production of chemical messengers, called cytokines, that regulate immune cell function.

- The use of imaging methods to evaluate the status of CNS responses in patients diagnosed with fibromyalgia compared with those diagnosed with another chronic pain disorder and pain-free controls.
- An investigation to understand how the activation of immune cells from peripheral and CNS sources triggers a cascade of events leading to the activation of nerve cells, chronic pain, and the dysregulation of the effects of analgesic drugs against pain.
- An intensive evaluation of twins in which one of the pair has chronic widespread pain and the other does not, along with twins in which neither has chronic pain, to help researchers assess physiological similarities and differences in those with and without chronic pain and determine whether those differences are caused by genetics or the environment.
- A study examining the effectiveness of cognitive-behavioral therapy in pain patients, which researchers hope will advance their understanding of the role of psychological factors in chronic pain. as well as provide a new treatment option for fibromyalgia.

Knowledge gained from these studies should enhance our understanding of the causes of fibromyalgia syndrome, as well as expand the number and effectiveness of the various treatment modalities.

Disclaimer

The views expressed in this chapter are those of the authors and do not necessarily reflect the official policy of the Department of the Navy, Department of Defense, or the U.S. government.

For More Information on the Topics Discussed:

American Society of Addiction Medicine (ASAM):

Covington EC, Kotz MM. Comorbid pain and addiction (Chapter 98). In RK Ries, DA Fiellin, SC Miller, R Saitz, eds. *The ASAM Principles of Addiction Medicine, Fifth Edition.* Philadelphia, PA: Wolters Kluwer; 2014.

Centers for Disease Control and Prevention (CDC):

Website: Fibromyalgia. (Access at: http://www.cdc.gov/arthritis/basics/fibromyalgia.htm.)

Fibromyalgia Network:

Information for patients and families. (Access at: www.fmnetnews.com.)

National Institute of Arthritis and Musculoskeletal and Skin Diseases (NIAMSD):
Questions and answers about fibromyalgia. July 2014. (Access at: https://www.niams.nih.gov/health_info/fibromyalgia/#h.)

References

1. Rahman A, Underwood M, Carnes D. Fibromyalgia: Clinical review. *BMJ*. 2014;348:g1224.
2. Abeles AM, Pillinger MH, Solitar BM, et al. Narrative review: The pathophysiology of fibromyalgia. *Ann Intern Med*. 2007;146:726–734.
3. Russell IJ, Orr MD, Littman B, et al. Elevated cerebrospinal fluid levels of substance P in patients with the fibromyalgia syndrome. *Arthritis Rheum*. 1994;37:1593–1601.
4. Elvin A, Siosteen A, Nilsson A, et al. Decreased muscle blood flow in fibromyalgia patients during standardized muscle exercise: A contrast media enhanced colour Doppler study. *Eur J Pain*. 2006 Feb;10(2):137–144.
5. Torgrimson-Ojerio B, Ross RL, Dieckmann NF, et al. Preliminary evidence of a blunted anti-inflammatory response to exhaustive exercise in fibromyalgia. *J Neuroimmunol*. 2014 Dec 15;277(1–2):160–167.
6. Deodhar P, Lorentzen A, Bennett R, et al. Growth hormone perturbations in fibromyalgia: A review. *Semin Arthritis Rheum*. 2007 Jan;36(6):357–379.
7. Arnold LM, Clauw DJ, Dunegan LJ, et al. A framework for fibromyalgia management for primary care providers. *Mayo Clin Proc*. 2012 May;87(5):488–496.
8. Centers for Disease Control and Prevention (CDC). Website: Fibromyalgia. (Accessed at: http://www.cdc.gov/arthritis/basics/fibromyalgia.htm.)
9. Vincent A, Lahr BD, Wolfe F, et al. Prevalence of fibromyalgia: A population-based study in Olmstead County, Minnesota, utilizing the Rochester Epidemiology Project. *Arthritis Care Res*. 2013 May;65(5):786–792.
10. Clauw DJ. Fibromyalgia: A clinical review. *JAMA*. 2014;311(15):1547–1555.
11. Weir P, Harlan G, Nkoy F, et al. The incidence of fibromyalgia and its associated comorbidities: A population-based retrospective cohort study based on International Classification of Diseases, 9th revision codes. *JCR*. 2006 Jun;12(3):124–128.
12. Berger A, Dukes E, Martin S, et al. Characteristics and healthcare costs of patients with fibromyalgia syndrome. *Int J Clin Pract*. 2007 Sep;61(9):1498–1508.
13. Verbunt J, Pernot D, Smeets R. Disability and quality of life in patients with fibromyalgia. *Health Qual Life Outcomes*. 2008;6:8.
14. Howard KJ, Mayer TG, Neblett R, et al. Fibromyalgia syndrome in chronic disabling occupational musculoskeletal disorders: Relevance, risk factors, and post treatment outcomes. *J Occup Environ Med*. 2010 Dec;52(12):1186–1191.

15. Schaefer C, Chandran A, Hustader M, et al. The comparative burden of mild, moderate and severe fibromyalgia: Results from a cross-sectional survey in the United States. *Health Qual Life Outcomes*. 2011;9:71.

16. Anderberg UM, Marteinsdottir I, Theorell T, et al. The impact of life events in female patients with fibromyalgia and in female healthy controls. *Eur Psychiatry*. 2000;15:295–301.

17. Cohen J, Neumann L, Haiman Y, et al. Prevalence of post-traumatic stress disorder in fibromyalgia patients: Overlapping syndromes or post-traumatic fibromyalgia syndrome? *Semin Arthritis Rheum*. 2002;32:38–50.

18. Hauser W, Galek A, Erbsloh-Moller B, et al. Posttraumatic stress disorder in fibromyalgia syndrome: Prevalence, temporal relationship between posttraumatic stress and fibromyalgia symptoms and impact on clinical outcome. *Pain*. 2013;154(8):1216–1223.

19. Hauser W, Kosseva M, Uceyler N, et al. Emotional, physical, and sexual abuse in fibromyalgia syndrome: A systematic review with meta-analysis. *Arthritis Care Res*. 2011 Jun;63(6):808–820.

20. Sherman JJ, Turk D, Okifuji A. Prevalence and impact of posttraumatic stress disorder-like symptoms on patients with fibromyalgia syndrome. *Clin J Pain*. 2000 June;16(2):127–134.

21. Arnold LM, Fan J, Russell IJ, et al. The fibromyalgia family study. *Arthritis Rheum*. 2013;65(4):1122–1128.

22. Wolfe F, Clauw DJ, Fitzcharles MA, et al. The American College of Rheumatology preliminary diagnostic criteria for fibromyalgia and measurement of symptom severity. *Arthritis Care Res*. 2010;62:600–610.

23. Canadian Pain Society. *2012 Canadian Guidelines for the Diagnosis and Management of Fibromyalgia Syndrome*. (Accessed at: www.canadianpainsociety.ca/pdf/Fibromyalgia_Guidelines_2012.pdf.)

24. Nuesch E, Hauser W, Bernardy K, et al. Comparative efficacy of pharmacological and non-pharmacological interventions in fibromyalgia syndrome: Network meta-analysis. *Ann Rheum Dis*. 2013;72:955–962.

25. White KP, Nielson WR, Harth M, et al. Does the label "fibromyalgia" alter health status, function and health service utilization? A prospective, within-group comparison in a community cohort of adults with chronic widespread pain. *Arthritis Rheum*. 2002;47(3):260–265.

26. Annemans L, Wessely S, Spaepen E, et al. Health economic consequences related to the diagnosis of fibromyalgia syndrome. *Arthritis Rheum*. 2008 Mar;58(3):895–902.

27. Goldenberg DL. Multidisciplinary modalities in the treatment of fibromyalgia. *J Clin Psychiatry*. 2008;69(Suppl 2):30–34.

28. Bernardy K, Fuber N, Kollner V, et al. Efficacy of cognitive-behavioral therapies in fibromyalgia syndrome—A systematic review and meta-analysis of randomized controlled trials. *J Rheumatol*. 2010 Oct;37(10):1991–2005.

29. Hauser W, Bernardy K, Arnold B, et al. Efficacy of multicomponent treatment in fibromyalgia syndrome: A meta-analysis of randomized controlled clinical trials. *Arthritis Rheum*. 2009;61:216–224.

30. Busch, AJ, Barber KA, Overend T, et al. Exercise for fibromyalgia: A systematic review. 2008 Jun;35(6):1130–1144.
31. Jones K, Adams D, Winters-Stone K, et al. A comprehensive review of 46 exercise treatment studies in fibromyalgia (1988–2005). *Health Qual Life Outcomes.* 2006 Sep 25;4:67. https://doi.org/10.1186/1477-7525-4-67
32. Hauser W, Klose P, Langhorst J, et al. Efficacy of different types of aerobic exercise in fibromyalgia syndrome: A systematic review and meta-analysis of randomized controlled trials. *Arthritis Rheum.* 2010;12(3):R79.
33. Jones KD, Clark SR. Individualizing the exercise prescription for person with fibromyalgia. *Rheum Dis Clin North Am.* 2002;28:419–436.
34. Mist S, Firestone K, Dupree Jones K. Complementary and alternative exercise for fibromyalgia: a meta-analysis. *J Pain Res.* 2013;6:247–260.
35. Langhorst J, Klose P, Dobos G, et al. Efficacy and safety of meditative movement therapies in fibromyalgia syndrome: A systematic review and meta-analysis of randomized controlled trials. *Rheumatol Int.* 2013;33:193–207.
36. Deare JC, Zheng Z, Xue CCL, et al. Acupuncture for treating fibromyalgia. *Cochrane Database Syst Rev.* 2013 May 31;(5):CD007070. doi:10.1002/14651858.CD007070.pub2.
37. Langhorst J, Musial F, Klose P, et al. Efficacy of hydrotherapy in fibromyalgia syndrome—A meta-analysis of randomized controlled clinical trials. *Rheumatology.* 2009 Sep;48(9):1155–1159.
38. Bernardy K, Fuber N, Klose P, et al. Efficacy of hypnosis/guided imagery in fibromyalgia syndrome—A systematic review and meta-analysis of controlled trials. *BMC Musculoskelet Disord.* 2011;12:133.
39. Tofferi JK, Jackson JL, O'Malley PG. Treatment of fibromyalgia with cyclobenzaprine: A meta-analysis. *Arthritis Rheum.* 2004 Feb;51(1):9–13.
40. Hauser W, Bernardy K, Uceyler N, et al. Treatment of fibromyalgia syndrome with antidepressants: A meta-analysis. *JAMA.* 2009;301(2):198–209.
41. Hauser W, Wolfe F, Tolle T, et al. The role of antidepressants in the management of fibromyalgia syndrome: A systematic review and meta-analysis. *CNS Drugs.* 2012 Apr 1;26(4):297–307.
42. Arnold LM, Hess EV, Hudson JI, et al. A randomized, placebo-controlled, double-blind, flexible-dose study of fluoxetine in the treatment of women with fibromyalgia. *Am J Med.* 2002;112:191–197.
43. Hauser W, Urrutia G, Tort S, et al. Serotonin and norepinephrine reuptake inhibitors (SNRIs) for fibromyalgia syndrome. *Cochrane Database Syst Rev.* 2013 Jan 31;(1):CD010292. doi:10.1002/14651858.CD010292
44. Arnold LM, Goldenberg DL, Stanford SB, et al. Gabapentin in the treatment of fibromyalgia. *Arthritis Rheum.* 2007 Apr;56(4):1336–1344.
45. Uceyler N, Sommer C, Walitt B, et al. Anticonvulsants for fibromyalgia. *Cochrane Database Syst Rev.* 2013 Oct 16;(10):CD010782. doi:10.1002/14651858.CD010782
46. Bennett R, Kamin M, Karim R, et al. Tramadol and acetaminophen combination tablets in the treatment of fibromyalgia pain: A double-blind, randomized, placebo-controlled study. *Am J Med.* 2003;114:537–545.

47. Fitzcharles MA, Ste-Marie PA, Gamsa A, et al. Opioid use, misuse and abuse in patients labeled as fibromyalgia. *Am J Med*. 2011;124:955–960.

48. Brummett CM, Janda AM, Schueller CM, et al. Survey criteria for fibromyalgia independently predict increased postoperative opioid consumption after lower extremity joint arthroplasty: A prospective, observational cohort study. *Anesthesiology*. 2013;119(6):1434–1443.

49. Russell IJ, Holman AJ, Swick TJ, et al. Sodium oxybate reduces pain, fatigue, and sleep disturbance and improves functionality in fibromyalgia: Results from a 14-week, randomized, double-blind, placebo-controlled study. *Pain*. 2011;152:1007–1017.

50. Spaeth M, Bennett RM, Benson BA, et al. Sodium oxybate therapy provides multidimensional improvement in fibromyalgia: Results of an international phase 3 trial. *Ann Rheumat Dis*. 2012 Jun;71(6):935–942.

51. Spaeth M, Alegre C, Perrot S, et al. Long term tolerability and maintenance of therapeutic response to sodium oxybate in an open-label extension study in patients with fibromyalgia. *Arthritis Res Ther*. 2013;15:R185.

52. Younger J, Noor N, McCue R, et al. Low-dose naltrexone for the treatment of fibromyalgia. *Arthritis Rheum*. 2013 Feb;65(2):529–538.

53. Younger J, Mackey S. Fibromyalgia symptoms are reduced by low-dose naltrexone: A pilot study. *Pain Med*. 2009 May–June;10(4):663–672.

54. National Institute of Arthritis and Musculoskeletal and Skin Diseases (NIAMSD). *Questions and Answers About Fibromyalgia*. Rockville, MD: NIAMSD, National Institutes of Health; July 2014. (Accessed at: https://www.niams.nih.gov/health_info/fibromyalgia/#h.)

Chapter 27

Pain and Addiction in Patients Who Smoke Cigarettes

LORI D. KARAN, M.D., DFASAM, FACP

Cigarette smokers are more likely than non-smokers to develop chronic pain, to report more intense pain, to request higher amounts of opioid analgesics, to experience depression and other mood disorders, and to suffer greater effects of their pain on their daily activities, including sleep, work, and recreation.

It is easy to ignore a patient's nicotine and tobacco use. Smoking cigarettes is not often on the patient's radar in terms of his or her pain. By fine-tuning emotions and medicating withdrawal, nicotine and tobacco use can be perceived by patients as providing comfort and serving as their best "false friend."

Because the usual doses of nicotine do not cause behavioral abnormalities associated with gross intoxication, and the health consequences of tobacco use are subtle and chronic, a patient's motivation to address cigarette smoking and other forms of nicotine and tobacco use often is deficient or lacking. However, instead of overlooking this problem, it is the clinician's duty to bring nicotine and tobacco use to the forefront. The clinician can make a major contribution by educating and motivating the patient, as well as assisting him or her with tobacco cessation.

Cigarette smokers inhale both nicotine and tobacco combustion products. Whereas nicotine is the psychoactive component that maintains addiction, it is the tobacco combustion products that produce the majority of the cardiovascular, pulmonary, and oncological morbidity and mortality that are experienced by cigarette smokers. Since the effects of nicotine and tobacco are not separated in many of the epidemiological studies cited in this article, it is difficult to know whether the use of e-cigarettes, which do not contain tobacco or result in its combustion, will have the same health effects as cigarettes so clearly do.

Incidence and Prevalence of Cigarette Smoking

The prevalence of cigarette smoking is 17–18% in the general population, 24–42% in chronic pain patients, and as high as 50–68% in patients enrolled in pain treatment programs [1].

One study found that, of 5,350 patients admitted to the Mayo Comprehensive Rehabilitation Center from January 1998 through December 2012, 25.2% (95% confidence interval [CI] 22.8–28.3) of patients with fibromyalgia, 22.8% (95% CI 21.3–25.9) of patients with low back pain, and 21.2% (95% CI 17.9–24.7) of patients with headache were current smokers.

Moreover, the prevalence of smoking did not decline in this patient population over the 15-year time span covered by the study. Whereas the overall prevalence of smoking among U.S. adults declined from 20.9% in 2005 to 15.1% in 2015 [2], the prevalence of cigarette smoking among patients enrolled in the Mayo Comprehensive Rehabilitation Center in 2000, 2005, and 2010 was 24.2%, 25.7%, and 28.3%, respectively [3]. The study thus illustrates the point that smokers are over-represented among pain patients. There are important reasons why this is so.

Patients who smoke are more likely to develop low back pain and other types of chronic pain. In one study, those who reported subacute back pain (i.e., no prior back pain, coupled with soreness that lasted 4–12 weeks) were three times more likely to report chronic back pain a year later than were nonsmokers [4]. In a longitudinal study in which 9,600 twins were followed for eight years, investigators found a dose–response relationship, in that study subjects who smoked more than 20 cigarettes a day at baseline were four times more likely to have low back pain at follow-up [5]. A number of studies also have associated smoking with the onset of fibromyalgia, chronic headache, rheumatoid arthritis, osteoarthritis, and other chronic pain conditions.

Clinical Effects of Cigarette Smoking

Smoking and the Musculoskeletal System

Smoking has a detrimental effect on the ligaments and tendons of the musculoskeletal system, as evidenced by the fact that smokers are 1.5 times more likely to suffer overuse injuries (such as bursitis and tendonitis) than are nonsmokers [6]. They also are more likely to suffer traumatic injuries such as sprains and fractures [7].

Smoking increases the risk for osteoporosis by reducing blood supply to the bones, slowing the production of osteoblasts, reducing calcium absorption from the diet, and breaking down estrogen more quickly in the body. Compared with nonsmokers, smokers have a 17% greater risk of hip fractures at age 60, which increases to a 71% greater risk at age 80. Not surprisingly, at age 80, smokers had a 6% lower bone mineral density than nonsmokers [8]. Jaramillo and colleagues [8] found that male smokers had a small but significantly greater risk of low volumetric bone marrow density and a larger number of fractures than female smokers. Jaramillo and colleagues suggest that male smokers should be screened with quantitative computed tomography (which is more sensitive than standard dual-energy X-ray absorptiometry) to facilitate earlier diagnosis of and treatment for osteoporosis [8].

A study of the effects of tobacco smoking on the degeneration of the intervertebral discs found that nicotine-mediated downregulation of cell anabolism reduced the glycosaminoglycan concentration at the cartilage endplate by 65% or more, thereby reducing the health of the discs. At the same time [9], the cell density and glycosaminoglycan levels in the nucleus pulposus were reduced by as much as half their normal values through smoking-induced vasoconstriction that reduced the exchange of nutrients and anabolic agents between blood vessels and disc tissue.

The same study found that quitting smoking had only limited benefit in terms of the regeneration of the degenerated intervertebral disc, whereas cell-based therapy in conjunction with smoking cessation provided significant improvements in disc health [9].

Cigarette smoke impairs oxygen delivery to tissues by increasing sympathetic outflow and carboxyhemoglobin levels [10]. Carbon monoxide, which may exceed 10% in smokers, binds to hemoglobin, reducing the amount available to carry oxygen. Carbon monoxide also shifts the oxyhemoglobin dissociation curve to the left, impeding release of oxygen from hemoglobin [11].

Smokers have a higher rate of postoperative infections than do nonsmokers [12], as well as poorer wound healing. In addition to problems with tissue oxygenation, microvascular disease caused by smoking also may interfere with angiogenesis through impaired release of substances such as nitric oxide that are important for wound repair [13].

Also, lower levels of bone mineral density in smokers lead to increased risk for fractures, heightened pain, complications in postoperative wound and bone healing, reduced rates of bone fusion, and postoperative complications in tendon and ligament healing [14].

Smoking Increases the Severity of Pain

Cigarette smoke triggers the release of proinflammatory cytokines, which increase inflammation and intensify pain [15]. For example, in a study of 4,259 smokers and 21,206 nonsmokers enrolled in the National Spine Network database, researchers found that smokers experienced more severe pain for a greater proportion of each day than did nonsmokers. Among patients with fibromyalgia, smokers reported greater pain intensity than nonsmokers, even after adjusting for education, employment, marital status, and history of abuse [16].

Smoking contributes to the onset and exacerbation of pain, which in turn motivates continued smoking. This results in greater pain and motivates the maintenance of tobacco addiction [17].

Smokers who report using cigarettes to cope with pain typically describe greater intensity of pain, pain interference, and fear of pain than do nonsmokers or smokers who say they have not used smoking as a coping strategy, even after controlling for relevant demographic characteristics, pain-related variables, depressive symptoms, and prescription opioid use. While causation cannot be determined from a cross-sectional study, those who smoked cigarettes to cope with pain did report poorer pain outcomes [18].

Smokers Are Prescribed Larger Doses of Opioid Analgesics for Longer Periods of Time

In another study performed at the Mayo Clinic, past or current tobacco use and substance abuse both were significantly associated with progression from a new opioid prescription to episodic or chronic opioid use one year later [19,20].

A study that compared military veterans of Operations Enduring Freedom/ Iraqi Freedom/New Dawn who smoked, with veterans of the same theaters who did not smoke (and which also controlled for age, service-connected disability, gender, obesity, substance abuse, mood disorders, and post-traumatic stress disorder), found that subjects who smoked reported greater pain intensity than did nonsmokers. In that study, current smokers were more likely than nonsmokers to receive an opioid prescription, even when their current pain intensity was controlled [21].

Persons with Tobacco Use Disorder Are at Increased Risk for Opioid Misuse

In one study, researchers examined 821,916 opioid claims in an insurer's national database, which were divided into those with (n = 6,380) and without (n = 815,536) a diagnosis of opioid use disorder (OUD). They found that individuals diagnosed with OUD were 1.45 times more likely to be smokers than nonsmokers [22].

Smokers Report More Associated Mood Disorders

Anxiety and depression have been related to the onset and maintenance of both chronic pain and tobacco dependence [23]. In addition, studies have found that co-occurring depression and anxiety are likely to mediate pain, smoking, and the pain–smoking interaction [24].

Smoking also can be part of the picture in depressed, overweight, sedentary patients, many of whom also have diabetes, cardiovascular ailments, chronic obstructive pulmonary disease (COPD), and/or sleep apnea. For example, smokers have a 30–40% greater risk of diabetes than do nonsmokers [25]. In part, this is because smoking increases inflammation and oxidative stress.

Smoking Promotes Addictive Behavior

Interactions between the nucleus accumbens, the amygdala, and the prefrontal cortex are thought to trigger the reinforcement of addiction [26,27]. Recent functional magnetic resonance imaging (fMRI) studies demonstrate that smoking predicts pain chronification (as in transitioning from subacute back pain to chronic back pain) by mediating the functional connectivity between the nucleus accumbens and the medial prefrontal cortex of the brain [4].

Chronic smoking also upregulates nicotinic acetylcholinergic receptors (nAChR) and greater nAChR availability during periods of abstinence from smoking has been associated with increased pain reactivity [28]. Nicotine withdrawal is associated with hyperalgesia in nicotine-tolerant rodents—a state that can be reversed by administering morphine [29].

Corticotropin-releasing factor (CRF/CRF1R) in the central amygdala has been shown to mediate nicotine withdrawal-induced increases in sensitivity to painful stimuli [30]. In mice, nAChR modulates nicotine analgesia and is central to the expression of anxiety and depression-like behaviors [31]. Rat models of nicotine self-administration implicate corticotropin-releasing factor 1 (CRF1) receptors in the manifestation of anxiety-like behaviors, as well as increased levels of pain during nicotine deprivation [32].

Metabolic Considerations

Smoking affects the metabolism of many medications, and these medications may need to be adjusted after smoking cessation occurs. For example, the polycyclic hydrocarbons of tobacco smoke induce predominantly CYP1A2 and possibly CYP2E1 & CYP450 enzymes. Interactions between smoking and methadone, duloxetine, ethanol, and acetaminophen need to be considered, because methadone is metabolized by CYP3A4 and CYP1A2, duloxetine is metabolized by CYP1A2, and ethanol and acetaminophen are metabolized by CYP2E1 [33].

Smoking reduces the plasma concentrations of alprazolam by up to 50% and of haloperidol by up to 70% [34]. It also may impede insulin absorption secondary to peripheral vasoconstriction, and trigger the release of endogenous substances that promote insulin resistance.

The concentrations in the patient's system of many psychiatric and other medications fluctuate with smoking as well as smoking cessation, when the requirements for opioid medications may decline. An improved therapeutic outcome can be achieved with medication levels that are more stable after smoking cessation [35].

Benefits of Smoking Cessation

Improvements in oxygenation, musculoskeletal health, and healing begin rapidly after smoking cessation and accumulate over time (see Table 27.1).

In a study that compared patients who continued to smoke during the course of treatment for painful spine disorders with patients who quit smoking, those who stopped smoking reported significantly greater improvements in pain in terms of "worst pain," "current pain," and "average weekly pain." The mean improvement in ratings on the visual analog pain scale was clinically important among patients who never smoked, those who were prior

TABLE 27.1 Physiological Improvements Following Smoking Cessation

Time After Last Cigarette	Physiological Change
20 minutes	HR/BP returns to normal.
12 hours	Blood CO levels decline.
2 weeks–3 months	Lung function improves.
1 month–9 months	Coughing and shortness of breath improve.
1 year	Added risk of CAD drops to half that of a smoker.
5–15 years	Risk of stroke is comparable to that of a nonsmoker. Risk of mouth/throat/esophageal cancer is half that of a smoker.
10 years	Risk of lung cancer is half that of a smoker.

Abbreviations: HR/BP = heart rate and blood pressure; CO = carbon monoxide; CAD = coronary artery disease.

Source: American Cancer Society, Inc.: *Benefits of Quitting Smoking Over Time*; 2016. Reprinted by permission.

smokers, and those who recently quit smoking. In contrast, patients who continued smoking during treatment had no clinically important improvement in reported pain [36].

The results of these studies indicate that smoking cessation may be a prerequisite for alleviating pain, and that delaying smoking cessation until a patient's pain has improved may be counterproductive. They also suggest that physicians who treat tobacco-dependent patients for pain should motivate them toward smoking cessation as soon as possible.

Motivating Smoking Cessation

Despite the fact that smoking cessation may reduce pain and promote bone health and healing, it is challenging to persuade tobacco users (even those experiencing pain) to commit to a smoking cessation plan.

Smoking affects health care as well as health outcomes. For example, patients who are to undergo orthopedic surgery require bone remodeling to heal. Similarly, surgery to address an underlying condition, or procedures such as spinal cord stimulators to assist with pain relief, depend on the oxygenation and health of tissue for a successful result. Smoking cigarettes increases the risk that bones will not heal properly, as well as the potential for post-operative infection. This is such an important factor that some surgeons and interventionalists require patients to stop smoking for three months before they will perform elective procedures.

In each of these situations, the motivation to stop smoking is clear. However, in cases involving chronic health problems for which a physical intervention is not planned, motivating a patient to stop smoking can be more difficult. The patient may be caught in a vicious cycle of using smoking to cope with anxiety, depression, and pain, all the while furthering hyperalgesia and the craving for a cigarette. In one study [37], daily smokers recruited from the community who experienced past-month pain typically reported less confidence in their ability to remain abstinent, as well as greater difficulty during their most recent attempt to quit smoking.

Conclusion

Smoking cessation is an accomplishment to be celebrated. The benefits of quitting smoking begin within minutes of smoking the last cigarette and accumulate over time [38].

Prospects for success improve when medications, cognitive-behavioral therapies, and addiction treatments are combined in a comprehensive approach. Addressing anxiety and weight gain, as well as providing continuing care, are important steps in preventing relapse.

Tobacco cessation and the treatment of tobacco use disorders are covered in many excellent references, such as http://www.chestnet.org/Publications/ Other-Publications/Tobacco-Dependence-Toolkit (also see the text box at the end of this chapter).

For More Information on the Topics Discussed:

American Society of Addiction Medicine (ASAM):

Hurt RD, Ebbert JO, Hays JT, McFadden DD. Pharmacologic interventions for tobacco dependence (Chapter 53). In RK Ries, DA Fiellin, SC Miller, R Saitz, eds. *The ASAM Principles of Addiction Medicine, Fifth Edition.* Philadelphia, PA: Wolters Kluwer; 2014.

Kahler CW, Bloom EL, Leventhal AM, Brown RA. Behavioral interventions in smoking cessation (Chapter 59). In RK Ries, DA Fiellin, SC Miller, R Saitz, eds. *The ASAM Principles of Addiction Medicine, Fifth Edition.* Philadelphia, PA: Wolters Kluwer; 2014.

American Academy of Family Physicians (AAFP):

Healthy Interventions: Tobacco and Nicotine Cessation Toolkit. (Access at: http:// www.aafp.org/patient-care/public-health/tobacco-nicotine/toolkit. html?cmpid=_van_915.)

American College of Obstetricians and Gynecologists (ACOG):

Smoking Cessation During Pregnancy: A Clinician's Guide. (Access at: http:// www.acog.org/~/media/Departments/Tobacco%20Alcohol%20and%20 Substance%20Abuse/SCDP.pdf?dmc=1&ts=20130123T1641376641.)

American College of Physicians (ACP):

Smoking Cessation Resources. (Access at: https://www.acponline.org/ gsearch/smoking?site=ACP_Online.)

Centers for Disease Control and Prevention (CDC):

The following CDC resources for clinicians can be accessed at: https:// www.cdc.gov/tobacco/campaign/tips/partners/health/hcp/.

- *Treating Tobacco Use and Dependence: A Quick Reference Guide for Clinicians*
- **FAQs for Health Care Providers** A printable, pocket-sized tobacco intervention card that lists steps for conducting a brief tobacco intervention with patients.

CDC resources for patients include:

- Handout for Patients: *Reasons to Quit Smoking.*
- *QuitGuide Mobile App.* QuitGuide is a free app that helps patients understand their smoking patterns and build the skills needed to become and remain smoke-free. For example, the app allows patients to track

cravings by time of day and location. It also provides inspirational messages for each craving to help patients stay focused on smoking cessation. (Access at: https://www.cdc.gov/tobacco/campaign/tips/quit-smoking/mobile-quit-guide/index.html?s_cid=OSH_tips_D9405.)

- Patients can obtain free help with quitting smoking by calling 1-800-784-8669 (or, for Spanish speakers, 1-855-335-3569).

National Institute on Drug Abuse (NIDA):

Drug Facts: Cigarettes and Other Tobacco Products (March 2017). This free guide provides an overview of the effects of smoking on the brain, other health effects, and approaches to smoking cessation. Also available in Spanish. (Access at: https://www.drugabuse.gov/publications/drugfacts/cigarettes-other-tobacco-products.)

References

1. Bastian LA. Cigarette smoking as a risk factor for opioid use. National VA Teleconference; Nov. 1, 2016.
2. Centers for Disease Control and Prevention (CDC). *Smoking and Tobacco Use Fact Sheet.* Atlanta, GA: CDC, U.S. Department of Health and Human Services; Dec. 2015.
3. Orhurhu VJ, Pittelkow TP, Hooten WM. Prevalence of smoking in adults with chronic pain. *Tobacco Induced Diseases.* 2015;13:17.
4. Petre B, Torbey S, Griffith JW, et al. Smoking increases risk of pain chronification through shared corticostriatal circuitry. *Hum Brain Mapp.* 2015 Feb;36(2):683–694.
5. Hestback L, Leboeuf-Yde C, Kyvik KO. Are lifestyle factors in adolescence predictors for adult low back pain? A cross-sectional and prospective study of young twins. *BMC Musculoskelet Disord.* 2006;7:27.
6. American Academy of Orthopedic Surgeons (AAOS). *Ortho Information: Smoking and Musculoskeletal Health.* (Accessed at: http://orthoinfo.aaos.org/topic.cfm?topic=a00192.)
7. Law MR, Hackshaw AK. A meta-analysis of cigarette smoking, bone mineral density and risk of hip fracture: Recognition of a major effect. *BMJ.* 1997;315:841–846.
8. Jaramillo JD, Wilson C, Stinson DJ, et al., and the COPD Gene Investigators. Reduced bone density and vertebral fractures in smokers. Men and COPD patients at increased risk. *Ann Am Thorac Soc.* 2015 May;12(5):648–656.
9. Elmasry S, Asfour S, de Rivero Vaccari JP, et al. Effects of tobacco smoking on the degeneration of the intervertebral disc: A finite element study. *PLoS One.* 2015 Aug 24;10(8):e0136137.
10. Narkiewicz K, van de Born PJ, Hausberg M, et al. Cigarette smoking increases sympathetic outflow in humans. *Circulation.* 1998;98:528–534.
11. Rietbrock N, Kunkel S, Worner V, et al. Oxygen-dissociation kinetics in the blood of smokers and non-smokers: Interaction between oxygen and carbon

monoxide at the hemoglobin molecule. *Naunyn Schmiedebergs Arch Pharmacol.* 1992:345:123–128.

12. Sorensen LT. Wound healing and infection in surgery: The clinical impact of smoking and smoking cessation: A systematic review and meta-analysis. *Arch Surg.* 2012;147(4):373–383.

13. Hashimoto H. Impaired microvascular vasodilator reserve in chronic cigarette smokers: A study of post-occlusive reactive hyperemia in the human finger. *JapanCirc J.* 1994;58:29–33.

14. Wright E, Tzeng TH, Ginnetti M, et al. Effect of smoking on joint replacement outcomes: Opportunities for improvement through preoperative smoking cessation. Instr Course Lecture #38; *American Academy of Orthopedic Surgeons.* 2016;65:509–520.

15. O'Loughlin J, Lambert M, Karp I, et al. Association between cigarette smoking and C-reactive protein in representative, population-based sample of adolescents. *Nicotine Tob Res.* 2008:10:525–532.

16. Vogt MT, Hanscom B, Lauerman C, et al. Influence of smoking on the health status of spinal patients: The National Spine Network Database. *Spine.* 2002;27:313–319.

17. Weingarten TN, Podduturu VR, Hooten WM, et al. Impact of tobacco use in patients presenting to a multidisciplinary outpatient treatment program for fibromyalgia. *Clin J Pain.* 2009 Jan;25(1):39–43.

18. Ditre JW, Langdon KJ, Kosiba JD, et al. Relations between pain-related anxiety, tobacco dependence, and barriers to quitting among a community-based sample of daily smokers. *Addict Behav.* 2015 Mar; 42:130–135.

19. Patterson AL, Gritzner S, Resnick MP, et al. Smoking cigarettes as a coping strategy for chronic pain is associated with greater pain intensity and poorer pain-related function. *J Pain.* 2012 March 13;(3):285–292.

20. Hooten WM, St. Sauver JL, McGree ME, et al. Incidence and risk factors for progression from acute to longer-term opioid prescribing: A population-based study. *Mayo Clin Proc.* 2015 July;90(7):850–856.

21. Volkman JE, DeRycke EC, Driscoll MA, et al. Smoking status and pain intensity among OEF/OIF/OND veterans. *Pain Med.* 2015 Sep;16(0):1690–1696.

22. Volkman JE, DeRycke EC, Bastian LA, et al. Smoking status and pain intensity among OEF/OIF/OND veterans. *Pain Med.* 2015 Sep;16(9):1690–1696.

23. Rice JB. A model to identify patients at risk for prescription opioid abuse, dependence, and misuse. *Pain Med.* 2012;13:1162–1173.

24. Shi Y, Weingarten TN, Mantilla CB, et al. Smoking and pain: Pathophysiology and clinical implications. *Anesthesiology.* 2010;113:977–992.

25. Zale EL, Maisto SA, Ditre JW. Anxiety and depression in bidirectional relations between pain and smoking: Implications for smoking cessation. *Behav Modif.* 2016 Jan;40(1–2):7–28.

26. Hooten WM, Shi Y, Gazelka HM, et al. The effects of depression and smoking on pain severity and opioid use in patients with chronic pain. *Pain.* 2011;152:223–229.

27. Centers for Disease Control and Prevention (CDC). *Smoking and Diabetes.* Atlanta, GA: CDC, U.S. Department of Health and Human Services; 2014. (Accessed at: https://www.cdc.gov/tobacco/campaign/tips/diseases/diabetes.html.)

28. DeBiasi M, Dani JA. Reward, addiction, withdrawal to nicotine. *Annu Rev Neurosci.* 2011;34:105–130.

29. Everitt BJ, Robbins TW. Neural systems of reinforcement for drug addiction: From actions to habits to compulsion. *Nat Neurosci.* 2005;8:1481–1489.

30. Cosgrove KP, Esterlis I, McKee S, et al. Beta2* nicotinic acetylcholine receptors modulate pain sensitivity in acutely abstinent tobacco smokers. *Nicotine Tob Res.* 2010;12:535–539.

31. Schmidt BL, Tambeli CH, Gear RW, et al. Nicotine withdrawal hyperalgesia and opioid-mediated analgesia depend on nicotine receptors in nucleus accumbens. *Neuroscience.* 2001;106(1):129–136.

32. Balamonte BA, Valenza M, Roltsch EA, et al. Nicotine dependence produces hyperalgesia: Role of corticotropin-releasing factor-1 receptors (CRF1Rs) in the central amygdala (CeA). *Neuropharmacology.* 2014 Feb;77:217–223.

33. Semenova S, Contet C, Roberts AJ, et al. Mice lacking the beta4 subunit of the nicotinic acetylcholine receptor show memory deficits, altered anxiety, and depression-like behavior, and diminished nicotine-induced analgesia. *Nicotine Tob Res.* 2012;14:1346–1355.

34. Cohen A, Treweek J, Edwards S, et al. Extended access to nicotine leads to a CRF1 receptor dependent increase in anxiety-like behavior and hyperalgesia in rats. *Addict Biol.* 2015;20:56–68.

35. Behrend C, Prasarn M, Coyne E, et al. Smoking cessation related to improved patient-reported pain scores following spinal care. *J Bone Joint Surg Am.* 2012;94:2161–2166.

36. Coffman BL, Rios GR, King CD, et al. Human UGT2B7 catalyzes morphine glucuronidation. *Drug Metab Dispos.* 1997;25:1–4.

37. Green MD, Belanger G, Hum DW, et al. Glucuronidation of opioids, carboxylic acid-containing drugs and hydroxylated xenobiotics catalyzed by expressed monkey UDP-glucuronosyltransferase 2B9 protein. *Drug Metab Dispos.* 1997;23(12):1389–1394.

38. Yoon JH, Lane SD, Weaver MF. Opioid analgesics and nicotine: More than blowing smoke. *J Pain Palliat Care Pharmacother.* 2015;29(3):281–289.

Chapter 28

Pain and Addiction in Adolescents and Young Adults

MICHAEL F. WEAVER, M.D., DFASAM

Adolescents and young adults experience acute and chronic pain just as adults do, but there are important differences between this population and adult patients in terms of available treatments. For example, because of ongoing development of the brain, adolescents are at elevated risk for misuse and abuse of opioid analgesics and related substances, as well as for serious and long-lasting consequences of such misuse.

On a positive note, treatment modalities for opioid use disorder that are appropriate for adolescents and young adults are available, including medication-assisted treatment with opioids such as methadone and buprenorphine.

This chapter will review the incidence of chronic pain and substance use disorders (SUDs) in adolescents, as well as treatment protocols whose efficacy is supported by the research literature.

Incidence of Chronic Pain in Adolescents and Young Adults

Experts have estimated that 15–25% of all children and adolescents suffer from recurrent or chronic pain [1,2]. Headache, abdominal pain, and musculoskeletal pain account for most of the recurrent painful states in this age group [2].

Children with recurrent headaches are at risk of developing additional physical and mental problems (such as anxiety and depression) as adults [3]. In addition, recurrent abdominal pain among children and adolescents not only affects physical and psychosocial aspects of daily family life, but also may predispose children to experience recurrent pain-related illnesses in adulthood [4].

In one study, 30–40% of children and adolescents who experienced pain reported that their pain had a moderate effect on their school attendance, participation in hobbies, maintenance of social contacts, appetite, and sleep. The study subjects' utilization of health care services also increased because of their pain [5]. In addition, the number of children who reported that they were unable to pursue hobbies because of pain increased with age [5].

Pain-related restrictions in daily activities also increased with age, as did utilization of health care services. Children and adolescents with abdominal, limb, and/or back pain reported visiting a doctor more often than those with headache pain. However, children and adolescents with headache were more likely to report taking medications for their pain [5].

These data underscore the reasons acute or chronic pain may lead to a child or adolescent's initial exposure to a mood-altering substance in the form of an opioid prescribed for pain relief.

Treatment of Chronic Pain in Adolescents and Young Adults

Treatment of specific pain syndromes in children and adolescents is beyond the scope of this chapter. Many basic principles of pain management in adults also apply to children, adolescents, and young adults. However, there are some specific considerations for use of pain medications in pediatric populations, including weight-based dosing and the immaturity of certain drug metabolism pathways. Many medications used regularly in adults have not been studied in pediatric populations, so little guidance on optimal dosing is available.

Some non-pharmacological treatment modalities, such as mindfulness therapy (see Chapter 21 of this Handbook) have been evaluated in pediatric populations, but they require that the age and maturity level of the patient be assessed. A systematic review has demonstrated the effectiveness of psychological outpatient treatments, especially for children and adolescents with chronic headache [5]. In adolescents, use of opioid analgesics can be appropriate for acute or chronic pain, but caution is advised because this population is vulnerable to misuse, as described earlier.

Incidence of Substance Use Disorders in Adolescents and Young Adults

The incidence of SUDs has increased steadily among adolescents in recent years, as have the associated risks of fatal and non-fatal drug overdoses, motor vehicle crashes, suicides attempted and completed, homicides, domestic violence, criminality, risky sexual practices, unintended pregnancies, and developmental problems that may have lifelong consequences [6]. Because adolescent substance use can be conceptualized as a continuum from experimentation to diagnosis of a full-blown SUD, it is more helpful to describe *use patterns* (behaviors that may influence health), rather than the *incidence of addiction* [7].

Adolescents and young adults have unique vulnerabilities and needs, stemming from their immature neurocognitive and psychosocial development. For example, recent studies show that the brain undergoes a prolonged process of development and refinement throughout the period from birth to early adulthood. During this process, a developmental shift occurs, as a result of which actions evolve from more impulsive to more reasoned and reflective. In fact, the brain areas most closely associated with aspects of behavior such as decision-making, judgment, planning, and self-control undergo a period of rapid development during adolescence [6]. The initial impulsivity associated with ongoing brain development helps explain why adolescents have such high rates of substance use.

There are several excellent sources of information about the prevalence of adolescent substance use, including the Monitoring the Future survey [8], Youth Risk Behavior Surveillance System survey [9], and National Survey on Drug Use and Health (Table 28.1) [10]. The source of information for this chapter is Monitoring the Future (MTF), a national survey of drug use that has been administered annually since 1975 and that offers a comprehensive view of the factors that influence drug use. In addition to surveying young people about their drug use, MTF addresses important factors such as survey subjects' beliefs about the dangers of nonmedical drug use and the perceived availability of drugs [11].

When MTF began in 1975, 55.2% of young people surveyed reported that they had used an illicit drug by the time they left high school. By 1980, this number had increased to 65.4%, before gradually declining to 40.7% in 1992. The proportion increased again in 1999 to 54.7%, then gradually declined to 47% by 2009, rising again to 49.1% in 2012 [11].

From the time eighth and tenth graders were first included in the survey in 1991, trends for that age group have paralleled those of twelfth graders, albeit at lower levels of use [11]. In 2012, 13.4% of eighth graders, 30.1% of tenth graders, and 39.7% of twelfth graders reported use of an illicit drug in the preceding year [12].

TABLE 28.1 Any Self-Reported Misuse of Drugs by Adolescents and Young Adults in Past Year and Past Month, 2015–2016

Drug	Time Period	Number Ages 12 to 17 (in thousands)		Number Ages 18 to 25 (in thousands)	
		2015	2016	2015	2016
Pain Relievers	Past Year	969	881	2,979	2,454
	Past Month	276	239	829	631
Heroin	Past Year	35	32	217	227
	Past Month	5	3	88	88
Tranquilizers	Past Year	394	434	1,874	1,844
	Past Month	162	121	582	536
Sedatives	Past Year	102	100	265	256
	Past Month	21	23	86	50
Prescription Stimulants	Past Year	491	427	2,537	2,578
	Past Month	117	92	757	767
Hallucinogens	Past Year	523	456	2,453	2,388
	Past Month	121	114	636	668
Marijuana	Past Year	3,137	2,982	11,246	11,401
	Past Month	1,752	1,609	6,921	7,184
Tobacco Products	Past Year	2,877	2,607	15,301	14,014
	Past Month	1,492	1,324	11,516	10,359
Alcohol	Past Year	5,652	5,385	26,355	25,720
	Past Month	2,392	2,289	20,367	19,754

Source: Adapted from Substance Abuse and Mental Health Services Administration (SAMHSA). *Results from the 2016 National Survey on Drug Use and Health: Detailed Tables.* Rockville, MD: SAMHSA, U.S. Department of Health and Human Services; September 2017. (Access at: https://www.samhsa.gov/data/sites/default/files/NSDUH-DetTabs-2016/NSDUH-DetTabs-2016.pdf).

"Nonmedical use" of prescription medications refers to use of a scheduled prescription medication (analgesics, stimulants, and tranquilizers/sedatives) outside of medical supervision. Although the proportion of twelfth graders who reported nonmedical use of prescription medications has remained stable since 2008, the annual prevalence in 2012 was still high, with 14.8% of twelfth graders reporting use of such agents in the preceding year.

Young people appear to believe that prescription drugs are less dangerous than illicit or "street" drugs and thus seem more inclined to use them [12]. Concerns have arisen regarding youth initiating opioid use with oral prescription medications and quickly becoming dependent on opioids, leading them to switch to intranasal and injectable drugs such as heroin out of economic necessity [6]. The sources of such prescription drugs remain primarily friends and (to a lesser extent) relatives [11], although recent surveys have implicated prescriptions from physicians and other providers [13].

For twelfth grade students, use of opioids other than heroin trended downward from 1977 through 1992. However, beginning in 1992, opioid use rose sharply, reaching an annual prevalence of 9.5% in 2004 [13]. In 2002, MTF included specific questions about use of OxyContin®, Vicodin®, and Percocet®. Since then, use of OxyContin has increased across all age groups, with annual prevalence rates of 1.6% for eighth graders, 3.0% for tenth graders, and 4.3% for twelfth grade students in 2012 [14]. Use of Vicodin has been steady at even higher levels, with annual prevalence rates of 1.3% among eighth graders, 4.4% among tenth graders, and 7.5% among twelfth grade students in the same time span [14].

Adolescents and young adults who seek treatment for SUDs typically present with complex treatment issues such as injection drug use, HIV risk related to sexual behaviors, abscesses, hepatitis C infection, school dropout, legal problems, and the like [15,16].

Adolescents' SUDs also are associated quite often with co-occurring mental disorders. These include attention-deficit/hyperactivity disorder (ADHD), oppositional defiance and conduct disorders, as well as depression and anxiety disorders [6]. Despite their relatively short addiction histories, patients younger than 18 years of age are at particularly high risk for serious complications of drug use, including overdose deaths, suicide, and HIV and other infectious diseases [16,17].

Treatment of Substance Use Disorders in Adolescents and Young Adults

Despite the growing number of adolescents and young adults who have opioid use disorder, the development and adoption of pharmacotherapies for this population has been slow [18,19]. One reason could be the practical and ethical difficulties involved in conducting drug trials in young people [20]. Moreover, some parents of adolescent patients object to agonist therapy. Also, young people with opioid use disorder may be ineligible for treatment with medication-assisted therapy because of governmental policies or regulations.

Nevertheless, a sizeable number of adolescents do present for medication-assisted treatment. According to the federal Treatment Episode Data Set (TEDS), opiates were involved in 2% of adolescent treatment admissions from 2004 to 2008 and 3% from 2009 to 2014. Opiates other than heroin represented 43% of adolescent admissions involving opiates in 2004. This increased to 67% in 2010, but fell to 42% in 2014. Over the same time period, the proportion of admissions for primary heroin use disorder increased by 36% (that is, from 262,518 in 2004 to 357,293 in 2014). In contrast, the proportion of heroin admissions for which the treatment plan included medication-assisted therapy (using methadone or buprenorphine) declined from 31% in 2004 to 28% in 2014 [21].

At present, most adolescents who enter treatment receive brief detoxification followed by psychosocial therapies (typically in outpatient and occasionally in residential settings), even though such interventions have not been well studied in this population. The degree of substance involvement is (and ought to be) an important determinant of treatment placement for adolescents, as are any co-occurring disorders, the family and peer environment, and the individual's stage of mental and emotional development [22].

Although buprenorphine is well-established as an effective treatment for adults, the empirical evidence for use of buprenorphine in adolescents and young adults is only now emerging. A randomized, multicenter trial of buprenorphine in youth aged 15–21 showed that the best outcomes occurred in adolescents who were randomized to the extended (12-week) regimen, with the dose tapered during the last four weeks of treatment [19]. A secondary analysis showed that compliance with various doses depended heavily on the adolescents' perception of pain [23].

Based on these studies, many addiction experts believe that buprenorphine is a viable treatment option for adolescent patients who have short addiction histories. Additionally, buprenorphine may be an appropriate treatment option for adolescent patients who have longer histories of opioid use disorder and multiple relapses, but who are not currently physically dependent on opioids [24].

Before beginning medication-assisted therapy, adolescent patients should have a complete evaluation, including a thorough substance use history, to confirm the diagnosis of opioid addiction. The evaluation also should include the patient's medical, mental health, and vocational and psychosocial histories, and must include a physical examination. All active problems should be addressed so that they do not interfere with recovery. Routine laboratory tests are recommended, particularly urine toxicology tests to confirm opioid use and to evaluate concomitant use of benzodiazepines (because of the risk they pose for death from overdose), and liver enzymes to assess hepatic function.

Whenever possible, treating physicians should engage parents or guardians in the treatment process to provide authority and structure, both of which improve adolescent treatment adherence, allow for prompt intervention when a relapse occurs, and minimize the risk of diversion [25].

Induction, Dosing, and Duration of Treatment

In treating adolescents and young adults, observed induction is recommended, accompanied by education of the patient and family about the importance of adherence. If possible, parents should be engaged in monitoring of medication adherence and for adverse effects such as drowsiness.

The relatively long half-life of buprenorphine permits once-daily dosing. In research studies, maintenance doses for adolescents have ranged from 2–24 mg/day, with 59% of patients stabilized on 9–16 mg/day. It is considered optimal to dose until the adolescent no longer reports withdrawal symptoms or craving for opioids. Since there is no scientific evidence regarding the optimal duration of buprenorphine treatment in adolescents, it is best not to hurry to wean such patients off buprenorphine. The length of treatment (which may be a year or longer) should be guided by the patient's progress, in consultation with the patient and a parent or legal guardian.

Even patients with short histories of opioid use disorder (less than one or two years) may relapse quickly after use of the treatment medication is stopped. For this reason, medications should be tapered slowly to avoid withdrawal symptoms and/or the resurgence of craving [16]. It also is appropriate to recommend that non-pharmacological therapies be continued.

A secondary analysis of a multi-center, randomized clinical trial in which 152 youth (ages 15–21 years) were treated for opioid use disorder compared a 12-week course of buprenorphine/naloxone with a two-week course of buprenorphine detoxification and weekly counseling [26]. Investigators found that adolescent subjects with advanced illness (for example, involving injection drug use and additional health problems) and those receiving ancillary treatments (such as counseling or mutual support group engagement) were the most likely to have reduced their nonmedical opioid use as a result of treatment [26].

Overall, the adolescent patients who were successful in the first two weeks of treatment with buprenorphine and those who completed the full 12 weeks of treatment had the best outcomes (defined by lower rates of relapse, as documented by urine drug tests) [26]. This analysis suggests that even adolescents with advanced opioid use disorder can achieve good outcomes from treatment with buprenorphine [27].

Family Involvement

Whenever possible, parents and family members should be involved in treatment. In many cases, parents are aware of their child's drug use. Therefore, the adolescent should be asked to give permission to the treating physician to discuss his or her diagnosis, treatment recommendations, and progress with his or her parents.

In order to protect the therapeutic relationship with the adolescent, it is best to avoid providing parents with details of the situation that do not affect treatment. Note that in some states, written parental consent may be required before medication therapy can be initiated; prescribers should be cognizant of the laws and regulations in their state, which typically can be accessed by contacting their state medical licensing board [27].

Conclusion

Adolescents and young adults comprise a critically underserved target population because of the epidemic of prescription opioid abuse and heroin abuse in their ranks. As a society, we seem to lack a sense of urgency and a coherent national response to this epidemic, although there are hopeful signs that an increasing sense of urgency in many communities and among health care professionals will move the situation forward. The growing body of evidence regarding treatment of chronic pain and opioid use disorder in adolescents and young adults is a most encouraging development.

For More Information on the Topics Discussed:

American Society of Addiction Medicine (ASAM):

Brooks TL, Knight JR. Screening and brief intervention for adolescents (Chapter 103). In RK Ries, DA Fiellin, SC Miller, R Saitz, eds. *The ASAM Principles of Addiction Medicine, Fourth Edition.* Philadelphia, PA: Wolters Kluwer; 2014.

Griffin KW, Botvin GH. Preventing substance use among children and adolescents (Chapter 101). In RK Ries, DA Fiellin, SC Miller, R Saitz, eds. *The ASAM Principles of Addiction Medicine, Fourth Edition.* Philadelphia, PA: Wolters Kluwer; 2014.

Simkin DS. Neurobiology of addiction from a developmental perspective (Chapter 102). In RK Ries, DA Fiellin, SC Miller, R Saitz, eds. *The ASAM Principles of Addiction Medicine, Fourth Edition.* Philadelphia, PA: Wolters Kluwer; 2014.

Weddle M, Kokotailo PK. Epidemiology of adolescent substance use (Chapter 100). In RK Ries, DA Fiellin, SC Miller, R Saitz, eds. *The ASAM Principles of Addiction Medicine, Fourth Edition*. Philadelphia, PA: Wolters Kluwer; 2014.

Whiteside U, Bittinger JN, Kilmer JR, Lostutter TW, Larimer ME. College student drinking (Chapter 38). In RK Ries, DA Fiellin, SC Miller, R Saitz, eds. *The ASAM Principles of Addiction Medicine, Fourth Edition*. Philadelphia, PA: Wolters Kluwer; 2014.

Winters KC, Fahnhorst T, Botzet A, Nicholson A, Stinchfield R. Assessing adolescent substance abuse (Chapter 104). In RK Ries, DA Fiellin, SC Miller, R Saitz, eds. *The ASAM Principles of Addiction Medicine, Fourth Edition*. Philadelphia, PA: Wolters Kluwer; 2014.

ASAM National Practice Guideline for the Use of Medications in the Treatment of Addiction Involving Opioid Use. Chevy Chase, MD: ASAM; June 1, 2015. (Access at: https://www.asam.org/docs/default-source/practice-support/guidelines-and-consensus-docs/asam-national-practice-guideline-supplement.pdf?sfvrsn=24.)

References

1. Perquin CW, Hazebroek-Kampschreur AA, Hunfeld JA, et al. Pain in children and adolescents: A common experience. *Pain*. 2000;87:51–58.
2. Goodman JE, McGrath PJ. The epidemiology of pain in children and adolescents: A review. *Pain*. 1991;46:247–264.
3. Fearon P, Hotopf M. Relation between headache in childhood and physical and psychiatric symptoms in adulthood: National birth cohort study. *BMJ*. 2001;322:1145.
4. Campo JV, Di Lorenzo C, Chiappetta L, et al. Adult outcomes of pediatric recurrent abdominal pain: Do they just grow out of it? *Pediatrics*. 2001;108(1):E1.
5. Eccleston C, Morley S, Williams AC, et al. Systematic review of randomised controlled trials of psychological therapy for chronic pain in children and adolescents, with a subset of meta-analysis of pain relief. *Pain*. 2002;99:157–165.
6. Roth-Isigkeit A, Thyen U, Stöven H, et al. Pain among children and adolescents: Restrictions in daily living and triggering factors. *Pediatrics*. 2005;115(2):e152–e162.
7. National Institute on Drug Abuse (NIDA). *Principles of Drug Addiction Treatment, 2nd Edition*. NIH Publication No. 09-4180. Rockville, MD: NIDA, National Institutes of Health; 2009.
8. Weddle M, Kokotailo PK. Epidemiology of adolescent substance use (Chapter 100). In RK Ries, DA Fiellin, SC Miller, R Saitz, eds. *The ASAM Principles of Addiction Medicine, Fifth Edition*. Philadelphia, PA: Wolters Kluwer; 2014.

9. The Regents of the University of Michigan. *Monitoring the Future, 1975.* Bethesda, MD: National Institute on Drug Abuse (NIDA), National Institutes of Health, 1976. (Accessed at: www.monitoringthefuture.org.)

10. Centers for Disease Control and Prevention (CDC). *Youth Risk Behavior Survey, 1991.* Atlanta, GA: CDC, U.S. Department of Health and Human Services; 1992.

11. Substance Abuse and Mental Health Services Administration (SAMHSA). *National Survey on Drug Use and Health, 1979* (Age 12–17). Rockville, MD: SAMHSA, U.S. Department of Health and Human Services; 1979.

12. Johnston LD, O'Malley PM, Bachman JG, et al. *Monitoring the Future National Results on Adolescent Drug Use: Overview of Key Findings; 2012.* Ann Arbor, MI: Institute for Social Research, The University of Michigan; 2012.

13. Johnston LD, O'Malley PM, Bachman JG, et al. *Monitoring the Future National Survey Results on Drug Use, 1975–2011: Volume I, Secondary School Students.* Ann Arbor, MI: Institute for Social Research, The University of Michigan; 2012.

14. Hertz JA, Knight JR. Prescription drug misuse: A growing national problem. *Adolesc Med.* 2006;17:751–769.

15. Johnston LD, O'Malley PM, Bachman JG, et al. The rise in teen marijuana use stalls, synthetic marijuana use levels, and use of "bath salts" is very low. Ann Arbor, MI: University of Michigan News Service; December 19, 2012. (Accessed at: www.monitoringthefuture.org.)

16. Substance Abuse and Mental Health Services Administration (SAMHSA), Office of Applied Studies. *Results from the 2011 National Survey on Drug Use and Health (NSDUH): Summary of National Findings,* NSDUH Series H-44, HHS Publication No. (SMA) 12-4713. Rockville, MD: SAMHSA, U.S. Department of Health and Human Services; 2012.

17. Subramaniam G, Levy S, for the Physician Clinical Support System for Buprenorphine (PCSS-B). *PCSS-B Guidance on Treatment of Opioid Dependent Adolescents and Young Adults Using Sublingual Buprenorphine.* East Providence, RI: American Academy of Addiction Psychiatry; March 27, 2010.

18. Sanchez-Samper X, Levy S. Opioid use by adolescents. In JA Renner, Jr., P Levounis, eds. *Handbook of Office-Based Buprenorphine Treatment of Opioid Dependence.* Washington, DC: American Psychiatric Publishing; 2011.

19. Woody GE, Poole SA, Subramaniam G, et al. Extended vs. short-term buprenorphine-naloxone for treatment of opioid-addicted youth: A randomized trial. *JAMA.* 2008 Nov 5;300(17):2003–2011.

20. Minozzi S, Amato L, Davoli M. Detoxification treatments for opiate dependent adolescents. *Cochrane Database Syst Rev.* 2009 Apr 15;(2):CD006749.

21. Statistics and Quality, Treatment Episode Data Set (TEDS). *National Admissions to Substance Abuse Treatment Services, 2004-2014.* BHSIS Series S-84, HHS Publication No. (SMA) 16-4986. Rockville, MD: Substance Abuse and Mental Health Services Administration; 2016.

22. Center for Substance Abuse Treatment (CSAT). *Treatment of Adolescents with Substance Use Disorders.* Treatment Improvement Protocol (TIP) Series 32. DHHS Publication No. (SMA) 99-3283. Rockville, MD: CSAT, Substance Abuse and Mental Health Services Administration; 1999.

23. Chakrabarti A, Woody GE, Griffin M, et al. Predictors of buprenorphine-naloxone dosing in a 12-week treatment trial for opioid-dependent youth: Secondary analyses from a NIDA Clinical Trials Network study. *Drug Alc Depend*. 2010;107:253–256.

24. Center for Substance Abuse Treatment (CSAT). *Clinical Guidelines for the Use of Buprenorphine in the Treatment of Opioid Addiction*. Treatment Improvement Protocol (TIP) Series 40. DHHS Publication No. (SMA) 04-3939. Rockville, MD: CSAT, Substance Abuse and Mental Health Services Administration; 2004.

25. Dasinger LK, Shane PA, Martinovich Z. Assessing the effectiveness of community-based substance abuse treatment for adolescents. *J Psychoact Drugs*. 2004 Mar;36(1):27–33.

26. Subramaniam GA, Warden D, Minhajuddin A, et al. Predictors of abstinence: National Institute on Drug Abuse multisite buprenorphine/naloxone treatment trial in opioid-dependent youth. *J Am Acad Child Adolesc Psychiatry*. 2011 Nov;50(11):1120–1128.

27. Federation of State Medical Boards (FSMB). *Model Policy on Opioid Addiction Treatment in the Medical Office*. Dallas, TX: The Federation; 2013.

Chapter 29

Pain and Addiction in Older Adults

NELLY A. BUCKALEW, M.D., N.D., M.S., M.S.L.,
RACHEL MAREE, M.D., M.P.H.,
ZACHARY MARCUM, PH.D., PHARM.D.,
AND DEBRA K. WEINER, M.D.

"Older adults" comprise a population typically defined as persons age 65 and older. Within this group, those ages 65–74 are referred to as the "young old," those 75–84 as the "middle old," and those 85+ as the "oldest old."

Perhaps more important than chronological age are changes in risk and resilience factors over the lifespan [1]. "Homeostenosis" refers to the inability of an aging organism's capacity to respond to stress and is in distinct contrast to "homeostasis," which is the capacity to maintain stability in the face of change [2]. A number of changes in an older adult's biopsychosocial reserves may contribute to the pathogenesis of pain conditions (e.g., sarcopenia and myofascial pain) as well as the degree to which pain interferes with function and quality of life (e.g., cognitive impairment and fear of pain). This chapter focuses specifically on chronic non-cancer pain.

Addiction in older adults has not been well studied, and there are significant gaps in the literature regarding prevention, identification of risk factors, and treatment methods. In chronic pain patients and older adults, it is particularly important to remember that misuse (defined as overuse, underuse, or irregular use) of prescription medications can lead to other conditions that impair a patient's health and ability to function, such as cognitive decline, increased risk of falls, exacerbations of other chronic medical conditions (respiratory and cardiac), and an increase in other psychiatric diagnoses, notably anxiety and depression [3,4].

Limiting exposure to potentially addictive substances is a key preventive measure for older adults with chronic pain. This begins with a comprehensive assessment of the older adult to identify contributors to pain and functional limitation, as discussed in this chapter.

Clinical Presentation

The Pain Signature

The presence of homeostenosis requires a comprehensive biopsychosocial assessment of the older adult who presents with chronic non-cancer pain, so as to identify the multiple contributors to pain and disability that are present in the vast majority of such patients [5]. Obtaining a thorough pain history requires asking questions that enable identification of key treatment outcomes.

While many patients are focused exclusively on reduction or elimination of pain, optimizing function for all patients who have chronic pain—and for older adults in particular—is the most important treatment goal. Each patient has his or her own unique "pain signature," which is defined as the functions with which pain interferes (see Table 29.1) [6].

TABLE 29.1 Example of an Older Adult's Pain Signature

Ask the patient: "Think about your pain over the past week. During that time, how has the pain affected your . . . :"	Not at all	A little	Somewhat	A lot	As much as I can imagine
Energy		X			
Mood			X		
Appetite					
Sleep		X			
Ability to do daily activities				X	
Ability to enjoy yourself					X
Ability to think clearly	X				

For some older adults, interference with their ability to concentrate and participate in pleasurable activities is the salient feature of the pain signature. For others, difficulty sleeping and loss of appetite are characteristic. At the time of the initial history, the clinician should identify the components of the patient's pain signature, which in turn will facilitate meaningful follow-up.

Evaluating Pain Contributors

Essential components of the patient history and the review of systems, social history, and physical examination are enumerated in Box 29.1. As part of this review, signs and symptoms of actual or potential addiction should be identified and recorded in the medical record.

Factors that complicate identification of substance-related problems in late life include the fact that addiction or intoxication may present in a manner difficult to distinguish from depression, delirium, or dementia. As such, the patient history and review of pain systems, the social history, and the physical examination are particularly important components of an older patient's pain evaluation.

It also is important to assess the patient for cooccurring or past substance use disorders (SUDs) and inadequately treated pain, as these are risk factors for misuse of medications. Misuse of prescribed medications can lead to the development of an SUD, which can be classified as mild, moderate, or severe according to the number of symptom criteria that are met [4].

Some indicators of an SUD are shown in Table 29.2 [7]. Additionally, as discussed in Chapter 10 of this Handbook, screening tools can be helpful in identifying the presence or future risk of opioid misuse in patients with chronic pain. While these measures are not specific to older adults, they have been used successfully in this population [8,9].

Assessing Pain and Addiction in Older Adults

Simply by virtue of the aging process, most older adults have a host of pathologies, such as vascular stiffness, skin laxity, and diminished water content of intervertebral discs. Such pathologies can create vulnerability to illness, even when they are not direct contributors to the patient's symptoms.

In most cases, a patient's history is the most powerful diagnostic tool for older adults who present with chronic non-cancer pain. Diagnostic testing should be guided by information learned from the patient's history. Table 29.3 presents common chronic non-cancer pain syndromes in older

BOX 29.1 Recommended Components of the Patient History in an Older Adult Who Presents with Persistent Pain

Answers to the following questions help define the older adult's pain signature and identify key treatment outcomes.

1. How strong is your pain (right now, worst/average over the past week)?
2. How many days over the past week have you been unable to do what you would like to do because of your pain?
3. Over the past week, how often has pain interfered with your ability to take care of yourself, for example with bathing, eating, dressing, and going to the toilet?
4. Over the past week, how often has pain interfered with your ability to take care of your home-related chores such as going grocery shopping, preparing meals, paying bills, and driving?
5. How often do you participate in pleasurable activities such as hobbies, socializing with friends, travel? Over the past week, how often has pain interfered with these activities?
6. How often do you do some type of exercise? Over the past week, how often has pain interfered with your ability to exercise?
7. Does pain interfere with your ability to think clearly?
8. Does pain interfere with your appetite? Have you lost weight?
9. Does pain interfere with your sleep? How often over the past week?
10. Has pain interfered with your energy, mood, personality, or relationships with other people?
11. Over the past week, how often have you taken pain medications?
12. How would you rate your health at the present time? Excellent, good, fair, poor, or bad?

Source: Based in part on Weiner DK, Karp JF, Bernstein C, Morone NE. Pain medicine in older adults: How should it differ? In: Deer T, Ray A, Gordin V, Buvanendran A, Kim PH, Panchal S. *Comprehensive Treatment of Chronic Pain by Medical, Interventional and Behavioral Approaches: The American Academy of Pain Medicine Textbook on Patient Management.* New York: Springer Publishing; 2013. Reproduced with permission of the American Academy of Pain Medicine.

TABLE 29.2 Recommended Components of the Review of Systems in an Older Adult Who Presents with Persistent Pain

This information helps the clinician identify key medical, psychological and social comorbidities that may affect treatment response.

Medical Comorbidities	Relationship to Treatment
Constipation	If present at baseline, a stimulant laxative should be prescribed (e.g., senna) at the same time that an opioid is started.
Lower extremity edema Hypertension	May be exacerbated by a nonsteroidal anti-inflammatory drug.
Congestive heart failure	Gabapentin and pregabalin can contribute to lower extremity edema.
Peptic ulcer disease	Renal insufficiency should be kept in mind when dosing various analgesics
Renal insufficiency	
Obesity	Some medications may contribute to weight gain, such as gabapentin, pregabalin, and tricyclic antidepressants.
Sleep disturbance	While pain may disrupt sleep, opioids also are associated with disruptions in sleep architecture.
Difficulty walking/falls	While pain itself can contribute to weakness, difficulty walking, and falls, older adults can have difficulty with mobility independent of pain. In these individuals, care must be taken to avoid medications that can contribute to mobility impairment, such as opioids, pregabalin, gabapentin, and tricyclic antidepressants.
Memory loss	As noted in the text, pain itself can cause decrements in multiple domains of neuropsychological performance. With effective pain treatment, memory may improve. Practitioners must be aware, however, that many pain medications may contribute to confusion, including opioids, pregabalin, gabapentin, tricyclic antidepressants, and others.

TABLE 29.2 Continued

Medical Comorbidities	Relationship to Treatment
Psychological Factors: Relationship to Treatment	
Depression Anxiety	Untreated depression and/or anxiety can impair top-down inhibition, so the older adult with comorbid depression and/or anxiety must be treated for these disorders as part of pain treatment.
Coping skills	Poor coping skills (e.g., a tendency to catastrophize) can inhibit the efficacy of pain treatment. While most cognitively intact older adults seem to cope well with chronic pain, the minority who do not should be referred for cognitive-behavioral therapy as a part of pain treatment.
Self-efficacy Confidence in mobility Fear of movement	Physical therapy reduces fear avoidance beliefs (such as fear of moving because of concerns about exacerbating pain) in older adults (Weiner, 2008). Older adults with a history of falls may exhibit fear of falling, have low confidence in their mobility, and may have low self-efficacy (i.e., lack of confidence in their ability to engage in certain behaviors to effect desired outcomes). For these individuals, referral to a pain psychologist and physical therapist should be part of pain treatment.
Treatment expectancy	Treatment expectancy must be established at the outset of pain evaluation. Patients who believe that treatment will work are more likely to improve (an example of the placebo effect). Those who believe that treatment will not work probably will not improve (i.e., nocebo effect) (Frisaldi, 2015).
Social Factors: Relationship to Treatment	
Social/caregiver support	Social isolation can interfere with older adults' ability to distract themselves from their pain and thus intensify the pain experience. This may be especially problematic for the older adult who also suffers from dementia.
Financial status	The practitioner always should consider the older adult's financial resources when prescribing treatments.

Source: Based in part on Weiner DK, Karp JF, Bernstein C, Morone NE. Pain medicine in older adults: How should it differ? In: Deer T, Ray A, Gordin V, Buvanendran A, Kim PH, Panchal S. *Comprehensive Treatment of Chronic Pain by Medical, Interventional and Behavioral Approaches: The American Academy of Pain Medicine Textbook on Patient Management.* New York: Springer Publishing; 2013. Reproduced with permission of the American Academy of Pain Medicine.

TABLE 29.3 Special Components of the Physical Examination of an Older Adult Who Presents with Persistent Pain

Component	Example
Cognitive function	Examiner gives the patient three unrelated words to remember. Then, s/he gives the patient a blank piece of paper and asks them to draw a clock with the hands pointing to a specific time. Then, the patient is asked to recall the three words. Patients who are able to recall all three words have a low likelihood of dementia. Those who recall zero words have a high likelihood of dementia. For those who recall 1–2 words, the examiner should assess the accuracy of the clock drawing test. If there are gross errors, the patient should be referred for evaluation of possible dementia.
Balance	Modified Postural Stress Test (Wolfson 1986): Examiner stands behind the patient with hands on sides of pelvis and states, "I am going to pull you backwards gently and try to throw you off balance. . . Do not let me. . . Are you ready?" Then, the examiner pulls the patient toward himself gently. If the patient is able to resist easily, try pulling a little more forcefully and observe response. The older adult whose balance is easily perturbed has decreased postural control and may be at heightened risk for falls.
Basic functional tasks	Chair rise, ability to pick up object from floor, ability to place hands behind neck and waist (movements needed for dressing), manual dexterity (e.g., ability to button and unbutton clothing, tie shoes).
Comprehensive identification of pain comorbidities	Knee/hip arthritis in patients with low back pain; Shoulder disease in those with neck/upper back pain; Myofascial pain in all patients, including those with neuropathic pain (Weiner & Schmader, 2006).

Source: Based in part on Weiner DK, Karp JF, Bernstein C, Morone NE. Pain medicine in older adults: How should it differ? In: Deer T, Ray A, Gordin V, Buvanendran A, Kim PH, Panchal S. *Comprehensive Treatment of Chronic Pain by Medical, Interventional and Behavioral Approaches: The American Academy of Pain Medicine Textbook on Patient Management.* New York: Springer Publishing; 2013. Reproduced with permission of the American Academy of Pain Medicine.

adults and important age-related considerations in ordering and interpreting diagnostic tests.

Although the table does not provide comprehensive information on the evaluation and treatment of these disorders, it does highlight issues of particular relevance to older adults.

Treating Pain in Older Adults

When developing a treatment plan for older adults with chronic pain, the following principles provide useful guidance:

1. *Aim to identify the multiple biopsychosocial treatment targets driving the patient's pain and disability.* For example, an older adult with chronic low back pain may identify back pain as the reason for his or her difficulty in functioning. In such patients, imaging almost always will reveal pathology. However, the main drivers of such a patient's disability may be depression and social isolation. In such cases, it is only by addressing those factors that the clinician can help the patient achieve meaningful improvement in his or her quality of life.

2. *Begin treatment with non-pharmacological interventions (NPIs) whenever possible.* As discussed later, many non-pharmacological treatments currently available can and do achieve positive outcomes, while avoiding deleterious drug–drug and drug–disease interactions.

3. *Remember that "slow and steady wins the race."* When non-pharmacological interventions are not sufficient to manage the patient's pain and the clinician decides to employ a pharmacotherapy, the adage "start low and go slow" should be a guide to treatment. It also is important to "keep going." Clinicians too often hesitate to titrate medications to effect because they fear harming an older adult. Yet, as noted elsewhere in this chapter, inadequately treated pain has many deleterious effects, so slow and steady titration of medications—coupled with ongoing assessment of risks and benefits—is crucial.

Non-Pharmacological Treatment Options

For most older adults, pain and disability are multifactorial and can be related to complications associated with poor nutrition, deconditioning, dysfunctional movement patterns, gait abnormalities, accidents, polypharmacy, cognitive decline, and comorbid psychological illness such as depression and anxiety. Given that the projected number of older Americans with SUDs is rising [10–12] and that physical dependence on alcohol and prescription medications is most prevalent among those aged 65 and over [13–15], a holistic, multimodal, multidisciplinary approach that begins with and is centered around non-pharmacological treatments is critical to success.

The choice of a therapy should be individually tailored to the patient's preferences and goals, as well as his or her ability to comply with the treatment regimen, taking into consideration patient characteristics such as cognitive status, level of functioning, family and social support, and access or transportation issues. For example, a multimodal approach might include working with a physiatrist, because physiatrists are specifically trained in methods that maximize function and treat pain through use of a multimodal approach. Another option is to work with a physician trained in Integrative Medicine, which involves a team approach that brings together health care professionals such as physical or occupational therapists, acupuncturists, myofascial or massage therapists, chiropractors (with caution), or a nutritionist, as well as those trained in spiritual guidance such as a minister, rabbi, or a professional trained in pastoral medicine. A multidisciplinary team approach requires coordinated care, in which the team leader maintains good communication with all the professionals involved, understands the services being provided by team members, has confidence in the competence of the team members, and periodically assesses the patient's progress and adjusts the overall treatment plan as needed.

Multimodal interventions may include pharmacological interventions if they can improve the patient's response to treatment [16,17]. It also is important not to under-treat pain, because to do so is unethical and poses a risk that the patient will self-medicate.

There is emerging evidence of the benefits in pain management for older adults using physical NPIs (such as exercise, acupuncture, trans-epidermal nerve stimulation [TENS], qigong, and yoga; see Table 29.3) and psychosocial NPIs (such as stress management, self-management education, cognitive-behavioral therapy [CBT], meditation/yoga, guided imagery, and listening to music), particularly for chronic pain [18,19].

Pharmacological Treatment Options

While non-pharmacological treatments for pain always should be considered as a first step, many older adults require pharmacotherapy to manage their pain. In fact, pharmacotherapy —mainly consisting of analgesics —is the most common management strategy for the treatment of pain [20]. However, pharmacokinetic and pharmacodynamic changes associated with aging (such as a decline in cytochrome P-450 function, overall liver and renal clearance), combined with frequent polypharmacy, places older adults at high risk for adverse drug effects (ADEs) [16,20,21]. Therefore, lower doses often are used to initiate therapy.

As a next step, analgesics should be titrated to response and often can be used safely in older adults, with appropriate monitoring [22]. As noted earlier, it is important to treat all underlying conditions that could affect pain and disability in an older adult, including depression, anxiety, and vitamin D deficiency.

Stepped care is routinely recommended for the treatment of both nociceptive and neuropathic pain in this population [9]. Multiple guidelines exist for the management of pain in older adults, but two of the most relevant and comprehensive are those issued in 2009 by the American Geriatrics Society (AGS) Panel on Pharmacological Management of Persistent Pain in Older Persons [9] and the British Pain Society and British Geriatrics Society Guidance on the Management of Pain in Older People (published in 2013) [22]. In these guidelines, analgesics (including opioids as well as non-opioids such as acetaminophen and non-steroidal anti-inflammatory agents [NSAIDs], and adjuvant medications), are recommended as the mainstay of pharmacotherapy for pain management.

Acetaminophen is recommended as a first-line analgesic for the management of symptoms of osteoarthritis and low back pain [9,22]. Given that its safety profile is better than that of NSAIDs, acetaminophen should be trialed first with an adequate dose. In order to assess acetaminophen's efficacy, it is important to begin by determining how much acetaminophen the patient is taking (before making any decisions to add an additional agent), including both prescription and over-the-counter products [9].

When inflammatory pain is present, NSAIDs may be needed. In addition, NSAIDs may be used to treat short-term pain [9,22]. However, older adults are at increased risk for NSAID-related adverse drug effects, including renal impairment, gastrointestinal bleeding, and negative cardiovascular outcomes. As a result, NSAIDs should be used with extreme caution in older adults (i.e., for the shortest period of time in the lowest effective dose) [9,22]. Moreover, topical NSAIDs may be used for short periods to minimize some of the system NSAID-related ADEs [9].

Opioid analgesics should be used in selected patients who have persistent moderate to severe pain and reduced functional impairment despite initial therapies [9,22]. The long-term safety and efficacy of opioids is largely unknown in older adults, so extreme caution should be exercised because of the potential for multiple adverse effects, most notably falls and resulting hip fracture, delirium, and constipation [9]. The clinician must juxtapose these risks against the multiple risks associated with untreated pain in older adults [23–28].

The decision to employ opioids for pain management in this population should be based on shared decision-making between the clinician and the patient, as well as a thorough risk–benefit analysis and monitoring plan.

Finally, tricyclic antidepressants and anti-epileptic medications have demonstrated efficacy in treating multiple types of neuropathic pain [22]. However, these agents have limited use in older adults because of their ability to cause adverse drug effects.

It is important to note that all pharmacological interventions should be paired with, rather than substituted for, non-pharmacological interventions in this population.

Beers Criteria

Certain medications are considered high risk, or potentially inappropriate, for use in older adults because of their unfavorable risk–benefit profile. Such medications are included in the Beers Criteria for Potentially Inappropriate Medication Use in Older Adults, which is published and updated by the American Geriatrics Society [29].

The Beers Criteria recommend against chronic use of analgesics, unless other alternatives are not effective and the patient can take a gastroprotective agent such as a proton pump inhibitor (PPI) [29]. However, caution should be exercised with PPIs, given their association with increased risk of osteoporosis and fractures (the U.S. Food and Drug Administration [FDA] has issued safety warnings about the risk of fractures of the hip, wrist, and spine) [29]. The NSAID indomethacin is not recommended for use in older adults due to its ability to cause adverse central nervous system (CNS) effects. Pentazocine—an opioid analgesic—is not recommended, also because of adverse CNS effects. Finally, meperidine is not recommended for use in older adults because it is not an effective oral analgesic in dosages commonly used and because it poses a relatively high risk of neurotoxicity [29].

Treating Opioid Misuse and Addiction in Older Adults

Treatments for opioid addiction associated with chronic non-cancer pain range from behavioral and therapeutic interventions to pharmacological therapies. The first step should involve evaluation of the patient's need for continued pain medication, as well as his or her desire for treatment of the SUD. Interventions that have been implemented successfully in older adults with SUDs include those associated with pain medications, including education about appropriate use, dosage, and potential misuse of medications.

Therapeutic interventions such as motivational interviewing, cognitive-behavioral therapy, and self-management methods also have been employed. Addiction treatment programs exist in a variety of forms (individual, group, intensive outpatient, 30-day rehabilitation, Narcotics Anonymous, etc.) and all are potentially appropriate options.

Other methods of treatment involve tapering patients from long-term analgesic therapy. Patients may undergo slow or rapid tapers, depending on the patient's and clinician's preferences and the care setting (inpatient vs. outpatient). Various schedules for tapers have been proposed in the literature. While no randomized trials to date have compared rapid vs. slow tapers in this population, smaller studies have shown that slower tapers—which are used more often in outpatient settings and sometimes with temporary maintenance therapy—are effective.

Various opioid maintenance therapies are available for opioid use disorders, including methadone, buprenorphine, buprenorphine-naloxone, and naltrexone. Some of these treatment modalities may be employed in combination at various points in a patient's treatment. Physicians should consult with their patients to determine the most appropriate course of action [30].

Conclusion

The difficulty in making recommendations about the use of pharmacotherapies in older adults is that important demographic characteristics that may influence outcomes are not consistently reported, such as age categories (young old, mid-old, or oldest old), ethnicity, and key clinical information (cognitive impairment, comorbidities, pain medication use) [18].

This kind of information may play a significant role in the safety and effectiveness of a broad treatment plan or a specific intervention. Again, the clinician is advised to work closely with the patient and/or the patient's caretakers in creating and executing the treatment plan.

For More Information on the Topics Discussed:

American Society of Addiction Medicine (ASAM):

Blow FC, Barry KL. Treatment of older adults (Chapter 36). In RK Ries, DA Fiellin, SC Miller, R Saitz, eds. *The ASAM Principles of Addiction Medicine, Fifth Edition*. Philadelphia, PA: Wolters Kluwer; 2014.

ASAM National Practice Guideline for the Use of Medications in the Treatment of Addiction Involving Opioid Use. Chevy Chase, MD: ASAM; June 1, 2015. (Access at: https://www.asam.org/docs/default-source/practice-support/guidelines-and-consensus-docs/asam-national-practice-guideline-supplement.pdf?sfvrsn=24.)

National Center for Complementary and Integrative Health:

The Center provides resources on complementary and integrative medicine for older adults, which are helpful in discussing non-pharmacological approaches with older patients. (Access at: (https://nccih.nih.gov/health/aging.)

National Institute on Alcohol Abuse and Alcoholism (NIAAA):

Alcohol use in older people. *Age Page: Health and Aging*. July 29, 2016. (Access at: https://www.nia.nih.gov/health/publication/alcohol-use-older-people.)

National Institute on Drug Abuse (NIDA):

Misuse of Prescription Drugs: Older Adults. August 2016. (Access at: https://www.drugabuse.gov/publications/research-reports/prescription-drugs/trends-in-prescription-drug-abuse/older-adults.)

Substance Abuse and Mental Health Services Administration (SAMHSA):

Substance Abuse Among Older Adults: Physicians Guide (TIP 26, Concise Desk Reference). Order number SMA12-3394. Published June 2012. (Access at: http://store.samhsa.gov/product/Substance-Abuse-Among-Older-Adults-Physician-s-Guide/SMA12-3394.)

References

1. Walco GA, Krane EJ, Schmader KE, et al. Applying a life-span developmental perspective to chronic pain: Pediatrics to geriatrics. *J Pain*. 2015 Sep;17(9 Suppl):T108–117.

2. Becker P, Cohen H. The functional approach to the care of the elderly: A conceptual framework. *J Am Geriatr Soc*. 1984 Dec;32(12):923–929.

3. Koechl B, Unger A, Fischer G. Age-related aspects of addiction. *Gerontology*. 2012;58(6):540–544.

4. American Psychiatric Association (APA). *Diagnostic and Statistical Manual of Mental Disorders, 5th ed*. Washington, DC: American Psychiatric Press; 2013.

5. Resnick NM, Marcantonio ER. How should clinical care of the aged differ? *Lancet*. 1997;350:1157–1158.

6. Weiner DK, Herr K. Comprehensive assessment and interdisciplinary treatment planning: An integrative overview. In DK Weiner, K Herr, TE Rudy, eds. *Persistent Pain in Older Adults: An Interdisciplinary Guide for Treatment*. New York: Springer Publishing Co.; 2002.

7. Douaihy A. Late-life substance use disorders. In MD Miller, LK Solai, eds. *Pittsburgh Pocket Psychiatry: Geriatric Psychiatry*. New York: Oxford University Press; 2013.

8. Kalapatapu RK, Sullivan MA. Prescription use disorders in older adults. *Am J Addict*. 2011;19(6):515–522.

9. American Geriatrics Society, Panel on Pharmacological Management of Persistent Pain in Older Persons. Pharmacological management of persistent pain in older persons. *J Am Geriatr Soc*. 2009 Aug;57(8):1331–1346.

10. Substance Abuse and Mental Health Services Administration (SAMHSA). *Results from the 2011 National Survey on Drug Use and Health: Summary of National Findings* (NSDUH Series H-44, HHS Publication No. [SMA] -4713). Rockville, MD: SAMHSA, U.S. Department of Health and Human Services; 2012.

11. Rosen D, Herberlein E, Engel RJ. Older Adults and Substance-Related Disorders: Trends and Associated Costs. *ISRN Addiction*. 2013: Article ID 905368.

12. Bamberger PA, Bacharach SB. *Retirement and the Hidden Epidemic: The ComplexLink Between Aging, Work Disengagement, and Substance Misuse—and What to do About It*. New York: Oxford University Press; 2014.

13. Substance Abuse and Mental Health Services Administration (SAMHSA), Drug and Alcohol Services Information System. *The DASIS Report: Older Adults in*

Substance Abuse Treatment. Rockville, MD: SAMHSA, Department of Health and Human Services; 2005.

14. Blazer D, Wu L-T. Non-prescription use of pain relievers among middle aged and elderly community adults: National Survey on Drug Use and Health. *J Am Geriatr Soc*. 2009;57(7):1252–1257.

15. Centers for Disease Control and Prevention (CDC). Vital Signs: Overdoses of prescription opioid pain relievers—United States, 1999–2008. *Morb Mortal Wkly Rep*. 2011;60(43):1487–1492.

16. American Geriatrics Society. The management of persistent pain in older persons. *J Am Geriatr Soc*. 2002;50:S205–S224.

17. Alexander LL. Palliative care and pain management at the end of life. *CME Res*. 2009;134:61–109.

18. Park J, Hughes A. Nonpharmacological approaches to the management of chronic pain in community-dwelling older adults: A review of empirical evidence. *J Am Geriatr Soc*. 2012;60:555–568.

19. Morone NE, Greco CM. Mind-body interventions for chronic pain in older adults: A structured review. *Pain Med*. 2007;8:359–375.

20. O'Neil CK, Hanlon JT, Marcum ZA. Adverse effects of analgesics commonly used by older adults with osteoarthritis: Focus on non-opioid and opioid analgesics. *Am J Geriatr Pharmacother*. 2012;10:331–342.

21. Kaye AD, Baluch A, Scot JT. Pain management in the elderly population: A review. *Ochsner J*. 2010;10:179–187.

22. Abdulla A, Adams N, Bone M, et al. British Geriatrics Society guidance on the management of pain in older people. *Age Ageing*. 2013 Mar;42(Suppl 1):11–57.

23. Leveille SG, Jones RN, Kiely DK, et al. Chronic musculoskeletal pain and the occurrence of falls in an older population. *JAMA*. 2009;302(20):2214–2221.

24. Tassain V, Attal N, Fletcher D, et al. Long term effects of oral sustained release morphine on neuropsychological performance in patients with chronic noncancer pain. *Pain*. 2003;104:389–400.

25. Jamison RN, Schein JR, Vallow S, et al. Neuropsychological effects of long-term opioid use in chronic pain patients. *J Pain Symptom Manag*. 2003 Oct;26(4):913–921.

26. Bosley BN, Weiner DK, Rudy TE, et al. Is chronic nonmalignant pain associated with decreased appetite in older adults? Preliminary evidence. *J Am Geriatr Soc*. 2004;52:247–251.

27. Weiner DK, Rudy TE, Morrow L, et al. The relationship between pain neuropsychological performance, and physical function in community dwelling older adults with chronic low back pain. *Pain Med*. 2006;7:60–70.

28. Rudy TE, Weiner DK, Lieber SJ, et al. The impact of chronic low back pain on older adults: A comparative study of patients and controls. *Pain*. 2007;13:293–301.

29. American Geriatrics Society, 2015 Beers Criteria Update Expert Panel. American Geriatrics Society 2015 Updated Beers Criteria for potentially inappropriate medication use in older adults. *J Am Geriatr Soc*. 2015 Nov;63(11):2227–2246.

30. Berna C, Kulich RJ, Rathmell JP. Tapering long-term opioid therapy in chronic noncancer pain: Evidence and recommendations for everyday practice. *Mayo Clin Proc*. 2015;90(6):828–842.

Chapter 30

Pain and Addiction in Women

MISHKA TERPLAN, M.D., M.P.H., FACOG, FASAM

Although much progress has been made in understanding the unique needs of women in the areas of pain management and addiction treatment, gender disparities still exist.

Women report a higher prevalence of chronic pain than do men [1] and are at greater risk for many pain conditions [2], a finding that persists across all racial and ethnic groups [3]. Gender differences have been described in pain perception, tolerance, and analgesic response (including the response to opioids), as well as in the likelihood of developing addiction.

Pain in women is not only more prevalent but less likely to be adequately treated. For example, 40% of women with chronic vulvar pain remain undiagnosed after three medical consultations [4]. This is due in part to the fact that health care professionals are more likely to dismiss women's pain, leading to a mental health diagnosis rather than pain treatment more frequently than in men [5].

General Principles

Different theoretical constructs have been used to explain gender differences in pain [6]. The principal theories include the following:

1. *Gender-role theory*, which describes the increased social acceptability of women reporting pain [7], as well as the negative gender stereotyping women experience when they report pain in a clinical context [8]. This is especially true for women who have chronic pain. When compounded by a clinician's lack of knowledge, gender differences in communication

[9], and bias, the situation can delay treatment and lead to unnecessary suffering (which may be considered unethical) [10].

2. *Exposure theory*, which suggests that women are exposed to more pain risk factors than are men. In fact, certain pain conditions do derive from women's reproductive capacity. Violence against women, particularly intimate partner [11] and sexual violence [12], are common and are associated with pain syndromes [13], as are substance use and substance use disorders (SUDs) in women [14].

3. *Vulnerability theory*, which proposes that women are more vulnerable to developing musculoskeletal and other forms of pain. The Institute of Medicine (IOM) considered this theory to be the "best supported by scientific evidence" [6], although much of that evidence is experimental rather than clinical. It involves the potential role of sex hormones in nociception, as well as physiological differences between men and women, such as body size and skin thickness.

Chronic pain conditions in women frequently overlap [15,16] and may be associated with co-occurring mental disorders and addiction [17], as well as with a history of childhood sexual abuse [18] and intimate partner violence [19,20]. For this reason, mental health issues, substance use and SUDs, and violence should be assessed in every woman who presents as a patient with pain.

Family planning needs are central for all women of reproductive age. Half of all pregnancies in the United States are unplanned, which also means they are more likely to be associated with poorer obstetrical and newborn outcomes [21]. All health care providers should screen women for reproductive health needs, including contraception, and either provide care or refer them to a clinician who can do so. Before initiating any therapy for pain syndromes, clinicians should screen women of reproductive age for pregnancy with a simple urine pregnancy test.

Screening for contraceptive needs can be accomplished using a simple question such as the One Key Question®: "Would you like to be pregnant in the next year" [22]? This question is patient-focused and non-judgmental and allows for triage of family planning needs. Women who answer "Yes" should be referred for pre-conception counseling. Those who say "No" or "I don't know" should be offered contraceptive counseling.

Clinical Presentation

This section is divided into two parts, one of which addresses pain and addiction in women of child-bearing age, and another that discusses pain and addiction in older women (including those in peri- and post-menopause).

Pain and Addiction in Women of Childbearing Age

The following conditions are among those seen most often in this population.

Dysmenorrhea: Pain with menstruation is common and is caused by uterine contractions leading to periodic ischemia. It is a leading cause of lost time from school and/or work in young women.

Primary dysmenorrhea begins at menarche and can be lifelong. Secondary dysmenorrhea is of later onset and due to another condition (see "chronic pelvic pain," following).

Limited data on the associations between dysmenorrhea and SUD (if any) suggest that women who engage in heavy alcohol consumption (defined as six or more drinks a week) experience greater discomfort [23].

Chronic pelvic pain is associated with several discrete syndromes and most commonly affects women during the reproductive years.

Such pain occurs below the umbilicus and is of at least six months' duration. It may be either intermittent or constant, and may or may not be related to menstrual periods. Possible causes include endometriosis, pelvic inflammatory disease, pelvic adhesive disease, as well as interstitial cystitis, irritable bowel syndrome, and fibromyalgia.

In general, alcohol and drug use disorders are associated with increased risk of non-cyclical pelvic pain [24].

Endometriosis is an estrogen-dependent disease characterized by the presence of endometrial glands and stroma outside of the uterus. It is a common disorder, affecting approximately 14% of all women of reproductive age, and is a major cause of infertility. Various theories have been advanced to explain the presence and implantation of ectopic endometrial tissue, including retrograde menstruation and coelomic metaplasia.

Symptoms of endometriosis range from mild to severe. There is no relationship between the extent of the disease observed during laparoscopy and the severity of symptoms. As many as 10 years can elapse between onset of symptoms and diagnosis.

There is an association between alcohol consumption and endometriosis, with a pooled odds ratio (OR) of 1.2 for any alcohol versus no alcohol, which may be due to the increase in circulating estrogens caused by alcohol [25]. There is no association between smoking and endometriosis [26] and no evidence regarding the effects of other substances on the disorder.

Fibromyalgia is a disorder of unknown etiology that is characterized by generalized pain, abnormal pain processing, fatigue, and sleep disturbances. A relationship between low opioid tone and fibromyalgia has been hypothesized [27].

Symptoms of fibromyalgia are classified according to criteria advanced by the American College of Rheumatology [28], which require that such symptoms are not explained by another condition and that they have been present for at least three months.

Low to moderate alcohol consumption is associated with less intense fibromyalgia symptoms and better quality of life, compared with no alcohol consumption [29]. Compared with other chronic pain patients, those with fibromyalgia tend to smoke more, and smoking is associated with more intense symptoms of pain [30]. There is no evidence to support an association between fibromyalgia and other SUDs.

Interstitial cystitis is a syndrome characterized by daytime and nighttime urinary frequency, urgency, and bladder/pelvic pain of unknown etiology [31]. There is no apparent associations between interstitial cystitis and SUDs.

Vulvodynia is characterized by chronic discomfort in the vulva, as well as dyspareunia. It can be present since coitarche, although more often symptoms appear after years of painless sex. It is not associated with sexually transmitted infections. Tenderness is present on examination with gentle pressure. There is no literature linking vulvodynia with substance use or SUDs.

Pregnancy is a time of marked biological and social transformation. The most common pain conditions that develop during pregnancy are musculoskeletal (back, pelvic girdle, and pubic symphysis pain) and headaches. Treating these conditions with opioids (or failing to identify a pregnant woman's use of non-prescribed opioids) can have serious consequences for the developing fetus, including fetal hypoxia and utero-placental insufficiency, resulting in elevated risk of prematurity, low birth weight, and fetal death (Box 30.1) [39,40].

For this reason, the American College of Obstetricians and Gynecologists (ACOG) has recommended that all pregnant women be screened for drug use (using urine testing if necessary) to reduce the growing number of infants born with opioid NAS [41].

Pain and Addiction in Older Women

Menopause, which is defined as the absence of menstrual periods for 12 months, is only one facet of the climacteric process that occurs as ovarian estrogen synthesis gradually declines over several years. The time from onset of menstrual irregularities to menopause is called the *perimenopause,* for which the median age of onset globally is 47.5 years. Among women in the United States, the mean age of onset of menopause is 51.

Common symptoms of menopause include vaginal dryness from atrophy (which is associated with dyspareunia) and joint pain. Osteoporosis is asymptomatic until a fracture occurs. Bone loss occurs more rapidly in trabecular than in cortical bone. Therefore, fractures occur earlier in the vertebral spine and distal radius (for example, among 25% of non-black women who do not receive estrogen by age 60) than in the femoral neck (as exemplified by data showing that 20% of white women who do not receive estrogen will develop a hip fracture by age 80).

BOX 30.1 Opioid Neonatal Abstinence Syndrome

Opioid neonatal abstinence syndrome (opioid NAS) is present in approximately 50–75% of infants exposed to opioids in utero [41–46]. Its presence and severity are influenced by multiple factors, including maternal smoking, use of substances other than opioids or certain medications (such as SSRIs), gestational age at delivery, and genetics [37].

The newborn with opioid NAS presents with central nervous system excitability, vasomotor signs such as seizures and tremors, and gastrointestinal signs that include vomiting and diarrhea. In addition, premature infants with opioid NAS may experience respiratory distress and need to be placed on ventilators [32].

While most—if not all—opioid-exposed infants experience some degree of NAS, the time to onset of symptoms varies. With infants exposed to heroin or other short-acting opioids, symptoms usually emerge in the first 48–72 hours after birth. In contrast, infants exposed to longer-acting drugs—particularly methadone or buprenorphine—typically exhibit symptoms later, but usually within the first four days [2]. The duration of symptoms also is variable, with some infants exhibiting subacute symptoms for weeks to months after birth [36,37].

As a first step, infants at risk for NAS should be assessed for signs of withdrawal 30–60 minutes after each feeding, using a standard scoring system such as the Finnegan Neonatal Abstinence Scoring System, a 31-item scale that is used to quantify the severity of NAS and guide its treatment [38]. Newborn urine and meconium toxicology screens also may be helpful in diagnosing opioid NAS [3].

Treatment depends on a differential diagnosis because of the non-specific nature of the signs and symptoms of neonatal opioid withdrawal. (Conditions that may produce symptoms similar to opioid NAS include sepsis, hypoglycemia, hypocalcemia, hyperthyroidism, perinatal asphyxia, and intracranial hemorrhage [36].)

The foundation of effective treatment is supportive, non-pharmacological interventions such as reducing stimulation, swaddling the infant or using skin-to-skin ("kangaroo") care, use of pacifiers, and frequent feedings on demand [3,39]. Some infants require intravenous fluids to maintain hydration.

In addition to supportive care, most infants with opioid NAS also will need appropriate pharmacological management. The goal of such therapy is to stabilize the infant so that he or she can eat, sleep, gain weight, and interact with caregivers, after which the medication dose can be gradually reduced [2].

The American Academy of Pediatrics [39–42] and other experts [43–49] agree that opioid replacement is the ideal pharmacological treatment for opioid NAS. An alcohol-free oral morphine sulfate preparation often is recommended as initial therapy, as is a morphine hydrochloride solution [50–56]. Other drugs used for treatment of opioid NAS include diluted tincture of opium and paregoric. (Paregoric was one of the first drugs used to treat NAS, but it is no longer recommended because of the potential toxicity of many of its ingredients [57–60].)

Discharge can be considered once the infant is clinically stable, feeding well, has begun to gain weight, and can be cared for by adults in a safe environment. While the recommended length of stay depends on the extent of *in utero* exposure to opioids, such infants generally should not be discharged before day 7, because the onset of withdrawal symptoms may be delayed for several days, particularly in breastfed infants [36].

Treatment Options

Although treatment options vary for each of the conditions described in this chapter, certain general principles apply to any treatment of a woman presenting with pain. These include:

- An empathetic and nonjudgmental approach that takes the patient and the pain complaint seriously.
- An emphasis on self-management and autonomy, which recognizes the individual's own capacity to control her pain.
- Realistic goals that focus on functional improvement rather than complete freedom from pain.

The goals of therapy typically differ for different women. Data reported in the literature indicate that some patients seek to have their pain legitimized even while the practitioner is focused on diagnosis and therapy [8]. Women in pain often are stigmatized by health care professionals, especially when the pain is caused by conditions that are gender-specific [32].

Patient assessment should begin with a complete history and a physical examination that focuses on the affected areas. Offering multidisciplinary care is important, including referral to a gynecologist for proper diagnosis and treatment of pelvic pain.

Self-management programs emphasize autonomy and have proved effective in reducing abdominal pain associated with irritable bowel syndrome (IBS) [33]. Similarly, exercise has been associated with improvement in symptom severity among women with fibromyalgia [34]. Programs such as these should be holistic and biopsychosocial in orientation.

Opioids should not be the first-line therapy for any condition. Whenever a patient *is* prescribed an opioid, risk mitigation strategies should be employed. These include—but are not limited to—a detailed assessment, with an individual and family history of addiction, use of state Prescription Drug Monitoring Programs (PDMPs) to determine whether opioids are being prescribed by other health care providers, discussion of overdose risk, and co-prescribing of naloxone (see Chapter 13 of this Handbook for additional information).

The best advice is to treat with non-pharmacological therapies first and to the greatest extent possible. Options include: physical therapy, massage, and complementary integrative medicine (CIM) approaches such as acupuncture, yoga, tai chi, xi gong, and mindfulness meditation [35].

Pregnancy is a time of marked biological and social transformation. The most common pain conditions that develop during pregnancy are musculoskeletal (back, pelvic girdle, and pubic symphysis pain) and headaches.

Pain in pregnancy should be taken seriously and an obstetrical consult obtained for any new symptoms. Untreated or undertreated pain in pregnancy is associated with poorer maternal and fetal outcomes. The same principles of pain management apply to the care of pregnant and non-pregnant women; however, special consideration should be given to medication decisions in pregnant women, particularly those involving use of opioids [36].

Opioids should not be the first line of therapy for chronic pain in pregnancy. However, for post-operative pain, pregnant women should receive analgesia in a manner no different than would be given to any other patient [37].

(The management of pain during labor and delivery is beyond the scope of this chapter, but is well addressed in several standard references [38].)

Conclusion

For reasons both biological (reproductive capacity) and cultural (gender-based violence), women are more likely than men to experience pain. Even so, health care professionals often minimize self-reports of pain from women, leading to a delay in diagnosis and treatment. Women who are experiencing pain benefit from an empathetic and nonjudgmental approach that takes the patient and her pain seriously.

Realistic treatment goals include functional improvement and emphasize non-pharmacological and non-opioid treatment modalities. Above all, care must be grounded in the principles of autonomy and respect.

Given the high prevalence of adverse childhood experiences and intimate partner violence among women with pain, assessment for these conditions should be a routine part of the overall plan of care.

Finally, assessment of the patient's intentions regarding pregnancy and reproductive health planning should be better integrated into women's health care for the sake of both women and their offspring.

For More Information on the Topics Discussed:

American Society of Addiction Medicine (ASAM):

Weaver MF, Jones HE, Wunsch MJ. Alcohol and other drug use during pregnancy: Management of the mother and child (Chapter 83). In RK Ries, DA Fiellin, SC Miller, R Saitz, eds. *The ASAM Principles of Addiction Medicine, Fifth Edition.* Philadelphia, PA: Wolters Kluwer; 2014.

ASAM National Practice Guideline for the Use of Medications in the Treatment of Addiction Involving Opioid Use. Chevy Chase, MD: ASAM; June 1, 2015. (Access at: https://www.asam.org/docs/default-source/practice-support/ guidelines-and-consensus-docs/asam-national-practice-guideline-supplement.pdf?sfvrsn=24.)

Campaign to End Chronic Pain in Women (CECPW):

Chronic Pain in Women (policy statement). Washington, DC: CECPW; 2010. (Access at: http://www.endwomenspain.org/.)

U.S. Department of Health and Human Services (DHHS):

National Pain Strategy: A Comprehensive Population Health-Level Strategy for Pain. (Access at: https://iprcc.nih.gov/docs/DraftHHSNational PainStrategy.pdf.)

References

1. Croft P, Blyth FM, van der Windt D. Chronic pain epidemiology: From aetiology to public health. In P Croft, FM Blyth, D van der Windt, eds. *Chronic Pain Epidemiology: From Aetiology to Public Health.* New York: Oxford University Press; 2010.
2. Fillingim RG, King CD, Riberio-Dasilva MC, et al. Sex, gender, and pain: A review of recent clinical and experimental findings. *J Pain.* 2009;10(5):447–485.
3. Hardt J, Jacobsen C, Goldberg J, et al. Prevalence of chronic pain in a representative sample in the United States. *Pain Med.* 2008;9(7):803–812.
4. Harlow BL, Kunitz CG, Nguyen RHN, et al. Prevalence of symptoms consistent with a diagnosis of vulvodynia: Population-based estimates from two geographical regions. *Am J Obstet Gynecol.* 2014 Jan;210(1):40.e1–e8.
5. Fishbain DA, Goldberg M, Meagher BR, et al. Male and female chronic pain patients categorized by DSM-III psychiatric diagnostic criteria. *Pain.* 1986;26(2):181–197.

6. Institute of Medicine (IOM). *Relieving Pain in America: A Blueprint for Transforming Prevention, Care, Education, and Research.* Washington, DC: National Academies Press; 2011.

7. Robinson ME, Riley JL 3rd, Myers CD, et al. Gender role expectations of pain: Relationship to sex differences in pain. *J Pain.* 2001 Oct;2(5):251–257.

8. Frantsve LM, Kerns RD. Patient-provider interactions in the management of chronic pain: Current findings within the context of medical decision-making. *Pain Med.* 2007;8(1):25–35.

9. Keogh E. Gender differences in the nonverbal communication of pain: A new direction for sex, gender, and pain research? *Pain.* 2014 Oct;155 (10):1927–1931.

10. Macpherson C. Undertreating pain violates ethical principles. *J Med Ethics.* 2009;35:603–606.

11. World Health Organization (WHO). *Multi-country Study on Women's Health and Domestic Violence Against Women: Summary Report of Initial Results on Prevalence, Health Outcomes and Women's Responses.* Geneva, Switzerland: WHO; 2005.

12. Black MC, Basile KC, Breiding MJ, et al. Prevalence of sexual violence against women in 23 states and two U.S. territories. *Violence Against Women.* 2014 May;20(5):485–499.

13. As-Sanie S. History of abuse and its relationship to pain experience and depression in women with chronic pelvic pain. *AJOG.* 2014;210:317.e1–e8.

14. Black MC. Intimate partner violence and adverse health consequences: Implications for clinicians. *Am J Lifestyle Med.* 2011;5:428–439.

15. Zolnoun DA, Rohl J, Moore CG, et al. Overlap between orofacial pain and vulvar vestibulitis syndrome. *Clin J Pain.* 2008;24(3):187–191.

16. Sinaii N, Cleary SD, Ballweg ML, et al. High rates of autoimmune and endocrine disorders, fibromyalgia, chronic fatigue syndrome and atopic diseases among women with endometriosis: A survey analysis. *Hum Reprod.* 2002;17(10):2175–2724.

17. Barry DT, Pilver CE, Hoff RA, et al. Pain interference and incident mood, anxiety, and substance use disorders: Findings from a representative sample of men and women in the general population. *J Psychiatr Res.* 2013 Nov; 47(11):1658–1664.

18. Spiegel DR, Chatterjee A, McCroskey AL, et al. A review of select centralized pain syndromes: Relationship with childhood sexual abuse, opiate prescribing, and treatment implications for the primary care physician. *Health Serv Res Manag Epidemiol.* 2015 Jan 26;2:2333392814567920. doi:10.1177/2333392814567920

19. Wuest J, Merritt-Gray M, Ford-Gilboe M, et al. Chronic pain in women survivors of intimate partner violence. *J Pain.* 2008 Nov;9(11):1049–1057.

20. Ellsberg M, Jansen HA, Heise L, et al., for the WHO Multi-country Study on Women's Health and Domestic Violence Against Women Study Team. Intimate partner violence and women's physical and mental health in the WHO Multi-Country Study on Women's Health and Domestic Violence: An observational study. *Lancet.* 2008 Apr;371:1165–1172.

21. Guttmacher Institute. *Unintended Pregnancy in the United States. Fact Sheet.* New York: The Institute; July 2015. (Accessed at: http://www.guttmacher.org/pubs/FB-Unintended-Pregnancy-US.html).

22. Oregon Foundation for Reproductive Health. *One Key Question (OKQ)*. 2012. (Accessed at: https://www.arhp.org/uploaddocs/RH13_Presentation_One_Question.pdf.)

23. Wilsnack SC, Klassem AS, Wilsnack RN. Drinking and reproductive dysfunction among women in a 1981 survey. *Alcohol Clin Exp Res*. 1984 Sep–Oct;8(5):451–458.

24. Latthe P, Mignini L, Gray R, et al. Factors predisposing women to chronic pelvic pain: Systematic review. *BMJ*. 2006 Apr 1;332(7544):749–755. https://doi.org/10.1136/bmj.38748.697465.55 (Published 30 March 2006)

25. Parazzini F, Cipriani S, Bravi F, et al. A meta-analysis on alcohol consumption and risk of endometriosis. *Am J Obstet Gynecol*. 2013;209:106.e1–e10.

26. Bravi F, Parazzini F, Cipriani S, et al. Tobacco smoking and risk of endometriosis: A systematic review and meta-analysis. *BMJ Open*. 2014 Dec 22;4(12):e006325.

27. Johnson B, Ulberg S, Shivale S, et al. Fibromyalgia, autism, and opioid addiction as natural and induced disorders of the endogenous opioid hormonal system. *Discov Med*. 2014 Oct;18(99):209–220.

28. Wolfe F, Clauw DJ, Fitzcharles MA, et al. The American College of Rheumatology preliminary diagnostic criteria for fibromyalgia and measurement of symptom severity. *Arthritis Care Res*. 2010;62(5):600–610.

29. Kim CH, Vincent A, Clauw DJ, et al. Association between alcohol consumption and symptom severity and quality of like in patient with fibromyalgia. *Arthritis Res Ther*. 2013 Mar 15;15(2):R42.

30. Goesling J, Brummett CM, Meraj TS, et al. Associations between pain, current tobacco smoking, depression, and fibromyalgia status among treatment-seeking chronic pain patients. *Pain Med*. 2015 Jul;16(7):1433–1442.

31. Hanno PM, Burks DA, Clemens JQ, et al. Diagnosis and treatment of interstitial cystitis/bladder pain syndrome. *American Urological Association Guidelines* (Published 2011; Amended 2014). (Accessed at: http://www.auanet.org/common/pdf/education/clinical-guidance/IC-Bladder-Pain-Syndrome-Revised.pdf.)

32. Campaign to End Chronic Pain in Women (CECPW). *Chronic Pain in Women* (policy statement). Washington, DC: CECPW; 2010. (Accessed at: http://www.endwomenspain.org/.)

33. Heitkemper MM, Jarrett ME, Levy RL, et al. Self-management for women with irritable bowel syndrome. *Clin Gastroenterol Hepatol*. 2004;2(7):585–596.

34. Busch AJ, Webber SC, Richards RS, et al. Resistance exercise training for fibromyalgia. *Cochrane Database Syst Rev*. 2013;12:CD010884.

35. Pennick V, Young G. Interventions for preventing and treating pelvic and back pain in pregnancy. *Cochrane Database Syst Rev*. 2007 Apr 18;(2):CD001139.

36. Broussard CS, Rasmussen SA, Reefhuis J, et al. Maternal treatment with opioid analgesics and risk for birth defects. *Am J Obstet Gynecol*. 2011;204:314.e1–e11.

37. American College of Obstetricians and Gynecologists (ACOG). *Opioid Abuse, Dependence and Addiction in Pregnancy* (Committee Opinion 524). Washington, DC: ACOG; 2012.

38. Jones HE, Deppen K, Hudak ML, et al. Clinical care for opioid-using pregnant and postpartum women: The role of obstetric providers. *AJOG.* 2014 Apr;210(4):302–310.

39. Johnston AM, Metayer HM, Robinson E. Section 4: Management of neonatal opioid withdrawal. In AM Johnston, TW Mandell, M Meyer, eds. *Vermont Obstetrical and Pediatric Guidelines.* Burlington, VT: Vermont Department of Health and Fletcher Allen Health Care; 2010:1–12.

40. Unger A, Metz V, Fischer G. Review article: Opioid dependent and pregnant: What are the best options for mothers and neonates? *Obstet Gynecol Intl.* 2012;195954. http://dx.doi.org/10.1155/2012/195954

41. American College of Obstetricians and Gynecologists (ACOG). *Pregnant Women and Prescription Drug Abuse, Dependence and Addiction. ACOG Toolkit on State Legislation.* Washington, DC: ACOG; 2014.

42. Osborn DA, Jeffery H, Cole MJ. Opiate treatment for opiate withdrawal in newborn infants. *Cochrane Database Syst Rev.* 2010a;10: Article ID CDDOO2059.

43. Osborn DA, Jeffery H, Cole MJ. Sedatives for opiate withdrawal in newborn infants. *Cochrane Database Syst Rev.* 2010b;10: Article ID CDDOO2053.

44. Tolia VN, Patrick SW, Bennett MM, et al. Increasing incidence of the neonatal abstinence syndrome in U.S. neonatal ICUs. *NEJM.* 2015 May 28;372(22):2118–2126.

45. Patrick SW, Davis MM, Lehman CU, et al. Increasing incidence and geographic distribution of neonatal abstinence syndrome: United States 2009 to 2012. *J Perinatol.* 2015 Aug;35(8):650–655.

46. Bagley SM, Wachman EM, Holland E, et al. Review of the assessment and management of neonatal abstinence syndrome. *Addict Sci Clin Pract.* 2014 Sep 9;9(1):9–19.

47. Queensland Clinical Guidelines. *Queensland Maternity and Neonatal Clinical Guideline: Neonatal Abstinence Syndrome.* Queensland, Australia: Queensland Health, originally published 2010; updated 2013.

48. Finnegan L, Connaughton J, Kron R, et al. Neonatal abstinence syndrome: Assessment and management. *Addict Dis.* 1975;2:141–158.

49. Johnson K, Gerada C, Greenough A. Treatment of neonatal abstinence syndrome. *Arch Dis Child Fetal Neonatal Ed.* 2005;88:F2–F5.

50. Jones HE, Fielder A. Neonatal abstinence syndrome: Historical perspective, current focus, future directions. *Prevent Med.* 2015 Nov;80:12–17.

51. Jones HE, Kaltenbach K, Heil SH, et al. Neonatal abstinence syndrome after methadone or buprenorphine exposure. *NEJM.* 2010;363(24):2320–2331.

52. Jones HE, Johnson RE, Jasinski DR, et al. Buprenorphine versus methadone in the treatment of pregnant opioid-dependent-patients: Effects on the neonatal abstinence syndrome. *Drug Alc Depend.* 2004;79(1):1–10.

53. Jones HE, Dengler E, Garrison A, et al. Neonatal outcomes and their relationship to maternal buprenorphine dose during pregnancy. *Drug Alc Depend.* 2014;134(1):414–417.

54. Colombini N, Elias R, Busuttil M, et al. Hospital morphine preparation for abstinence syndrome in newborns exposed to buprenorphine or methadone. *Pharm World Sci.* 2008;30(3):227–234.

55. Ebner N, Rohrmeister K, Winklbaur B, et al. (2007). Management of neonatal abstinence syndrome in neonates born to opioid maintained women. *Drug Alc Depend*. 87(2–3):131–138.

56. Liu R, Bjorkman T, Stewart C, et al. Pharmacological treatment of neonatal opiate withdrawal: Between the devil and the deep blue sea. *Int J Pediatr*. 2011;Article ID 935631. http://dx.doi.org/10.1155/2011/935631

57. Dryden C, Young D, Hepburn M, et al. Maternal methadone use in pregnancy: Factors associated with the development of neonatal abstinence syndrome and implications for healthcare resources. *Int J Obstet Gynaecol*. 2009;116(5):665–671.

58. Abdel-Latif ME, Pinner J, Clews S, et al. Effects of breast milk on the severity and outcome of neonatal abstinence syndrome among infants of drug-dependent mothers. *Pediatrics*. 2006;117(6):e1163–e1169.

59. Lindemalm S, Nydert P, Svensson JO, et al. Transfer of buprenorphine into breast milk and calculation of infant drug dose. *J Hum Lactat*. 2009;25(2):199–205.

60. Hunt RW, Tzioumi D, Collins E, et al. Adverse neurodevelopmental outcome of infants exposed to opiates in-utero. *Early Hum Dev*. 2008;84(1):29–35.

Chapter 31

Pain and Addiction in Military Personnel and Veterans

ILENE R. ROBECK, M.D., FASAM., STEPHEN C. HUNT, M.D., M.P.H., LUCILE BURGO-BLACK,M.D., FACP, JEREMIAH MCKELVEY, PHARM.D., AFREEN SIDDIQUI, M.D., AND ANTHONY J. MARIANO, PH.D.

Deployment to combat theaters frequently results in physical injuries that evoke chronic pain. In many cases, co-occurring mental disorders and the psychosocial stresses of deployment complicate the assessment and clinical management of that pain.

Although many military personnel and veterans receive all of their health care within the Department of Defense (DoD) or Veterans Administration (VA) systems, others may receive no health care in those systems, or receive care that is co-managed in the private sector as well as military or VA facilities. Therefore, it is important for all clinicians to understand the impact of military service on the sources, intensity and prevalence of chronic pain, as well as the resources available to patients in the military or VA systems [1].

Pain and Addiction in Active-Duty Personnel and Veterans

During deployment, active duty personnel are exposed to life-threatening situations in which hypervigilance is necessary for survival. Service members frequently are exposed to high noise levels, physical injuries, infectious diseases, deaths of friends and team members, as well as prolonged separation from family, friends, and other support systems.

Military families also face unique stressors involving frequent relocations, separation from and irregular communication with loved ones, and constant shifting of roles within the family, depending on whether the service member is present or absent. If a service member is severely injured, further stress is placed on the family as they attempt to provide care to that individual.

The situation can be even more stressful for members of the National Guard and Reserves, who are likely to have less job security, to face potential loss of benefits, and to enjoy less support from their community than families of service members who continue on active duty. As a result, binge and problem drinking are significant problems in this population [1].

Post-Deployment Care

Experts estimate that as many as half of male service members and up to three-fourths of female service members seen in VA primary care settings report the presence of pain and pain-related disability [1].

The most prevalent combat-related conditions following all conflicts are musculoskeletal injuries. More than half of recent combat veterans present with musculoskeletal problems, which often are linked to multiple deployments, accidents in service, blast exposures, and the weight of combat gear. These frequently are accompanied by pain and functional impairment, mental health problems, and non-specific symptoms, which include fatigue, chronic pain, and cognitive disturbances involving memory, attention, and concentration.

Conflicts in the Middle East have produced an unprecedented number of blast injuries. Because of improvements in protective gear and battlefield medical care, a growing number of personnel survive their injuries, but go on to live with serious long-term consequences such as amputations, spinal cord injuries, traumatic brain injuries (TBIs), and severe burn injuries.

The experience of pain often co-occurs with post-traumatic stress disorder (PTSD) and persistent post-concussive syndrome. Also, comorbid mental health disorders or psychosocial stressors may lower the pain threshold and augment the pain experience. Moreover, chronic pain rarely occurs in just one part of the body. In fact, patients often report pain at multiple sites. Overall, chronic pain usually is associated with poorer physical and psychosocial function. For all of these reasons, the biomedical model of pain is inadequate to address the complexity of chronic pain in military personnel and veterans, and a more comprehensive biopsychosocial approach is recommended [1].

Diagnosis

Clinicians who care for returning military personnel should focus first on providing appropriate medical care and diagnosing conditions common in civilian patients with similar demographic and risk factors.

Clinical Presentation

Pain syndromes in combat veterans typically involve headache, low back pain, shoulder pain, and knee pain. It is essential to screen these patients for comorbid conditions and substance use disorder or SUD (especially alcohol use disorder [AUD], PTSD, TBI, depression, and suicide risk). A standard history and physical should be conducted, incorporating a biopsychosocial focus on pain conditions and a comprehensive assessment of pain generator(s), overall function, and comorbidities, including mental disorders.

Taking a Military History

Health care for those who have served in the military, whether delivered in DoD facilities, VA facilities, or in the community at large, should include a basic military and deployment history. Such a military history serves three purposes:

- It creates a more meaningful bond between the clinician and the patient.
- It affords an opportunity to acknowledge and express appreciation for the patient's service.
- It gathers information on service-related health concerns or risks that call for specific interventions, health monitoring, or access to VA benefits for the patient.

A military history should gather the following information about the patient:

1. Branch of service (Air Force, Army, Coast Guard, Marine Corps, Navy)
2. Enlistment or commissioning date
3. Current duty status; e.g., National Guard or Reserves, Active, Retired
4. Rank/rate
5. Educational level attained

6. Training, jobs in the military, and actual duties performed
7. Deployments and duty stations (dates, locations, activities during deployment)
8. Health concerns related to military service (including environmental exposures and heat/cold stress)
9. Impact of military service and deployment on spouse and family
10. Positive and negative aspects of military service
11. Quality of post-military life (including education, family, and work).

Close attention should be paid to combat exposure, blast exposure and concussive injuries, illnesses, as well as all injuries and treatments during service. In addition, patients should be queried about tinnitus/hearing problems; dental concerns; chronic pain; sleep disturbances; tobacco, alcohol and other substance use; depression; PTSD; and suicide risk.

Physical Examination

A standard examination should include attention to any service-related injuries, illnesses, or environmental exposures.

Treatment and Support

It is important to verify that the patient is aware of VA benefits and registry examinations (such as those for burn pit and Agent Orange exposure), and to help the patient access needed care.

Develop a Treatment Plan

Development of a patient-centered, integrated, evidence-based plan of care is essential, as are ongoing assessment of the plan's effectiveness and adjustment of the plan as indicated.

Acute pain relief needs to be approached by appropriately addressing the pain generator and using a holistic approach to alleviate suffering, including self-care, self-management (ice/elevation/activity adjustment), physical manipulative strategies, acupuncture, cognitive strategies, and pharmacological modalities (reserving opioids for severe pain and using time-limited/low-dose prescriptions with close follow-up). For this population, the primary goals are symptom relief, avoiding reinjury, maintenance of function, and avoiding progression from an acute to a chronic condition [2].

Chronic pain is *not* an emergency and should be approached from a functional, rehabilitative perspective that employs pharmacological, behavioral, and alternative treatment modalities. These include physical therapy, massage, transcutaneous electrical nerve stimulation (TENS), thermal and aqua therapy, encouragement of regular exercise, chiropractic treatment, and acupuncture. Incorporating behavioral strategies into a comprehensive, collaborative treatment plan that involves a psychologist (for cognitive behavioral therapy, biofeedback training, and stress management), as well as alternative techniques (such as deep relaxation training, meditation, and yoga) have been shown to improve pain outcomes [3–5].

Opioids should be used with caution and reserved for acute, short-term, severe pain, and with even greater caution for refractory chronic pain conditions. Comorbid mental health conditions compound the risk of inappropriate use of opioids and self-medication of "psychological pain." A diagnosis of PTSD has been found to be associated with increased prescribing of opioid prescriptions, high-risk opiate use, and associated adverse events [3].

Lifestyle Modification

The evidence is clear that chronic pain can be an overwhelming life experience. Thus, patient care should address the whole person and all the problems the individual experiences because of pain, rather than focusing only on the symptom of pain. Supportive self-care involves exercise, relaxation/meditation, and community- and web-based social supports [3].

Post-Traumatic Stress Disorder (PTSD) and Traumatic Brain Injury (TBI)

Prolonged symptoms of PTSD or TBI in the active-duty and veteran populations may be associated with substance use disorders (SUDs), in which case both disorders must be treated simultaneously in order to achieve the best results [6–9].

In addition, many Vietnam veterans received chronic therapy with benzodiazepines, which now are recognized as ineffective for long-term treatment of PTSD; in fact, they may worsen other symptoms in addition to creating dependence on benzodiazepines [10]. (See the discussion of PTSD in the Sidebar to Chapter 24 of this Handbook, as well as the discussion of TBI in the Sidebar to Chapter 25 [11–15].)

Referral for Specialized Care

It is wise to consider partnering with a VA facility in the assessment and management of pain concerns, both through co-managed approaches and by ensuring that the veteran is aware of, and knows how to access, VA resources and benefits. Every VA facility has a transitions care manager who can assist with care coordination/case management and who is knowledgeable about community, VA, and DoD resources [16–19].

Concerns Specific to Personnel Deployed to Iraq and Afghanistan

The hallmark injuries among service members returning from Iraq and Afghanistan are related to blast injuries, which often result in TBI, PTSD, and chronic pain. Problems observed in these personnel also are related to multiple deployments, which increase the risk of PTSD, family disruption, and SUDs. Individuals who experience repeated deployments are more likely to engage in recent-onset heavy drinking and binge drinking, to suffer alcohol- and other drug-related issues, and to misuse prescribed opioids and benzodiazepines. They also are more likely to begin smoking or to relapse to use of nicotine products [17,18,20,21].

One study found that 25% of service members returning from Iraq and Afghanistan reported symptoms of a mental health or cognitive disorder, while one in six reported symptoms of PTSD. Both of these problems are strongly associated with SUDs. Another factor is wide availability of marijuana and other cannabinoids in Iraq and Afghanistan, coupled with a perception of low risk inherent in use of those substances [1].

Post-deployment sleep disorder is another common problem. Prazosin has been used off-label for nightmares, as have cognitive-behavioral therapy (CBT) approaches such as CBT-Insomnia, which is available through the VA [22]. An app titled CBT-I is available at Apple and Android app stores.

Concerns Specific to Veterans Deployed in the First Gulf War

While the incidence of PTSD is significantly lower among Gulf War veterans than in personnel who served in Iraq or Afghanistan, there are stressors unique to that war. Such stressors serve to increase the risk of chronic pain and stress-related illnesses that may complicate the picture, especially when these problems co-occur with SUDs. Stressors include:

- Exposure to oil pit fires;
- Exposure to pesticides (including lindane, DEET, organophosphorus pesticides, and permethrin);
- Concerns about immunizations; and
- Medically unexplained but persistent symptoms [23].

Concerns Specific to Vietnam Veterans

As Vietnam veterans reach an age at which they may have Medicare as well as VA benefits, an increasing number seek care in the private sector. This requires case management and, where possible, partnership with a VA facility so as to coordinate care and obtain the best results.

All personnel who served in Vietnam or who were exposed to equipment used in Vietnam may have been exposed to Agent Orange, which increases their risk of developing chronic pain related to:

- Amyloidosis
- Chronic B cell leukemias
- Chloracne (or similar acneform disease)
- Diabetes mellitus type 2
- Hodgkin's disease
- Ischemic heart disease
- Multiple myeloma
- Non-Hodgkin's lymphoma
- Parkinson's disease
- Peripheral neuropathy (acute and subacute)
- Porphyria cutanea tarda
- Prostate cancer
- Respiratory cancers (including lung cancer)
- Soft tissue sarcomas (other than osteosarcoma, chondrosarcoma, Kaposi's sarcoma, or mesothelioma)
- Amyotrophic lateral sclerosis (ALS).

Veterans who have symptoms related to any of the foregoing disorders should register with the VA for a review of available benefits and treatment options [19].

Mental Health Problems

In addition to PTSD, the mental health problems seen most often in Vietnam veterans are:
Males (lifetime risk):

1. Alcohol abuse
2. Alcohol dependence
3. Generalized anxiety disorder
4. Antisocial personality disorder.

Females (lifetime risk):
1. Generalized anxiety disorder
2. Depression
3. Alcohol abuse
4. Alcohol dependence

Cannabinoid use is common in this population and, with recent increases in availability, may complicate treatment of underlying medical problems as the Vietnam veteran population ages. In addition, many Vietnam veterans received chronic therapy with benzodiazepines, which now are recognized as ineffective for long-term treatment of PTSD; in fact, they may worsen other symptoms in addition to creating dependence on the benzodiazepine [21,22].

Concerns Specific to Women Service Members and Veterans

The Women's Armed Services Integration Act of 1948 granted women permanent status in Regular and Reserve forces of the Army, Navy, Marine Corps, and Air Force. As a result, 90% of all service positions are now open to women, with duty limitations under constant revision.

Women also compose the fastest growing segment of the veteran population and have a high prevalence of pain. Musculoskeletal conditions are a leading contributor to their health profile. Women in the 45–64 age group, who constitute the largest subgroup of women veterans, also have the highest rates of musculoskeletal, substance use, and mental health disorders. Of these, depression, PTSD, and anxiety are the mental health conditions most often diagnosed in women veterans. In fact, mental health and substance use disorders are diagnosed more frequently in female than in male veterans.

Musculoskeletal pain also is seen more often in female than male veterans, especially in the over-45 age group, in whom spine and joint disorders are exceptionally common. Between 2002 and 2009, 47% of 51,344 women veterans treated in the VA system had a medical diagnosis of musculoskeletal disorder, while 44% presented with mental health problems. Connective tissue diseases also are seen more often in female than male veterans, suggesting that these multi-system diseases contribute to both pain and a decline in functional status.

Women veterans also have very high rates of clinically relevant headache. However, the use of prescription medications for their headaches has been associated with poor mental health status, higher incidence of psychiatric symptoms, and higher rates of traumatic events.

Experts have theorized that women veterans may hide their physical and psychological issues out of a fear that revealing such problems may lead to a perception that they are "weak" in comparison with their male counterparts. Others have hypothesized that women may conceal their physical and psychological issues in order to negate the notion that they are unable to handle military duties.

Specialists and primary care providers need to adopt a team-based approach that facilitates coordination of mental health and rehabilitative services. Studies consistently find that addressing persistent pain along with other conditions may improve adaptive coping and functioning in these patients. Many VA facilities have developed clinics designed to meet the particular needs of women veterans, while others are seen in the VA's "medical home" model that treats all veterans, male and female, in the same clinic environment.

Innovations in Pain Care

The VA has adopted innovative models and new technologies to improve the care of veterans who suffer from chronic pain. This section briefly outlines strategies being employed and technologies that have been adopted to support a cultural change in VA pain care, with opioid safety as a central concern.

- *National VA Pain Website:* A redesigned website can be accessed at: http://www.va.gov/painmanagement/. The website acts as a public portal to resources, tools, and general information about pain management in the VA.
- *New Models of Collaboration Between the VA and DoD:* The Joint Pain Education Project is working to standardize clinical training and patient education across the VA and DoD systems. These materials are available to the public on the national pain website: http://www.va.gov/painmanagement/.
- *New Models of Access to Specialty Care:* Video-conferencing is widely used within the VA. The SCAN-ECHO program provides opportunities for health care teams to access subject matter experts for didactic instruction and individual case consultation, on a national basis and in real time.
- *New Models of Collaboration Between Pain and Addiction Services:* Several VA facilities have developed clinical programs to care for veterans with both pain and substance use disorders.
- *Online Learning:* The VA offers online patient education for a variety of life skills that support self-management of pain. The website, http://www.veterantraining.va.gov/, provides links to free, confidential, and easy-to-access online training. Courses include (1) AIMS: Anger and Irritability Management Skills; (2) Moving

Forward: problem-solving skills; (3) Veteran Parenting: parenting skills to help veterans deal with family issues; and (4) PTSD Coach: skills training for veterans with PTSD and anyone coping with stress and trauma.

Online training that encourages shared decision-making and collaborative care within a biopsychosocial model of pain is available on the VA national pain website. The companion Veterans Integrated Service Network (VISN) 20 provider training module provides conceptual, clinical, and communication skills for professionals.

Opioid Safety in Veterans

The Veterans Administration is not immune to the current opioid "epidemic." Indeed, the Veterans Health Administration (VHA) has experienced a similar increase in opioid prescribing and related adverse events, including overdose [3,21–23]. Veterans are at an elevated risk for accidental overdose compared to the general U.S. population, and those with PTSD, TBI, and/or SUDs have a higher prevalence of adverse outcomes [20,23]. Veterans on chronic opioid therapy also are at increased risk for suicide.

The VA is committed to a multimodal approach to the effective management of pain, which includes the safe use of opioids. As part of this approach, it has developed and implemented the following services:

- The Opioid Safety Initiative (OSI) Dashboard, as well as STORM (Stratification Tool for Opioid Risk Mitigation) and Opioid Therapy Risk Report (OTRR), which generate reports on opioid utilization and identify patients for whom interventions are recommended.
- The OSI Toolkit, which provides evidence-based materials to aid in clinical decision- making.
- Academic Detailing, which serves as an educational outreach program to provide support and resources to VA staff, with the goal of improving patient care and health outcomes (https://www.pbm.va.gov/academicdetailingservicehome.asp).

Mobile Apps

Dozens of apps are available to patients, families, and professionals, many of which can be accessed at www.mobile.va.gov. The DoD website www.afterdeployment.dcoe.mil offers a wide range of materials, including online self-management workshops and mobile apps that address problems such as depression, substance use, and stress management, as well as family concerns and work adjustment.

Conclusion

The Department of Defense and Veterans Administration are committed to developing innovative methods to promote patient-centered pain care that emphasizes collaborative treatment and self-management. One aspect of this approach is web-based access to numerous patient and provider educational materials, as well as clinical tools and resources, some of which are highlighted in this chapter and the accompanying text box.

For More Information on the Topics Discussed:

American Society of Addiction Medicine (ASAM):

Lewis DC, Beale RR, Falco M, McCarty D, O'Brien CP, Weisner C. Preventing and treating substance use disorders in military personnel (Chapter 114). In RK Ries, DA Fiellin, SC Miller, R Saitz, eds. *The ASAM Principles of Addiction Medicine, Fifth Edition.* Philadelphia, PA: Wolters Kluwer; 2014.

Zweben JE, Storti S. Risk factors for military families (Chapter 114S). In RK Ries, DA Fiellin, SC Miller, R Saitz, eds. *The ASAM Principles of Addiction Medicine, Fifth Edition.* Philadelphia, PA: Wolters Kluwer; 2014.

Blow FC, Barry KL. Traumatic injuries related to alcohol and other drug use: Epidemiology, screening and prevention (Chapter 81). In RK Ries, DA Fiellin, SC Miller, R Saitz, eds. *The ASAM Principles of Addiction Medicine, Fifth Edition.* Philadelphia, PA: Wolters Kluwer; 2014.

Veterans Administration (VA):

Substance Use Disorder Clinical Practice Guidelines. Washington, DC: VA/DoD; 2017. (Access at: http://www.healthquality.va.gov/guidelines/MH/sud/.)

VA Public Health Exposure website. (Access at: http://www.publichealth.va.gov/exposures/index.aspx.)

VA Academic Detailing Home Page (Access at: https://www.pbm.va.gov/academicdetailingservicehome.asp.)

VA National Center for PTSD. (Access at: http://www.ptsd.va.gov.)

References

1. Department of Veterans Affairs and Department of Defense (VA/DoD). *Substance Use Disorder Clinical Practice Guidelines*, 2017. (Accessed at: http://www.healthquality.va.gov/guidelines/MH/sud/.)
2. Department of Veterans Affairs (VA). Public Health Exposure website, n.d. (Accessed at: http://www.publichealth.va.gov/exposures/index.aspx.)
3. Bohnert KM, Ilgen MA, Rosen CS, et al. The association between substance use disorders and mortality among a cohort of veterans with posttraumatic stress disorder: Variation by age cohort and mortality type. *Drug Alcohol Depend.* 2013 Feb 1;128(1–2):98–103.
4. Seal KH, Cohen G, Waldrop A, et al. Substance use disorders in Iraq and Afghanistan veterans in VA healthcare, 2001–2010: Implications for screening, diagnosis and treatment. *Drug Alcohol Depend.* 2011 Jul 1;116(1–3):93–101.
5. Park TW, Saitz R, Ganoczy D, et al. Benzodiazepine prescribing patterns and deaths from drug overdose among U.S. veterans receiving opioid analgesics: Case-cohort study. *BMJ.* 2015;350:h2698.
6. Department of Veterans Affairs (VA). National Center for PTSD. (Accessed at: http://www.ptsd.va.gov.)
7. Ciechanowski P. Posttraumatic stress disorder in adults: Epidemiology, pathophysiology, clinical manifestations, course and diagnosis. *Up to Date.* 2015. (Accessed at: www.uptodate.com.)
8. Stewart MO, Karlin BE, Murphy JL, et al. National dissemination of cognitive-behavioral therapy for chronic pain in veterans. *Clin J Pain.* 2015 Aug;31(8):722–729.
9. Phifer J, Skelton K, Weiss T, et al. Pain symptomatology and pain medication use in civilian PTSD. *Pain.* 2011;152:2233–2240.
10. Vieweg WV, Julius DA, Fernandez A, et al. Posttraumatic stress disorder: Clinical features, pathophysiology, and treatment. *Am J Med.* 2006;119:383.
11. Yehuda R. Post-traumatic stress disorder. *NEJM.* 2002;346:108.
12. Monson CM, Fredman SJ, Macdonald A, et al. Effect of cognitive-behavioral therapy for PTSD. A randomized controlled trial. *JAMA.* 2012;308:700.
13. Kroenke K, Bair MJ, Damush TM, et al. Optimized antidepressant therapy and pain self-management in primary care patients with depression and musculoskeletal pain: A randomized controlled trial. *JAMA.* 2009;301:110.
14. Otis JD, Keane T, Kerns RD, et al. The development of an integrated treatment for veterans with comorbid chronic pain and posttraumatic stress disorder. *Pain Med.* 2009;10:1300–1311.
15. Fareed A, Eilender P, Haber M, et al. Comorbid Posttraumatic stress disorder and opiate addiction: A literature review. *J Addict Dis.* 2013;32(2):168–179.
16. Outcalt S, Yu Z, Hoen MS, et al. Health care utilization among veterans with pain and posttraumatic stress symptoms. *Pain Med.* 2013;15:1872–1879.

17. Seal KH, Shi Y, Cohen G, et al. Association of mental health disorders with prescription opioids and high risk opioid use in U.S. veterans of Iraq and Afghanistan. *JAMA*. 2012 Mar 7;307:940–947.
18. Seal KH, Maguen S, Bertenthal D, et al. Observational evidence for buprenorphine's impact on PTSD symptoms in veterans with chronic pain and opioid use disorder. *J Clin Psychiatry*. 2016 Sep;77(9):1182–1188.
19. Department of Veterans Affairs (VA). Public Health Exposure website. (Accessed at: http://www.publichealth.va.gov/exposures/index.aspx.)
20. Department of Veterans Affairs (VA). Recently updated clinical practice guidelines for the management of traumatic brain injury. (Accessed at: http://www.healthquality.va.gov/guidelines/Rehab/mtbi/.)
21. Department of Veterans Affairs (VA). National Center for PTSD. (Accessed at: http://www.ptsd.va.gov.)
22. Spelman JF, Hunt SC, Seal KH, et al. Post deployment care for returning combat veterans. *J Gen Intern Med*. 2012 Sep;27(9):1200–1209.
23. Burgo-Black AL, Brown JL, Boyce RM, et al. The importance of taking a military history. *Public Health Rep*. 2016;131(5):711–713.

Index

Note: Page numbers followed by *b,* f, or *t* indicate a box, figure, or table.